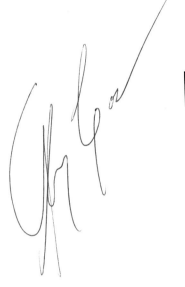

D1195843

# BRAIN INJURY

— • —

A Message from the Publisher

In keeping with White Knight Book's mandate
to bring great titles of social value to the reading public
across North America, we feel fortunate as a dedicated
non-fiction publisher to have been closely involved
with this important publication that will be part of
White Knight's latest genre,
"The White Knight Health Series"

# BRAIN INJURY

The riveting, true story about a promising young
person who becomes severely brain injured, and the
total picture as revealed in the 25 years that follow,
leading up to a final determination.

by

## Alan J Cooper

WHITE KNIGHT BOOKS
2006

Published in 2006 by
White Knight Books, a division of Bill Belfontaine Ltd.
Suite 103, One Benvenuto Place, Toronto Ontario Canada M4V 2L1
T. 416-925-6458 F. 416-925-4165 • e-mail whitekn@istar.ca
Web site: www.whiteknightbooks.ca

Ordering information

| CANADA | UNITED STATES |
|---|---|
| White Knight Book Distribution Services Ltd. | APG Distributors |
| c/o Georgetown Terminal Warehouses | (Associated Publishers' Group) |
| 34 Armstrong Avenue, | 1501 County Hospital Road |
| Georgetown ON, L7G 4R9 | Nashville, TN, 37218 USA |
| T: 1-866-485-5556 F: 1-866-485-6665 | T: 1-888-725-2606 F: 1-800-510-3650 |

First printing: August 2006

**Library and Archives Canada Cataloguing in Publication**

Cooper, Alan John, 1947-
Brain-injured : the riveting, true story about a promising young person who becomes severely brain injured, and the total picture as revealed in the 25 years that follow, leading up to a final determination / Alan John Cooper.
ISBN 0-9780570-0-7
1. Cooper, Alan John, 1947- —Health.
2. Brain damage—Patients—Canada—Biography. I. Title.
RA645.B73C66 2006     617.4'81044092     C2006-902059-0

EDITING
Sharon Crawford

COVER AND INTERIOR DESIGN
Karen Thomas Petherick, Intuitive Design International Ltd.

PRINTED AND BOUND IN CANADA

Dedicated to
my two true sons

# Table of Contents

The foreword to this book has been prepared by Douglas Henderson Hopp, DVM, DipCompMed, CD, MMW.

Dr. Hopp is a consultant in experimental medicine and surgery, a former research animal clinician in several schools of medicine and teaching hospitals in the United States and Canada, including The Johns Hopkins University School of Medicine, Toronto Western Hospital, The Addiction Research Foundation of Ontario, Mount Sinai Hospital and The Hospital for Sick Children in Toronto, The University of Ottawa, Washington University in Saint Louis School of Medicine, Saint Luke's Hospital in Chesterfield, Missouri, and Saint Michael's Hospital in Toronto. He was clinical coordinator with regional burn centers throughout the U.S. Midwest for the Tissue Research Laboratory in Maryland Heights, Missouri and currently is coordinating an extensive publication project on the subject of BioTransmission, linking the fields of evolutionary biology, neurobiology, genetics, sexology, anatomy, and behavioral psychophysiology with other disciplines. He completed his postdoctoral fellowship in Comparative Medicine at the Johns Hopkins University School of Medicine in Baltimore, Maryland, in 1980, as a Fellow of the Ministry of Health of the Province of Ontario. Dr. Hopp was a doctoral candidate in neurobiology at Purdue University, is a collaborator and co-author in work being conducted at The University of Arizona, and has lectured at Arizona State University. At present he divides his time between Toronto, Saint Louis and Tucson.

Foreword by
Douglas Henderson Hopp, DVM,
DipCompMed, CD, MMW

## ORIENTATION

Brain damage is a bit like cancer—one never knows precisely whom it might afflict, when it may occur, or how this condition may manifest itself or progress. In this way, it is not like infectious diseases, nor like trauma to mere structural, motor, or non-neuronal physiologically-functional components of the body. The frontiers for discovery, and understanding of the causes of, pathogenesis, treatment and prognosis of these latter conditions formed the foundation of twentieth-century medicine, and even cancer received immense attention over the last one-third of that century. We know much about the features of metabolic, infectious, autoimmune and degenerative disease and how to modify the course of these types of conditions in all other areas of our beings. Healing in general is relatively straightforward for non-neoplastic and non-neurologic afflictions. But in the case of Alan J Cooper, a once-brilliant orator/debater, gifted musician, and consummate specialist in the field of marketing, it was closed damage to the brain which was to be his fate, as opposed to one of the more treatable maladies.

As someone who previously knew Alan Cooper, as well as several of the other figures in his story, generally bearing pseudonyms for what will become obvious reasons, I can attest to the alarming truths contained herein. This account of damage to Alan's brain, incurred in an accident when he was hit in a blinding snowstorm by a heavy car driven by an unstable individual, is actually two stories in one.

In the first, it chronicles the immense, but in some ways quite subtle, effects of severe damage to the left, frontal lobe—a lobe responsible for certain verbal or linguistic associations, formation or retention of short-term memory, thought processes involving problem-solving, intellect, and along with associated areas, regulation of certain bodily functions. The author's recounting of the effects of this traumatically-altered brain on his physiology and faculties is graphic, exhaustive, and on occasion, deeply affecting. The other story, the one which in its own way is even sadder than the direct changes which the brain injury has inflicted on Alan's life and abilities, shows the reflexive effect of how his changed capacities and persona, as perceived and responded to by those with whom he has contact, impact back upon him in most anguishing and unpredictable ways.

We see through our victim's eyes, in an anthology of significant episodes from his early and then later shattered life, often presented through vignettes, samples from his frequently-expressed hobby of writing throughout the years, both before and subsequent to that fateful car accident. Alan's story is not without moments of mirth, owing to the author's fortunate retention of at least a modicum of his obviously well-developed and deeply-ingrained sense of humor.

A general effect of left frontal lobe dysfunction, as frequently observed, and most certainly present in this case, is its propensity to induce a change in personality, leading the afflicted individual to criticize, eventually alienate and hence lose acquaintances, fall prey to addictions, and unfortunately to antagonize those who possess the wherewithal to make life even more miserable for an already-victimized patient. Unable to restrain brain-damage-induced intermittent antisocial remarks or behaviors, Alan manages to irritate, or enrage on occasion, critical persons from all sectors of society. He thus alienates his family, friends, associates and superiors at work, and those who hold key positions in formal organizations within our society, such as religious and educational institutions, potential employers, insurance investigators, and finally those in our legal or (in)justice system. All of the foregoing successively abandon and/or attack him in their response to his altered self. Alan J Cooper truly becomes more severely affected by the resultant actions of these others, than he has been through the direct manifestations of the intrinsic trauma-induced alterations within his brain.

In summary, this is a truthful and frightening look inside the head and the life of a victim of traumatic brain injury (TBI) and at our society's inability to deal appropriately with this problem.

This book is intended, in the method and spirit proposed to Alan by "Doctor Fisher," as you will come to know him, as an example of how a brain-injured person might think and write about his own situation. In order to preserve this special character-istic of the manuscript, the choice of words, their punctuation, and their placement or usage is totally created by the author. Any changes to spelling or syntax have occurred solely through sugges-tion at most by others, and integrated by and at Alan's option only if such recommendations seemed better to him upon reflection.

Before you proceed with his story, you should be alerted to note, understand, and perhaps learn to appreciate some of the idio-syncrasies which characterize Alan's now-altered (i.e. "post-TBI") style of writing or communication. Alan lost a serious proportion of some of his special abilities as a result of the permanent brain damage due to the car accident. His ability to quickly find "the right word" when speaking, for example—one of his great skills as an accomplished debater and public speaker, was not only dimin-ished almost to non-existence, this faculty became highly unpre-dictable. Periodically "out of the blue" he became capable of inserting or interjecting an incorrect or on occasion entirely inappropriate word, this bizarre characteristic being particularly noticeable with respect to selection of adjectives, or other modifiers of a concept. Another was a tendency when speaking to interchange consonants quite frequently. In conversation he is now prone to reverse the order of the consonants in a "consonant blend" within a single word, as in saying "gagrle" instead of "gargle", and often commits a "spoonerism" involving parts of two words as in saying "brood plessure" instead of "blood pressure". Syntax errors crept into his speech, and short-term memory became very significantly impaired.

Although the previously-listed changes may not show in his writing style, the following aspect of his "re-wired" brain will. An interesting feature of Alan's modified capacities, is that his ability to use numbers has been far less diminished by the injury, than has his ability to use words. Owing to this relative shift in his ability with numerical data, Alan became preoccupied with numbers, and for example, found that he could repeat, in reverse order, a list of eight numbers which had been read to him. Consequently, he began to perceive aspects of the world around him with numerical, rather than verbal or pictorial modes of assisting him in keeping track of things. He could recognize, use, and remember numbers better as Arabic numerals (e.g. 1, 2, 3...) than as written out letter-equivalents (e.g. one, two, three...) or the acoustic sounds of the numbers when spoken. His brain seemed to visualize the "shape" of the numbers, and retained recollections of seemingly insignificant numbers which he had learned before the accident. In his writing, he started using numerals exclusively, as opposed to the written-out forms, when referring to numbers, since that was the way his brain was now relating to numbers.

One hope Alan had in producing this book, was that it might serve as an example for brain-injured persons, their families or close associates, and those who deal with them, as a means of better understanding the range of faculties which can be affected by such a condition. Not all persons with brain injury, whether acquired traumatically or otherwise, can communicate for themselves in the way that the author can, thus his writing may be able to serve in part as a voice for many others.

Although this book may read at times like fiction, it is all too true, and may prove to be a pillar of self-help for some. This work could be an invaluable resource or inspiration to the millions of persons whose lives or those of a loved or close one have been affected by brain injury. As well, health care or legal professionals and students, social workers, and other caregivers could benefit greatly from a read.

Tucson, Arizona

# BRAIN INJURY

# FRIDAY, APRIL 26, 2002

My student teacher year is almost complete and I have an A average. I am being told by an adjudicating committee that I have failed.

The committee has gathered in the school office of Principal King, a senior woman whose face radiates the wisdom and kindness of an old bloodhound. She will be the deliverer of my failure message and is sitting ceremoniously behind her desk. Seated silently facing her and several seats around a curve of chairs directed toward the front of her desk, is my university supervisor Katy Bard. As Ms. King utters the last word of her one long sentence, supervisor Bard hands back to me without eye contact, my copy of Harold Minden's *Two Hugs for Survival*. Bard's boss is there too, the one who has already told students, "You will all pass, you will all get jobs." Now she begins to talk about what a crush this meeting must be for me, "...having put my heart and soul into the entire school year." Bard's boss is offering me psychological counseling back at the University of Toronto and softly adds that help is waiting there for me.

Though much of the meeting moves along as if it had been cued, the producer, director and choreographer has yet to utter a decipherable sound.

I then pose an unanticipated question, "May I have it in writing, Ms. King?"

The principal seems momentarily at a loss but the producer-mastermind Ms. Coy, who is the director of practice teaching, eases in with an answer representative of her agility with the use and abuse of words. She finishes with, "It's over."

I am finished in minutes and though it is still lunch time, I am out of the school and none of my students see me leave. I am in shock but not surprise. My associate teacher has been openly happy with me as have the children, and I have shared with Ms. Bard my confidence that this is a school in which I would very much like to teach. But I have had over 20 years of such sudden firings, failures and dismissals, and each time that I have heard the words anew, I have turned increasingly mute.

I bus home that Friday, unaware of the shield that my brain has created around itself. Noise is brushing by. My mind is shooting through the past 5 days of practice teaching and how frantic they must have been for the firing's mastermind. Only the Friday before had I been forced to slip my letter of protest under her office door, after her leaving early. More likely than not, she would have thought she had closed the door on her personal compromise, and by the Monday following, I would already be practice teaching.

The producer-mastermind, Ms. Coy, had offered me the makeup Practicum only 2 days before my entering it, thus making a mockery of my intended appeal. She had advised me at the time that if I wanted to appeal the sham of 2 months earlier, I would not be able to enter the makeup practice teaching on Monday. For over 6 weeks I had been requesting from Ms. Coy, the college's position from which to appeal. In the end, Coy had finagled me into a trap in which I could not appeal and still graduate in June. Legally, she had pulled off a masterful stroke.

My letter of protest to Coy had made it clear I was not appealing my case but had made mention that supervisor Katy Bard had given me no warning of changing her reference on me. Bard had changed it from a promised excellent to an outright refusal to give one, after having heard Coy's overview of my failing 2 months earlier.

At the time, a substitute supervisor under Coy had directed my in-class teacher to change her assessment on me from "pass" to "fail." The substitute had done so only 20 minutes before the end of the term, without so much as witnessing my practice teaching that week. Within days of the failing and despite my being told earlier by a Toronto School Board interviewer that the TSB was eager for me to become a teacher within it, I had received from them a 2-sentence "not-interested" letter. As for Ms. Bard's changed reference, she had been alerted by her boss about Bard's not forewarning me of a reference change. I had then been given by Ms. Bard the saying I had been given so often—to put the issue behind me and concentrate on the future.

I have worked 100 hours per week for 8 straight months since September. My papers and class work have been regarded as outstanding—but an issue, one that continues looming every hour for the past 20 years and 4 months—is center again. Despite my A average, Toronto Teacher's College is determined not to allow me to teach. Its written response will list a litany of behavior patterns that betray my severe and permanent brain damage.

Mid-Friday afternoon, I reach home and am beyond exhaustion. I collapse into an heirloom chair in my little living room and ponder what to do next. There is always suicide as I have contemplated so many times before. But suicide seems so much overdone as is also true of its prime motivator, the need to punish. I look at the air and the walls, and wonder what, if anything, I will ever do again. Nothing seems left, not even pain. Where anger and indignation once boiled, there is not even despair. It is as if I have been in prison for many years and face nothing but prison yet to come, with all its new pains and injustices for a sentence that was never mine.

I move from chair to toilet to tap water and this ritual goes on for hours. I feel like a drowned towel and the thought of going to sleep is one I cannot endure. I keep looking at nothing, biding my prison time and awaiting some clue as to the reason for my being.

Around hour 4, I find my mind turning, as it has done so many times over the past 20 years, to writing. I search for paper, for a place to start. Though my home is ultra-organized to aid in using my battered brain, the sheer number of coded files, cabinets, drawers and briefcases feels overwhelming. As has happened so many times before, my right brain has begun to signal for something the left side can't find.

I descend steep steps into the cellar and in the abandoned dank of a former coal storage room, start to probe through old papers from my Master of Education. My personality knows one brain side is deranged and the other driving, and I feel I have no choice but to follow my right brain's signal while the left side plods on. I come across a piece I wrote for my 2 sons' school, and at some point I must have considered it important enough to have slotted it later into a massive binder of formal learning. It is an opinion paper, based not so much on formal learning as on my gut feeling at the time from watching, playing and working for 2 years as prime caregiver with my sons James and Robert. The handwritten piece talks of child development and how critical it is for children's physical development to precede their intellectual development and spiritual development to precede the physical. I warn that spiritual development is not religious development but is the opposite, to me.

I remember now how James and Robert had not only read, written and spelled before the age of 2 but had also swum, skated, bicycled, climbed trees, danced and from their daddy's many lessons, had known how to fall. Both were happy with their father looking after them and had proven out, hour to hour, that children can develop sooner—much sooner—than even the most progressive elements of our Canadian educational society had allowed. I had taken them to the library, had written them stories and listened to their letters. Their paintings had been displayed throughout our home, along with their writings, cartoons and architectural constructs.

I find myself digging into papers going back years to my earlier Master of Religious Education. Religious I am not, but curiosity keeps driving my wondering how religiosity spins spirituality and skews human behavior. I find from 7 years earlier an essay which summed up some of my values. It was a review of the Christian bible's *Book of James*, purportedly written by James, brother of Jesus of Nazareth. The *Book of James* is crisp, clear and reflective of a single writer. I was once told that the original Greek is also of the highest order. Not bad, I think to myself, for a person whose prophet brother spoke only Aramaic. I begin reading.

# A Review of *The Letter of James* and its Contribution to Ongoing Spiritual Education

**Professor Ken Bradley**                    **U. of T. Course  WYP 2567S**

The integration of faith and learning is an issue fraught with dissent. The very words "faith" and "learning" contain connotations possibly too numerous to list and their actual denotations have been historically shaped to meet the expediencies of time, place and power. In reading about faith/learning integration, one can have difficulty conceiving of the subject's being free of controversy.

*The Bible's Letter of James* deals with both faith and learning and the integration not only of the two but each in relation to life's living. Not surprisingly, it has never been free of controversy and perhaps was so designed. As a source document, how can *The Letter of James* make a meaningful contribution to the faith/learning subject?

James deals first with the testing of one's faith, a trial which he believes should be greeted with joy, since such testing produces endurance that in turn leads to maturity and integrated wholeness. 'If one feels lacking in wisdom, one need only ask for it from a generous god and wisdom will be given; provided, however, one asks in faith, not doubt.' Doubt in the sense used here, is the duplicitous doubt espoused by the apostles in *Luke* 24:11 and is not to be confused, (it is suggested), with the doubting in good faith, ever captioned by poet Tennyson,

> *There lies more faith in honest doubt,*
> *believe me, that in half the creeds.'*

Material wealth is cut down to size in James' *Letter* as are those myopic and self-centered souls who wallow in it—'The rich...will wither away'. Temptation is said to be of one's own making, and blessings are given to those who endure it. Alternatively, generous acts of giving are always outflows of God's love.

The author assigns critical importance to listening within any communications process, with the learned person's always being ready to remain silent to learn more. Being quick to anger is admonished as betraying ill will. Strong and repeated emphasis is placed upon those acts which carry through the word of God versus illusive hearing of that word. The one ascribed "perfect" law, the only one needed for anyone's pursuing the path of principles, is the 'law' of perfect liberty. Those people who are only professedly religious, have suspect faith. Those who care for the needy and try to steer clear of temptation, have true faith.

James continues. 'Gauge a person's substance or worth not on the magnificence of his car. Exercise a hermeneutics of suspicion on anyone insecure or pagan-like enough to wear his wealth on his sleeve—did he acquire such material gain through the oppression of others? Love others as you would be loved. Do not compromise in your living out that love. Do not profess to have faith if you do nothing to demonstrate that faith; don't pride yourself on not being adulterous, if your behavior regularly contributes to life in the inner city being ruinous.'

'Few people should become teachers, for teachers help mold minds and are thus to be held accountable with greater strictness. All of us are human and capable of making honest mistakes. The teacher, though, is like the rudder on a ship—capable of unwavering, strategic guidance or of running us amuck. The tongue is one of the greatest rudders. One should never lose mind of its awesome potential for doing good and evil. If one is wise, one can show it with the gentleness of works born of wisdom. If, however, one is envious or consumed with self-centered ambition, one should not compound those spiritual afflictions with hypocrisy. Once allowed to take hold of a person, envy and self-ambition lead to other disorders and wickedness of every kind. But wisdom from God is free from hypocrisy and partiality. Those who glean such wisdom from God are eager to help others and are full of mercy and peace.

'What are the sources of conflicts and disputes among people? Are not the sources actually cravings at war within oneself? One can enter into every conceivable wrongdoing to satisfy those earthly cravings and in so doing, one separates oneself further from God, becoming a self-exalted creature of pride. Ironically, the truly exalted are the unassuming who see in the first place, the illegitimacy of such cravings and the moral undoing in trying to satisfy them. One should thus resist devilish temptations and they will flee. If one draws near to God, He too will draw near.

'Do not speak of evil against one another, because to do so is to make one an illegitimate judge of a law that only God can judge. To pretend to become that kind of judge, one becomes incapable of carrying out that law. For trying to be god-like, one loses one's own freedom. Nevertheless, if one understands both God's law and the right thing to do in a specific instance but fails to do it, one still commits sin. Those of us who have spiritually raped people and the land in pursuit of our own luxuries, need to look at the temporality and the quality of the booty—withered clothes; rusting gold and silver. Yet the expensive trinkets remain as evidence against us and will cause our ultimate downfall.

'Above all, we should not make insincere oaths. Our "yes" should mean "yes" and our "no" a true-to-ourselves "no". We should pray, and if joyful, should sing prayers of thanks. If sick, we should exercise our faith and trust, and God will care for us. If we have done wrong and we ask in true faith for forgiveness, we will receive it. If any of us helps another out of spiritual sicknesses or back from the plagues of wrongdoing, we will have helped save that person from a hell on earth.'

It is not surprising that The Letter of James continues to create discomfort for many of us today. James says what is often not said in university faculties and his points bear relevance for even the agnostic or atheist. There is in The Letter of James, arguably not one thought that does not penetrate our consciences and our way of living now. The Letter is predicated on principles that are timeless and universal. The fact that the Letter comes packaged in a Christian message or reflects classical Jewish thinking should be of only moot concern. A careful reading through *The Letter of James* from time to time in any educational process cannot but help realign our inevitably out-of-balance sets of values. James' reminders of our human frailties should also underscore to us the never-ending need for spiritual as well as mental and physical growth, as part of the educational process.

Alan J Cooper, July 24, 1995.

*(Professor's note:*
*"Alan: You have pushed the class and me in good ways with this.")*

## Next day: Saturday

Strange for me but in my dreams I am reaching out for help. I fear help, for I fear the damage that anyone operating under its guise may do. Trusting others has been so damning for 20 years. Bach may lend strength in his music as he has in the past but in ways that I do not want now to understand. The university's Hart House has helped too, if only by its architecture and reason for being, but I feel Hart House now could remind me too much of old pains.

I need nature. I have to get out of Toronto. Hart House sits mid-city in the University of Toronto, but Hart House has a farm out in the Caledon Hills, an hour's drive northwest. Once I get past farm keeper Gord and wife, there will be no-one there and its ravine's ponds will be cold, clear, and I guess, clean. I could bicycle, bus or hitchhike.

Two hours and 5 pees later, I am being dropped off in the hamlet of Cheltenham, 4 miles south of the farm. With a half-full jug of water, I begin to hike up through the hills of pampered countryside, past the horses, cedar and post beams that reek of gentle country wealth. In less than an hour, after 2 more stops to urinate and subsequently quench my thirst, I reach the stone fence of Hart House Farm.

It is a 6 minute walk up the driveway to the farmhouse and another 30 down the ravine to the ponds, and I make my way past the house and amble onto the tree-cathedral path sloping away to the rear. I reach the top of a trail that winds down this part of the Niagara Escarpment and as I start to descend, my eyes are met everywhere with green, brown and a dabbling of stone gray. I arrive at the bottom, which is enwrapped in dark forest, brown earth and huge ridges of limestone. At the first pond, I stop on the dock long enough to search for the swing rope. It is still there, a sweet yet hurtful reminder of times past when James, Robert and I each took turns doing Tarzan yells, lunging outward and plopping into the pond.

I walk along the last 4 minutes of path, pause as I pass pond 2 for yet another needed pee, then saunter on to the sauna alongside the last pond.

There is a little pile of cut wood to start the oven but I opt not to fire it up. Instead, I walk onto the giant dock, stand and gaze at the massive stone wall of the Niagara gorge in front of me. On the dock, facing the pond and wall beyond, I peer at the pine trees rising out of the needle-covered earth sloping up the hill, and the air all around is full of sweet breath. As I stand alone and stare, I feel the god within me trying to make contact with the god beyond.

"God dear servant, it's been over 20 years of this stuff. I do not always try my best but I think this time my best is not enough. You know God, I was just about to ask you for help but noticed no-one ever asks you how *you* are doing. We are so caught up in ourselves that when we turn to you, we begin with a mercenary tit-for-tat. First, in some neurotic need we have for determinacy, we label you as perfect. Then we butter you up, lavishing upon you earthly phrases we regard as praise. We often call you "Lord" as if you were some sort of landowner up on a hill or we say "The Almighty" as if you have an ego that needs to be told you can out-power all. Then we want our slates cleaned, so we tell you we've sinned and ask your forgiveness, then we say thank you for all sorts of things that we ourselves judge good, then we get around to the asking part.

As you know, doctors will not help me and suicide will hurt James and Robert too much. They have no way of knowing what has gone on with their dad during these last 2 decades. A dog might help but I cannot afford a dog. God, I sense you're busy but I need to turn to you—you know me better than I. Please help me discern what you are wanting and asking me to do. I know you cannot tell me, because your doing so would kill my freedom, but please, God clue the god within me. I'm asking with as much as I can."

I am dehydrated and grope at my jug for one last taste of water. For over 20 years, I have had over 15 cups per day to offset vast volumes of urination but now I am stuck with a 30-minute hike up the ravine to drinkable water. What will happen, I wonder, if I drink from the pond? It is embedded in limestone and has been cleansed from the winter snow. Or so I figure. I fill a little from the pond, take a drink, fill a little again and drink.

— • —

Since my brain was deranged, I have almost never remembered my dreams but this night back in Toronto I do. I do not believe in epiphanies, perhaps because I sense in them their theatrics. Why then this dream? My short term memory is shot and retrieval is unpredictable; is my mind diving deeper into old mind files, searching for source help?

I draw on earliest memory and my mind finds a story. I am again a toddler, little more than a year in age but have died. I enter a room misty on all sides, yet with a clear sphere in its middle. Toward the back of the sphere are a few grownups. When they first see me enter, they halt all murmuring and turn and look down on me with loving smiles. In the midst of these grownups and slightly to the left is a woman, younger than the others, who speaks to me in a musical, healing voice.

"Hello, Alan. We've been waiting for you."

Marg Moray, my favorite babysitter. Over 50 years ago, I was a one year-old, unable to sleep after being put in my grandfather's bed while he wintered in Florida. I began to think of things frightening. It is doubtful that Marg heard me from her place downstairs and more likely that she had been planning later a routine check. My sniffling had thus become louder. When Marg at last creaked up the stairs and entered the room, she could see I was unhappy and asked me what was the matter.

"I am going to die some day, Miss Moray."

She then gave me something I can never remember receiving from my mother, father, brother or any member of my childhood family—Marg gave me a hug. "Oh Alan, that won't happen until you are 84."

The hug felt safe and I suddenly felt secure. "84 is a long way…Are you sure, Miss Moray?"

Her huge hug held. "Yes Alan, I'm sure."

I felt more secure than anything I had ever known and I hugged her back. Then she lay me back down in my grandfather's double brass bed and I fell asleep.

## Sunday Morning

I do not have Beaver fever but do have a rash. The pond. Other than that, I feel rested, like someone who has been running for a long time and is now finally caught. I am not guilty but am sure I'll get sentenced anyway. That's the third world way in first world countries more often than our stomachs allow. Bullshit baffles brains and much of messaging lies in the delivery. Bush's backers know that, have oiled the world and it is no longer safe to be educated in the land of the non-free. Canada seems a little safer and at least *liberal* has not yet lost its meaning but I do not know now what I will do.

As I ease down the narrow stairs into the little living room, I catch a glimpse of an old photo on the wall at the bottom. The photo is of a gleeful toddler, me, and reveals—what 14 years ago no-one would allow to be found—that my eyes did not always have pupils of 2 different sizes. I stay stuck on the bottom rung, staring into my former eyes.

Suddenly, feedback jolts back my head. I seem to have set off some communications loop between the eyes in the toddler photo and 54 year-old me—Marg Moray and my dream, Saturday's supplication, this photo...my big white boots of babyhood, the bird that I as a baby kept visualizing on the floor, Allie Thompson calling me "Bright Eyes", my swimming at 8 months, my huge need for oxygen, my mother always saying how proud she was of me. I feel I am tracing life all over again, looking at that third of a century before an erratic driver smashed into me head-on in a snowstorm.

Jacob Brownoski, I think my shattered memory recalls from *The Ascent of Man*, said there are few things that can retard the advance of civilization but one is brain damage. Well, I still have an imaginative right hemisphere and that right is beginning to race.

---

## Monday, April 29, 2002

Why need there be such a thing labeled as "The Truth" rather than a series of truths through which we move, their becoming refined over time? For that matter, why need there be "The" anything, for any thing keeps changing over time? Is not God a process, the many manifestations of which occasionally cool down enough to be seen? Is not life some order of magnitude over being inanimate and only a manifestation of one of the billions of big bangs going on all the time? Is not humanity's most far-reaching form about helping others and taking no credit other than understanding good acts to be part of that far reach? Are not good acts thus selfish, distinguishable from self-centeredness by their focus on what is most far reaching? If maturity means being responsible for truth, if truth is critical to communications and communications should always involve love, then truth and love make possible the self worth necessary for living in the furthest reach of maturity's manifestations, that being heaven on earth.

I feel like an infant once again, yet with an appreciation that the smothering of curiosity in our children constitutes human beings' greatest act of inhumanity. Authority should stem from knowledge, not might. We have mothers who have abused power to lord it over their children and under the delusion of love, carry down tyrannical teaching to the youngest learner. It thus becomes impossible for those learners ever to recognize that they are in a prison of their thoughts—young learners carry forward the dictates and learn to see society itself as a prison with a pecking order for all power. Toss in original sin, stew it all in perceived persecution and we have become puppets for at least 2 millenniums.

I am in a Monday of my understanding, with so much daring to be looked at.

## Tuesday, Wednesday and Thursday with Brain Racing

In the beginning, that is to say 8 thousand years ago in Earth's 10 billion years, came the plough, and along with the plough came private property, territorialism over freedom, capitalism over economics, slavery, prisons, wars, rules over principles and religion over spirituality. And so a group of mightier and wilier people got to the top of this new deal first and set up a series of systems tapping into fear, guilt, awe, bird envy, superstition, mother power, determinacy and the suffocation of curiosity. We didn't yet have Einstein and we wanted desperately for answers on which we could stub our toe. Out of a desire for absolute answers came perfection, a concrete concoction for our prefab god.

We human-centric landlubbers don't get it yet. Other forms of life are here not to serve us but we are here to serve them. We are more knowing and, therefore, must help as does God our servant. Our egos keep getting in the way, made worse by both over-mothering and the power brokers' appeals to fears and short-term cravings.

Heaven and hell are human expediencies as are people demonized or made saints. Genius is another far flung word and seems ascribed to anyone who can sum up some of what we are trying to see in ourselves. Then there is that word "natural." It is not natural, some say, to be homosexual; does not such a skew of the word "natural" betray an emphasis in that post-plough religion on being fruitful and multiplying? Are not cows, penguins and rams sometimes homosexual to ensure a control on growth?

No-one has the right to judge. By so judging, are we not abrogating our responsibility? Once we affix the label of devil, saint, genius or deviant, can we not shrug off what we should or should not do, and compartmentalize further the judged person?

Are rules needed? How about rules of thumb, like the 3% rule? How often is it heard that only 3% of alcoholics are street people, 3% of people on welfare are malingerers, 3% of homosexuals pedophiles, 3% of alcoholics make it to AA, 3% of North Americans listen to classical music, 3% to jazz, 3% go to public libraries. How about the notion that only 3% of dish cleaning is due to the dishwashing liquid, 3% of laundry to the detergent or that 3% of diamonds have any use beyond cosmetics? The list could come to good use but what would it do to the inventions and our need to create necessities for them?

We use cell phones 30% of the time to say we are going to be late for the meeting but our ability to drive is impaired by the cell phone. In Toronto often, in New York, London, and Hong Kong more, the quickest way to get somewhere is to walk, the 2nd is bicycle, the 3rd public transit, the 4th taxi and the 5th one's own car. If we use a car because we have too much to carry, do we not ask ourselves if we are consuming too much? Is not the automobile's petroleum-fed engine, the #1 polluter? The most efficient way to communicate is in person with body language, next by postage to lend time to thought, next by phone to get feedback, and lastly by e-mail where we get listed.

I happen to meet on the street at 3:00 a.m., night person Fleming and I tell him I am thinking of writing a book. He says that is a coincidence because he once thought of reading one. A moment's relief.

Since part of my brain was smashed, I have been shut out by other people. I cannot live with anyone but cannot live with myself. I go back home.

There seems little symmetry to what I am thinking. My anger has no focus and a series of truths stay submerged.

There is a small dried flower that our Scottish nanny called *sweet honesty* and my wife called *silver dollar*. *Silver dollar* summed up much of what my wife was made. Before I met her mother, Maria had betrayed confidence about my esophagitis and her mother Yolanta had then lectured me with pointed finger "Alan, we know about you people, and you must watch your ulcers". Before marriage, Maria and I had been pedaling through Toronto's posh Kingsway area and she had confessed she could not feign not wanting all of that. When years later I had taken her to one of the ritziest rooms in Ottawa's Chateau Laurier hotel, she had proclaimed, "*This* is where we belong." When I had taken her to Tokyo's Imperial Palace Hotel, she had sniped that she could have done better by marrying someone else.

My wife Maria had invaded my Boy Scout leadership and concluded how good it would look on my résumé. She had pushed me to date her gorgeous cousin Miranda and had tried to entrap me with Miranda's feedback. When earlier, I had returned home after work and had told her how a pre-marriage girlfriend had offered me $100,000 to procreate a child for her, my wife had yelled, "Take it! We need the money." Maria had teased a repair guy for 3 weeks, while he had kept coming to fix her car window and she had repeatedly invited him in for coffee. She'd had the hots for my celebrity lawyer Adam Stone too and would have ditched me, had there been any indication he would have taken her on in her further claw up.

I find myself descending into the little cellar, following a brain bleep to another damp file.

There is a mildewed satchel called *Marital* and stuck to its bottom is a letter, 4 years old.

January 10 1998

Dear Maria:

## Re: Ongoing Conflict of Interest

You mentioned to me before the new year that "It was too bad about Women's University Hospital, Bev and Stefan, eh; it looks as though they're going to lose their jobs." I was shocked at your knowledge of my relationship with Stefan. He, Stefan Kellar as you then pointed out, was and is a Women's University doctor, a sexologist and Bev works with him. A year ago, Bev had officially removed herself from my file, her telling Dr. Kellar that she was a close friend of yours. It's now obvious that you've spoken to her about me and my extremely confidential doctors' meetings.

This is not the first time that this sort of thing has taken place. Only 2 years ago and after we had separated, I confided to my younger brother Donald, that I had fathered an out-of-wedlock child in 1967. Again to my shock, Donald said he knew, because his ex-wife Jenn had told him after your telling her. Jenn, a biological out-of-wedlock-and-adopted child herself, had gone to you when you were a social worker at Children's Aid and had asked you for your assistance in tracking down her biological parents. You had then taken it upon yourself without your employer's knowing and without my permission or knowledge, to penetrate the City of Wentworth Children's Aid's system to find out about my child and his traceability (I had confided to you, my fathering the child on our 3rd date, 2 years before we had married). After your communicating at some length with Wentworth, you had later told me without your mentioning your conversation with Jenn, that my child was not interested in contacting me, nor was the child's biological mother interested in communicating with him or me.

Maria, I said nothing in 1987–1988 when you defrauded the Unemployment Insurance Commission out of a year's benefits while you openly told relatives, neighbors and fellow school-moms that you planned to stay home with your children so that they "wouldn't have to be raised by some Phillipina nanny." Nor did I say anything when you failed to inform Unemployment Insurance of your won severance. But I must ask you to stop using your office, station and professional status to seek inroads into my personal life and, when suited to your own gain, make them public.

*Alan*

---

## Still Searching By Thursday

Half of those 20 broken-brained years have passed since in 1992 I met with my kind, old Doctor Fisher. He was a 78 year-old psychiatrist, an Austrian Jew schooled in Vienna and he had the look of Freud. He had been a Holocaust victim, pulled by the Nazis en route to a concentration camp, forced to work for them, then captured by the Allies and imprisoned in Canada. There he had used his devotion to humankind to help all those around him, and within the world community, had grown to be one who worked all the waking hours to help the world's living.

"Alan, you are a remarkable human being. Yes, these tragedies did happen, the brain damage is there to stay and you have been horribly wronged. But in your lifetime, you have been hit by many trucks...I think it would take a Himalayan mountain..."

I dropped my head and began doing what had become for me an almost physical impossibility, that of forming tears. My eyes turned back to his.

"You are very kind, Doct' Fiscsher."

I did not appreciate the slurred nature of my speech nor had I ever, post-brain injury, sensed such slurring. Any drug would do it and no-one now knew but I, how I had functioned before.

It was in the wee hours before dawn and I was not in his office but in his home, an old mansion next to a back yard of apple trees and green ravine. I was with Doctor Fisher on the 3rd floor in a small room nestled into the mansion's northeast corner. One would have seen within a few hours, the sun rise through the east Palladian window. The room was paneled on all 4 walls with books from floor to ceiling. There was one cloth chair that had a look of patient neglect as if it had been waiting for someone for a long time but was resigned to under use. There was one other chair, Dr. Fisher's own, with lumbar support to aid his ailing back, and next to his chair sat a desk drawerless and empty, save a single book. The desk rested inward toward the northern wall and if one sat and worked at it and then looked to the right, one would look out through the window, over the big back yard and into the green ravine.

The sole book on the desk was entitled *Alcohol and Alcoholism* and had been introduced by another doctor, Sir Martin Roth, who had been President of the United Kingdom's Royal College of Psychiatrists. The book was open to a page on brain injuries and the likelihood of a victim's developing alcoholism within 12–24 months post-injury.

Dr. Fisher was awaiting 2 phone calls from England, one from Sir Roth and the second from Geoffrey Fellowstock, also a doctor and head of all medical and science faculties at the University of London.

I had been seen for 9 years by Dr. Fisher and my staying standing at that moment to defy my Ativan was not known to me to be in vain. I stood fast, feet wide apart, looking directly down at Doctor Fisher who was sitting upright and trying to ease, from time to time, his aching back. From where I stood at the southern edge of the room, I could look out through the window's paneled darkness and fantasize my being in a Barbizon school of vision, eyeing black treetops and the roofline of my college's former poet, E. J. Pratt. My eye had a kind of wishful overlay as if I longed to round out the sharp edges of reality.

Dr. Fisher's wife and grandchildren were asleep on a floor below but somehow I had known he would be awake when I had telephoned. He had agreed to see me and had left the front door open. I had already taken the 6 milligrams of his prescribed night-time Ativan but could still not sleep and had marched the 30 minutes to his house, climbed the wide front stairs and found his little room at the back.

"Alan, I'm glad you could come. It seems the traumatic brain injury has not hurt your sense of direction."

I was still puffing from the speed walk, stair climb in my winter clothes and Ativan.

"I was a Cub Scout leader, Dr. Fishch. In fact, I …"

Doctor Fisher was smiling gently. He knew of my need to compensate and of my rewired brain's often breaking off into mega-bites. I stopped the bragging litany.

"Alan, I'm not surprised at your continued rage. Yes, what happened remains a disgrace and a scandal…Have you taken the Ativan yet?"

"Yes, 6 millillgrams, Dr. Fishsher and the 'est r in my pocket."

"Remarkable…I suggest best, Alan if you pass on taking any more today."

Feeling some comfort in his knowing the amount of sedative in me, I sat down and lowered my head to stare at the bare oak floor.

"Dr. Fishsher, you're a 24th hour survivor of t' Holocaust and you know my family ss been in Canada for 200 years."

I raised my eyes to meet those of a tearful Dr. Fisher.

"But Doctor Fishsher, I feel I know how a Jew felt 50 years ago in a German courtroom."

"You are not dead, Alan."

"M' I nnot worse, Doctor Fisher?"

"I have given a great deal of thought over the years to your situation, Alan, and your call tonight heightened my thinking."

Dr. Fisher's eyes lowered to the floor, and mine followed as if trying to find the spot where he focused.

"Alan, you have permanent brain damage. You incurred bleeding in your left frontal lobe, hypothalamic disturbance, diabetes insipidus, hormonal and organic personality change, memory, speech and balance loss, impotence and a more diffuse ripping of your brain."

In all the time spent with me, Doctor Fisher had never been so categorical. Our eyes met again and his face changed to a fatherly smile.

"Alan, you have talents that you have not yet begun to tap and those talents remain."

"But Foctor Disher, I was in the Mendelssohn Choir and now cannot even get out the notes, artic'late or r'member t' words. And my mouth is so visshcous, it feels like old milk!"

"But the musical ability remains, Alan. It taught you how to speak again, granted in a slower and more approximate way."

"Speak? Doctor Fishsher, I love you and I'm not yelling at you now but, Dr. Fishsher, I was a champion elocutionist. I could ar-ti-cu-late with John Cleese speed! I was a master mimic of any sound! Now I can't find th' words, mixm nup and can't pronounce sher-tain conshonants. I can't tongue with the letters 't' and 'k' the way I was known for, when I played French horn. The top of my t'mouth is dead and so is the tip of my tongue!"

"All that is true, Alan and perhaps those problems constitute one reason why you write so much now. You have told me that with the pen, you have time to retrieve or correct your words...Alan?" His eyes focused straight on mine.

"Yes, Doctor Fishsher."

"Alan, since you were a tiny child, you have felt responsibility for the good of the world."

"How...I guessh it takes one to know one."

"I am thankful to have come to understand so many parts of you, Alan."

"But what can I do now, with a crusshed brain?"

"The same as a great contributor to our 20th century, with a crushed country."

I looked for long seconds into Doctor Michael Fisher's eyes. In front of me was sitting a 78 year-old ex-Viennese Jew, a student of Freud, a man who knew Einstein and so many others. His eyes never left me.

"Gorbachev."

All stopped. I had loved discussing international affairs in another life and my mind started running wild, wondering from where this vision of a wise old doctor had come.

"He has saved as many lives as Stalin took and as many as those before."

I tried to bring the talk back to my perceived here and now.

"But Dr. Fishsher, what could I ever hope to do, especially now that much of my brain is dead?"

"Now, especially because much of your brain is dead, Alan."

"Sho. You finally admit it, Dr. Fishsher?"

"I never doubted it."

"I guessh you never did say otherwise."

His eyes stayed focused on mine.

"Write, Alan."

"Write?"

"You have shown over a period of time that you can weave thoughts together to write a document or powerful piece of fiction. Now Alan, I hope you will feel you must, write something never written before. A complete account of a closed brain injury and all the neurological, psychological and sociological sequelae related thereto, from the patient's perspective."

"And incur more savagery?"

"Change the names to protect the guilty."

"...Then?"

"Give it to the world. The next steps will unfold for you, Alan."

I looked at the little man, then my eyes scanned the desk and wooden wall behind him. The daylight was still some time off but I sensed some threat from its illumination. I wanted to stay in the present with this world doctor who was trusting to share with me something he felt I would understand.

"Doctor Fishsher, you make me proud to say that I am a member of the human race."

It was 5:00 a.m. and Dr. Fisher was late for a house call. He graciously left. Shortly I departed, leaving in a haze to walk the 2 miles home.

For a week I tortured every thought, but I now think there was never any truer feeling than the one which kept coming back. I was going to say "yes" to Doctor Fisher and for all that he stood. I wanted to sense his confidence in my knowing.

— • —

I was once again in a giant old Dr. Fisher house but this time his midtown office, full of many doctors. I was in his waiting room.

"Excuse me. Mister Cooper?"

"Alan. Yes?"

"I am Dr. Atlas...Doctor Fisher died 4 hours ago. I don't know anything about your relationship with Dr. Fisher but I have been asked to tell you."

The next words I barely got out. "He was my mentor."

Doctor Atlas put her arm on my shoulder. "I'm sorry," then left.

I remained alone in the empty waiting room, not conscious of why. It was as if I still had to stay my full hour, hoping to glean some assurance that Dr. Fisher would still be there. I had grown to love him and had for years felt parented by the physically little man who knew me. I waited for his slow footsteps to come down the hall and for his gentle face to appear once again, asking me quietly to come in.

I heard steps on the carpet leading to the waiting room and the familiar groaning of hardwood underneath. But the groans did not have that measured predictability that I had long associated with Dr. Fisher. It was Dr. Atlas who was coming to deliver the news to the next scheduled patient.

"Oh! Sorry, Mr. Cooper. I thought...Are you all right Alan?"

She smiled as if not to rush me, and then stepped out. Alone again, I stood and for the last time, went through Doctor Fisher's waiting room door.

A day later, I went to the funeral on Bathurst Street in Beth Tzedec synagogue and was invited to a Shiva at the Fisher home. Among the many dignitaries, I was made to feel welcome and to my later surprise, found myself lecturing Dr. Fisher's daughter Liva over her don't-care comment about work.

"We need to carry on and help others. Doctor Fisher must know that we will. Otherwise..."

I became louder and more animated. "...the poor man will probably roll over!"

The nod by Doctor Fisher's daughter, herself a doctor, built confidence in me. I told her of her father's request and she became eager to learn parts of her father she had never known. Then without warning, my broken-brained indecision struck and I started to stall. "The book would often ramble, with my now-rambling brain."

"It would help me understand to see such rambling. I'm a doctor."

Twelve months passed and I wrote only 12 lines of what I never had an opportunity to promise Dr. Fisher. His wife phoned me on the first anniversary of her husband's death and invited me to speak at a special memorial. It was at an expensive home on Toronto's Bridle Path and if there were any other non-Jews present, I was one of the few. I spoke without microphone to 100 friendly faces, my wanting to feel closer to these Dr. Fisher friends I did not know. They listened in silence with all eyes fixed upon me and afterward congratulated me on my tribute, talking of my story as if they could feel some sense of empathy with the dilemma of my unjust condition.

## My Sensing Some Clarity by Friday, Day 7 Post-failure

alanjohn.cooper@utoronto.ca
104 Helendale Avenue
Toronto, Ontario M4R 1C7
(416) 488-0228

Dear James and Robert,                    Friday May 3, 2002

It is nearing Father's Day and like the 2 Father's Days past, you probably won't be allowed to see me. Anyway, what is important now is that you both carry forward in life from wherever I leave off. No, I am not dying. I don't have time. I am on a mission, passionately pleaded for by my sweet old Dr. Fisher. I did not know at the time that one week later when I was scheduled to see him again, he would be dead at 78. Your mother knew Doctor Fisher, saw him with me for a while in the first few years after my brain injury, and I feel I must have seen him 100 times. He was a world famous psychiatrist, held in awe by some of the most senior international people I have ever seen, whisking in and out of his office. Dr. Fisher represented to your Goy

Boy Dad, the best of what the Jewish mind can contribute and I loved him dearly. Here is what he said to me.

'Alan, please, you must do this. There are many millions of people on this planet with brain damage and they can not speak for themselves. We medical practitioners, whether we be neurologists, neurosurgeons, psychiatrists or any of the thousands of cretins hacking money out of this system, don't understand brain injuries or the brain-injured person. We have never had a patient who could so precisely and comprehensively articulate to us the symptomatology. For you to be able to do so means that you must not only have been extraordinarily gifted before but also about equally developed in both right and left hemispheres. Your Dentist Dr. Kockman is right. The tooth configuration that you have, with 2 eye teeth punching down and 2 other teeth missing, is *extremely* rare and indicative of an equally rare intelligence. Your eyes too, in the toddler photo that you have shown me, radiate that penetrating, backlit intelligence.'

James and Robert, I am going to try to write a book, with names changed to protect the guilty. I don't know how I'm going to pull it off with no money.

I was on student loans over the last year and was going to Teacher's College. Despite my working every waking minute since September, Teacher's College just failed me. I am appealing but the way the College is playing the appeal game, it is timing it so that it is logistically impossible to graduate in June or go for teaching job interviews. In fairness, they do not know what they are doing.

Anyway, your university costs are taken care of, if you go to the University of Toronto at Victoria College and first take there an undergraduate degree in as mind-broadening a discipline as you can. The bursaries will be even bigger for you both if you go into residence, starting in year one. Thereafter, you will still both be on bursaries, to specialize in whatever area you choose. U. of T. is financially strapped but the College, I'm told is rolling in it. It is landlord to some of the plushest land on Bloor Street. Your godparent Regis Waters says just keep your marks up.

James, you were given by your aunt when you were a toddler, a book illustrating why your middle name is Franklin. Your great grand-father Papa was Arthur Franklin Cooper, and every generation gets the Franklin name since Benjamin Franklin.

Robert, you may not know this but after we had all come back from visiting your mother's cousins in Buffalo, your 3 year-old brother James was making non-hurtful fun of their accents. James was saying "Oh my Gad, oh my Gad means you are going crazy." You put down your knife and fork, looked across the table at James and said "No, James. 'Oh my God' does not mean you are going crazy; 'Oh my God' is just an expression." I looked at you, then at Mommy, then back at you. Then I said to you "It's lonely at the top, Robert. All you hear is your own echo." Robert, you were 22 months old.

Dr. Fisher once said to me of our ancestors, 'Alan, don't rest your shoulders on them, let them rest their shoulders on you.' James and Robert, I love you more than I thought one human being could ever love another, and so soon I would like to rest on your shoulders. I am going again to that shack at Round Lake for 2 weeks, from June 29th to July 13th. I would love to have you join me, like we did in happier times.

Love forever,
*Dad*

And so, from the 12 lines I wrote after Dr. Fisher died 10 years ago, I start again my story.

# NEAR THE CLOSE OF 1981

The morning after Christmas, Maria and I tore out of Toronto, heading north 200 miles to the village of Sundridge. Before leaving the city, we picked up Constantine after his mother had fed him, then raced up the highway for 3 hours, landing before noon at my parents' village cottage.

The snow was waist deep in front of my parents' summer home and we had to wade our way to the front door, leaving the ski stuff in the car. Our little German sedan sat passively along the main ploughed road and looked somewhat out of place in rural Canada.

The home's heating had been pre-set above freezing, before my mother and father had set out for their 4 months wintering south of Tampa. We turned on the furnace, unzipped our parkas and laid out our lunch. Thirty minutes later, we were back in the car, setting out for a little local slope to do some light afternoon skiing.

The cold clear air felt welcome after both the 3-hour drive and previous night's pig-out, and it became hard to recall that only a half-day earlier, Maria's father had been ramming straight vodka down my sizzling esophagus. My wife had not noticed, since she too had been imbibing while listening slavishly to the unending incantations coming out of her mother's mouth. Even Maria's younger brother Constantine had been into the sauce and the whole house had meandered over the evening in a state of disintegration. Presents had been opened and broken, sweet grandmother Babcia had sat in silence, food had poured forth and noise and alcohol had covered all.

After 3 hours of get-in-shape skiing, we headed back to the cottage. Maria started whisking from kitchen to bedrooms, eventually settling herself solely in the kitchen, while Constantine and I played darts in the basement. Mother-in-law Yolanta made her mandatory phone call some time before 6:00 p.m. and would have stayed on longer but for hearing that daughter Maria was making us supper. We sat down and ate, then ate again and when Constantine and I tried to pry ourselves away, Maria popped up to offer more. She then started scurrying back and forth, not allowing me in front of Constantine to do my customary dishes and kept up the showbiz long enough to prepare bedding for Constantine and unpack his clothes. After TV, we all went to bed at 10:00.

## December 27, 1981

Saturday kicked off early, our feeling in high spirits after the previous day's workout and long night's sleep. We skied away the sunshine at Nipissing Ridge, south of the little city of North Bay but far north of any Torontonian. By 4:30 in the afternoon, we began seeing shadows on the hill and sensed our skiing would have to stop.

We departed Nipissing Ridge and drove a couple of curvy miles east along the snow-packed road leading back to main Highway 11. It was already starting to darken and the sun on the rear of the road was falling below the snow banks behind us. Once we were back on Highway 11, instead of turning right to head south the 30 miles back to Sundridge, we veered north to try searching for some new eating place in North Bay.

We arrived in the beginning of a snow squall and in the hopes that the storm would soon blow over, opted to turn off Highway 11 down to Lake Shore Road for a quick dinner. After schnitzels, salads and some herbal tea, we left the restaurant, only to find fluffy snowflakes filling the air all around us and the 6:30 p.m. a December night's black.

We whisk-broomed the snow off our little car, wedged ourselves in against the ski equipment and slowly drove southeast along snow-smothered Lake Shore Road. The snowstorm was semi-blinding by then and was producing the odd whiteout where for seconds at a time, nothing could be seen.

"Looks like last year, Alan, when your hiatus hernia forced you to overnight in North Bay."

"You drove in this?"

"It seemed as bad, and all I could think of was getting back to Sundridge to phone."

We reached the junction with Highway 11 and found the snowed-over ramp to head right and south. We had wanted to see the 1930s birthplace of the Dionne quintuplets just 2 miles down the road but such was not to be. We were alone going south but for 2 red tail-lights 100 yards ahead of us. We were driving at the maximum speed we could, 20 miles per hour in the increasingly thick snow, and coming north was a long train of traffic, 10 cars or more, crawling in procession through the dark night and new, white snow blanket.

We were rounding a long lazy turn when suddenly a pair of wide headlights appeared directly in front of us. A huge car was pounding north, straight up our southbound lane. As Maria screamed, I swerved the sports sedan as far right as it could go into the southbound shoulder but the lights kept coming, in fact, swerved to face us, off in the shoulder. The last vision I had that night was of a big old full-sized Buick with its angry Wildcat grill, heading at high speed right for my driver's door. I don't recall at all the cannon-like sound that followed—by then, the world had turned soundless and black.

This story is being re-started on Saturday May 4th, 2002. I put down 12 lines of it 10 years ago after that plea from world famous

Doctor Fisher. Twenty years have passed since a cognitively challenged and unemployable man drove his estranged wife's $300 Buick Wildcat into the driver's door of my little car.

The 20th century is behind us now and the world is changing with blinding speed. To some immeasurable degree, Canadians still feel themselves morally purer than their American cousins and continue to vocalize outrage at them and their leaders. But Canadian people in power, Canadian leaders, do they really behave differently than the tyrants of our planet's most oppressive regimes?

Back to my story. I have written these first pages in over 300 hours with extreme difficulty. The primary reason for that difficulty is the key result of that car accident 20 years ago when that giant old Buick Wildcat hit my car, squashed it and changed my life forever. The car accident has left me permanently, irretrievably, brain damaged and it is now only through exhaustive repetition and note-taking that I keep track of day-to-day living. Physical, neurological damage is the number one reason why these first pages have taken so much agony and work.

Now I begin the next 300 or more pages. They will be much more difficult to produce and much more painful, since I now have to deal with the aftermath across these past 20 years. Though my absorption of new information is and forever will be severely impaired, since that erratic driver broke my brain more than 2 decades ago, I have learned much about life, about people, that I would rather not have learned.

But I must write down what has happened, for in Canada alone where over 30 million people live, 50 thousand per year incur traumatic brain injury. In the United States with 300 million people, 500,000 per year get badly brain injured. Quick arithmetic suggests that on planet Earth with its 6 billion people, 10 million annually get closed head injured. In poorer countries, many die, but in Earth's economically advanced nations, most brain-injured people still live.

Doctors have not scratched the surface of understanding the vast unknown of the human brain, let alone one broken. There are billions, multiplied by more billions of kinds of brain injuries and one of the biggest enemies we broken-brained people suffer from is the notion that so-called experts of any kind understand what it is like. Brain-injured people almost to the person, cannot communicate their problems to any doctor or anyone. Within this ignorance, many medicinal pimps live off a system which, like religion to the spiritually hungry, distorts things to every evil end.

Just as an alcoholic may help another alcoholic, so too must we brain-injured people begin to help ourselves. Damned difficult because the helping mechanism can be the very thing broken, the depression-fighting apparatus the very thing depressed, the injury repair control center the thing damaged and the communications control center part of the very thing crushed. But we are all broken in different ways, and like the alcoholic, are shattered mentally, physically and spiritually. If an alcoholic whose condition is unlike that of another alcoholic, can still help that other, then maybe a brain-injured person whose condition will always be different from that of another, can be of some help, too. In any event, can we broken-brained people afford to continue dependency on non-empathetic people who claim to have our best interests at heart?

It has to fall to some broken-brained person to try to help us. The problem is not going to go away, it is rather going to get worse and while so far, we have not been able to communicate well our dilemma, no one knows the depth and scope of the problem so well as a brain-injured person. This situation could go on for another generation or more as 21st century medicine ironically improves brain-injured people's chances to keep breathing. But if we are ever to hope for a life more than mere survival, we must create some breakthrough way to speak for ourselves.

I have perhaps gone through over 2 decades of hell and snuck under some wire of life to undertake now, that work which constitutes some meaning. The brain is a bigger frontier than the deepest depths of our oceans or the farthest reaches of outer space and any understanding of the brain broken may help us understand the brain unbroken. Maybe too, in unraveling the brain, we begin to unravel much else.

At any rate, never again must any closed brain-injured person have to undergo what I have been through. I must honor Doctor Fisher, do what he knew I could do and stop the preposterous injustice that is being perpetrated on every brain-damaged person.

## Toronto, 5 1/2 Years Later in 1987: Trying to Explain to James, Age 3 and Robert 1

"You see boys, before you were born, a dangerous driver such as you've heard about in Ms. Wilmott's Nursery School, came cruising up our cottage highway, at night, in a snow blizzard, on the wrong side of the road."

I was acting out every part to my toddlers' enchanted eyes. "I swerved and thus saved Mommy and Uncle Con's lives but the little car I was driving was no match for his 2-ton Buick. Its big, saw-toothed grill crashed into my door and knocked me out."

I fell to the lawn and pretended to be unconscious. James and Robert fell to the ground too and started imitating what they thought I was doing. They rolled over toward me and I gathered my 2 sons under each arm. Together, we lay on our backyard lawn, all looking up at the sky.

"Mommy went with me by ambulance to the hospital in North Bay and then taxied back to Sundridge with Uncle Con. In Nana's house, she happened to see on your Papa Cooper's desk, the phone number for their doctor.

The doctor was really angry when he heard about the hospital doing nothing in North Bay. He ordered an ambulance-airplane to fly me to Toronto's Flanders Hospital. You know, James, the big one near here with its neurological intensive care unit."

"What does noorelojens care mean, Daddy?"

"Help, James for people like me with broken brains."

"Wasyr brain broken, Daddy?"

"Yes, Robert."

"Did turt, Daddy?"

"I don't know, Robert. I was like this."

I went back to playing a sort of semi-consciousness. James followed suit and Robert followed James.

"Like this, Daddy?"

"Yes, James."

"Ike 'is, Daddy?"

"Yes, Robert."

"I was like this for 7 days and I couldn't talk the way we are talking now. I didn't seem to know much of anything."

James was puzzled. "Why do you know everything now, Daddy?"

I felt a moment's gratitude. "Thank you, James, but Daddy doesn't know everything, just a few more things than you do for now."

"W' we know more tomorrow, Daddy?"

"Yes, Robert and more in the tomorrows after that."

"Did you have to have stitches, Daddy? I had to have stitches at Sick Children's Hospital."

"No, James. My bleeding was internal. I mean inside."

"So that doesn't hurt as much?"

"Well, I don't think I felt much but the damage was pretty bad. The main blood splotch was called mild, leading some people to be confused and call the whole brain injury mild. There was a ripping and tearing over all of my brain."

I took my 2 hands and pretended to rip cardboard, with a

tearing sound. I then scratched my fingers across my shirt, in imitation of an airplane making a hard touchdown.

"Mommy was told my brain damage was severe."

James and Robert were still looking up at the sky but when they heard the word "severe," James sensed some recognition, perhaps from context and tone. He let out a gentle "Ohhh" and Robert followed. James, then Robert, rolled over and hugged me.

"I love you, Daddy."

"I love you, Daddy."

"I love you, James. I love you, Robert."

"When will Mommy come home from work?"

"In about 2 hours, boys, at around 6:00. Until then, it's just us."

They both rolled closer and again gave me a loving hug. We stayed huddled together, with all of us looking up at the clouds lulling by overhead.

"Will we ever learn, Daddy about your car accident?"

"I hope so James and Robert, for you both are extremely intelligent and can help give us brain-injured people some understanding of who we are."

Robert was only 20 months old and rarely asked a question before 3 year-old James. This time, I guess he felt he had to. "B' Daddy, you already know who you are."

I hugged Robert more closely to me and squeezed his little toddler self.

"Robert, you are a sweetheart. Eager to know but always kind in asking."

We were in our old North Toronto backyard that day in May of 1987, one day of almost 200 I spent that year with my sons James and Robert. Never since the brain injury had I known such happiness.

"Daddy, tell me what happened with that car accident and the hoser driver Barry Lewis."

"Mommy was told by the brain doctor, Schwantz that I was

undergoing a remarkable recovery and would be back to 100% in 3 months."

"What is 100 pure sent, Daddy?"

"Sorry, Robert. It's an expression meaning all better, if used that way."

"So your brain would be all better again in 3 months, Daddy?"

"That is what I was told, James. Mommy was pleasantly surprised, given I was still blurry after a whole week. She took me out of Flanders Hospital after only 9 days, on condition that I stayed under her direct care. Mommy insisted she was a professional social worker who knew what to do, and the hospital did not follow up."

"After only 9 days, Daddy with a broken brain?"

"Yes, James. There was a strange doctor who kept asking about me and telling my own doctor wrong things. The strange doctor said he knew me but didn't. He was not from the hospital but was still going into my hospital records. Outside doctors could do that then."

Robert skipped over the unknown word "records" and asked "Were you all better aft' 3 muns, Daddy?"

"No, Robert I wasn't but I didn't dare let my place of work know that. My whiplash ached, my speech slurred unless I spoke Texas-style and I couldn't seem to remember anything new. I felt I had to pretend I would be all better soon and return to work by the end of February."

"Were you all better by then, Daddy?"

"No, James. Near the start of February, I began to see the horrible things that had happened to my brain forever. In front of Mommy, I collapsed in tears."

Just then, Robert also broke down in tears. "It's all right, Daddy. We'll take care of you. We love you."

## The Devastating Reality of January–February 1982
## After the December 27, 1981 Crash

I recall those days, perhaps because they penetrated me like the death of a spouse. In Intensive Care, I screamed for Maria during a fleet of consciousness and her mother later decreed how I had so proved out my love. Beyond that emotion in those first 9 days in Flanders, I felt no depression or anger or sorrow.

Maria repeatedly told me I was to be fully recovered within 3 months and I may have found some solace in so knowing. She later told me, however, I had not seemed to care about anything. I did not seem to feel much other than a deep wish to go home and get more than the badly broken sleep in Flanders Hospital.

While I was in hospital in this semi-coherent state, I kept getting phone calls from work, all from boss Willy Cork. When word first reached the Ministry of Food that I was in hospital, Assistant Deputy Minister Cork began sourcing information about brain injuries from the ADM at Health. Cork went on to circulate stories about my brains being scrambled. He was particularly intrigued by the Health Assistant Deputy's saying I might now be unable to get an erection—Cork and his wife for years had assumed I had been fornicating my pretty female staff. The concept of androgynous management was foreign to both Corks and Willy in one of his many variations on a lie, had spread across the Ministry that I had been sexually compromising my underlings in exchange for their promotions. Cork himself had tried to get a piece of the perceived action but had failed gracelessly.

While Willy Cork worked his way through the Food Ministry, manipulating all possible angles against me, a Doctor Malthrop was at work in Flanders Hospital. Malthrop was a psychiatrist and had documents substantiating his accreditation in many areas of formal learning. Totally unbeknownst to half-conscious me, Malthrop was already changing things in Flanders, working for the other side in a legal battle to which I had not yet given a thought. Flanders doctors and other health workers were made to believe that Malthrop was working for me, and that I was hiding things and more coherent than pretending. The poisonous misconception would spread without end.

During the final 3 weeks of January 1982, alone at home, my "miraculous recovery" began to experience a locomotive slowdown. I think my first doubts were sewn then that I would not have a full recovery. My balance was so bad that I had to stagger the 10 city blocks to physiotherapy in extreme bowleggedness. My speech improved but it still slurred badly and my consonant blends would frequently reverse themselves. Getting my "mords wixed" and saying "shuhi sef" was the norm of the day. In the mirror, my eyes looked crossed as if I had Down's syndrome and my pupils remained at 2 different sizes. I felt the acuity of my hearing worsened. I found it exceedingly difficult to smell anything and often confused those things I did smell. My saliva was viscous and I could not whistle. The extremities of my lips and tip of my tongue felt dead, and any thought of my speaking French again or resurrecting French horn playing was gone, as was as yet-to-be known my singing. I had no hunger for food; I had no hunger for sex. I kept finding it extraordinarily difficult to locate, sort and retrieve words from my brain's library, and would call water "black" when I meant "hot."

New information became exceptionally difficult for my brain's left hemisphere to absorb and retrieve, and proper names were almost impossible. If I did absorb new information, I could still find recall of it impossible or slow-to-come or incorrect but similar in sound. Odd to me but numbers, not names, stayed easy to retain. As I became increasingly aware of this exception, I began to cling to numbers, quantifying things wherever possible and showing off to others who questioned my memory, my skill at recalling statistics, phone numbers or numbers of any kind. I began to write numbers always in their non-verbal form as I do now in this true story. This sudden, new preoccupation with numbers was never explained to me, and my inconsistency between recall of numbers and names would play a pivotal role in further destruction.

The direct hit had been to the left, frontal lobe and there had been a diffuse ricochet-ripping across the entire brain. Those parts that I thought were intact became increasingly exasperated with the shattered parts and I felt a war breaking out inside my mind. My personality, itself riveted and rewired by the accident, seemed to be in the middle of a lopsided war between once 2 equals, like a sensitive child witnessing the separation between 2 loved and respected parents and unable to do anything about it.

Most difficult for me to understand then or express now is that physically deranged personality, because I express that change now with the same altered personality. Dr. Fisher told me I was a symphony gone sour. Formerly an outgoing person, I wanted no well-wisher to hear my crushed communicative abilities, none to see my insidious depression, no-one to suspect the permanency of my brain damage. I would try camouflaging my injuries with humor, but unlike my pre-accident wit which friends had applauded, my humor was suddenly *witzelsucht*, off color and inappropriate.

My parents had telephoned once in early January to Flanders Hospital but the conversation had bordered on the impossible. I could not be understood and was passing in and out of semi-consciousness. My parents tried again in mid-January 1982, when they received a long note from Maria. Then Maria and my parents tried to talk about lawyers. Maria told them that she planned to pay off our $68,000 mortgage, but I retorted that I was expected to have a full recovery. My biological parents made it plain that the accident was having a severe impact on them, their health and their emotional well-being. At my urging, they did not visit.

To allay suspicions, I felt that I had to carry through on

returning to work early. My loyal secretary phoned and warned that ugly rumors were flying, particularly after I had a number of sympathy visits from Cork. I thus committed to a premature February 22nd return and then realized I had to build myself up quickly—my weight had plummeted from 170 to 147 pounds and my physical appearance was that of a war prisoner who could not sleep. I had no appetite and could not taste what little food Maria forced me to eat. Across the first 7 days of February, I attempted to put on calories, stimulating my appetite by drinking one, then 2, 3 or as many as 4 pints of Guinness stout during each 24 hours. To no avail—I continued to look like a concentration camp inmate. My face was chalk-white but for 2 black holes that held my crossed and fear-filled eyes. My cheeks were sunken and my cheekbones jagged out. My broken clavicle and whiplash kept me in almost constant pain and my nights were spent tossing and turning to find a comfortable spot for my shoulder and neck.

With each new day of February 1982, some new manifestation of my brain damage revealed itself. Appetite for sex was gone but a new one grew for misplaced anger. I knew nothing of those crashed brain parts that govern social inhibitions and I would stagger into Toronto's sin area, bang off people's shoulders, shove skin heads out of my way and hurl insults, all the while feeling invincible.

One night we had a minor house fire and a deep sleeping Maria was the one to awaken. Maria thus came to realize I could not smell much at all. Other parts of the brain that had controlled addictions seemed uprooted. A non-drinker of caffeine pre-accident, I was suddenly addicted to coffee. A former cardiovascular fanatic, I was suddenly smoking pipes, cigars and cigarettes. Those neurologically deadened parts of my palate became so burnt that my mouth's roof went white like a spent fireplace, and I began developing nicotinic stomatitis. A former health food freak, I was suddenly taking in vast quantities of salt, in an attempt to stimulate my appetite. At night I ate mounds of monosodium glutamate in

Bar-B-Q potato chips, one of the few foods I could taste. The ends of my lips were numb and now suddenly chapped in the cold. My fingers too were numb and on a not-so-cold day in that dreadful February 1982, I almost got frost-bite.

---

## Lawyer Dour and My Wife Maria

I could remember events in my life prior to the brain injury. In that sense, I was not unlike many stroke-plagued patients who can often recall songs from early childhood. The moments leading up to the actual accident seemed clear.

Maria and I finally met a lawyer in late February. Gordon Dour had not been Maria's first choice. She had developed a list from her social work contacts and her first choice had been the law firm of Timpson Cable that specialized in personal injuries, specifically brain injuries. That firm had refused her, citing some conflict, but Maria had gone on for weeks still trying to secure it. Like me, Maria had no idea that Timpson Cable had long been on the case. Dour had come almost by default when I remembered him from years earlier. At the time, my former business law professor had recommended him to me on another issue.

Dour did not remember me at all. When we met, he started by asking my wife and me to describe the accident, and Maria went first. In serious demeanor and professional tone, she began describing in detail, events leading up to the actual crash. As I sat in silence, my jaw dropped and I started wondering about my ability to remember events even before my brain injury. My wife recited full and false details of a clear night with no snow, no traffic and good visibility. She then went on. Not only was her description wrong, each of her details was the exact opposite of what had happened. When litigation lawyer Dour then asked me to relay events,

I did not know what to say, so I simply said Maria's description was totally wrong. As I refuted her statements, detail by tiny detail, she kept interjecting with a quick but theatrical, "Oh yes, that's how it happened." As I continued, Maria kept interjecting while an increasingly skeptical Dour kept looking at me, with his bi-focals lowered and a Lyndon Johnson straight-eye.

While the accident report would prove out everything I said and show Maria 100% wrong, the damage would be done. So much so, that lawyer Dour from that first meeting on, would not believe a word I said and repeatedly told me so. He did not bother to retrieve the accident report and he would go through pre-trial Discoveries, still believing my lying wife, whose interjecting made it look as if I had coached her.

Odd, like another piece that to this day I cannot fit into the puzzle. At the time of my wanting to escape Flanders Hospital, neurosurgeon Dr. Schwantz had told Maria that he had been reluctant to allow me to leave, "...since (I) had been giving (him) a consistently wrong recollection of how the accident had actually happened." When Dr. Schwantz had relayed my description as I later gave it to lawyer Dour, Maria had loudly proclaimed "That's exactly how it *did* happen," and I had immediately been released from Flanders. What false accident details were in the hospital file? Who had been misrepresenting me?

## Grace

Mid-February, I was invited by the Deputy Minister's secretary to attend a formal dinner. All my staff was present as well as a solid complement of Ministry personnel, about 500 in total. I was to sit at the head table, on stage with senior staff but no speeches were expected. While I had been a speaker in demand before the accident, none of the public and few work persons had heard or seen me since. Late in the meal, Willy Cork unexpectedly rose to go to an on-stage microphone. I found his move surprising, since Cork was not a good speaker and had spoken in public only when forced.

"We're all glad to see Alan Cooper back and want him to say a few words."

I was stunned. Impromptus I had always handled with alacrity and Cork had often quashed my doing them. Maybe, only to me was Cork's game plan clear—I had drunk nothing but my slurred speech and loss for words would be picked up by all.

The large audience gave me a welcome cheer. To hide my bad balance, I John Wayne walked to the microphone. "Thank you... I guesh shome of you...carss... a Buick can..." It got worse. I never completed one sentence. I couldn't remember what the preceding clauses or phrases were. My attempts went on for 7 long minutes. The audience was hushed and then a polite applause emerged, but along with it there was a low murmuring.

I have a 1994 edition of *The Chambers Dictionary* (Chambers Harrap Publishers Ltd., Edinburgh. 1994). On page 724, it contains a definition of the word "grace". Grace can mean the undeserved mercy of God but it can also mean any unassumingly attractive or pleasing personal quality, favor or kindness.

---

## "I Am Fine and Will Be 100% in 3 Months"

A week later I returned to work, hobbling into hostility. I tried to perform my senior job and pretended that, except for a broken clavicle, nothing was wrong. I was Director of Marketing in charge of promoting Ontario foods at home and abroad. Neurosurgeon Dr. Mark Schwantz had advised against my going back early but I had insisted: I understood the "100% recovery in 3 months" to mean the end of March. Before returning, however, I saw Dr. Schwantz and he changed his prognosis from a 100% recovery in 3 months to 6. In a panic, I knew I could not credibly change the prognosis for my place of work. Dr. Schwantz demanded that for the first 8 weeks back at work, I was to limit myself to half-days but I feared that my working such slack hours would signal deeper troubles and fuel the rumors of which I had been warned. I intended to build quickly to a full day.

Inside week one I found the normal tasks draining. I handled relentless questions and varnished concern about my well-being with increased fatigue. I kept impeccably groomed but wondered how I was going to pull it all off. I tried to appear my former high-energy self but I looked like an immaculate, white faced zombie.

At the start of week 2, an assignment required my meeting new people from 2 incoming trade missions and part of my Director job was to head both. One mission involved a revamp of Ontario's agricultural trade with emerging Eastern Europe and the other constituted little more than niceties to a pasta trade already completed with the city of Boston. I chose to let junior staff play with the Boston job, while I tackled Eastern Europe hands-on. I was going to try to show off creative, right brain powers and camouflage left brain deficits. At least that was my plan to display I was normal.

Before meeting the 5 mission people, I knew that to avoid being exposed, I would have to memorize their names. I spent an hour alone in my office, repeating them to myself, but to my horror, found I could not recall the 5 people's first and surnames. I was misplacing them, hitting words close to them or losing them entirely. My stomach knotted with the thought that after the upfront handshake and related repeating of names, I would lose them. Having no time to rehearse any longer, I detailed the names into my appointment book, swamping the whole page for that day. That moment marked the birth of my infamous 'black book' where

I learned to store every act I did and all information related thereto, every day for the rest of my life.

Come the introductory portion of the mission, I uttered my name first with apparent confidence, then tried to repeat each person's first name aloud, only to forget it moments later when I repeated the process for the next person. I correctly surmised I would fail even my own people's names and thus committed the forgivable faux pas of leaving Ministry professionals to introduce themselves. When it came time for person #3, I got the names reversed and told the delegate he was Alan Cooper. The delegate then gave me an odd look as if he did not understand that use of English, and I seized the opportunity to make it seem some sort of parody on diplomatic protocol.

Creativity flowed within the loudness and in the days and weeks ahead, I found myself trying to use the same combination of right brain imagination and exhaustively detailed black book to hide my left brain's deadness. I flaunted these spins of creativity and tried juxtaposing myself as an eccentric genius who need not bother recalling unimportant information. "Renaissance Man" one group had coined me years earlier and I tried resurrecting the title to legitimize my new veneer.

Physically, I returned to the University of Toronto squash club, and as part of the Renaissance package, clung to my still being seen as an athlete. In new games with old squash partners, once my even match, I discovered my eye-to-hand coordination was gone. My balance, which had improved dramatically since January, was now put to a different test and on the court I quickly became dizzy and off-balance. I kept the membership to try to show I was healed, but dropped the game forever, as well as hockey, jogging, 10-speed bicycling, indeed all other sports, except for walking and the inter-mittent swim.

My repulsive exaggerations of my abilities, my egocentricities, were there for all to see. Except for me, everybody knew about my brain injury and could witness the damage. My cover-ups and slave-like work forced me to be alone almost every non-working hour. What kept me going was the fact that Flanders Hospital's neurosurgeon and neurologist Doctor Mark Schwantz had done a second prognostication of a 100% recovery, now changed from 3 months to 6.

## I Tried to Get My Wife to Listen

Dear Maria,

It is nearing the end of month 3 in my recovery and Dr. Schwantz as you know, has adjusted his prognosis to a 100% recovery by 12 midnight, June 26th 1982. I have felt no change except for balance, since I returned to work 19 1/2 days ago.

I think I am fooling most everybody at work into thinking I am normal. It's a frenetic scramble but I seem to be pulling it off...

Maria, it seems the only way I can now fairly express myself is on paper and I know that communication too has its deficits and difficulties. The thing though, that writing in pencil gives me—in fact printing, since my cursive writing is no longer artistic or even legible—is time and sight to find words, to recall, to correct misplaced words, to record non-sensible sentence structure and to correct the multitudinous mixing up of words, consonant blends, letters, spelling and slurring of speech that plagues my spoken language so many times daily. If I could write everything I said, my functioning would I guess be vastly improved but I would have to be essentially a mute who could take the time to create and maintain a huge library, more than even the exhaustive note-files I now have, and communicate to others virtually always on paper. And I would have to have a master retrieval command post for sorting and selecting all the information, since I could never rely as I cannot now, on my own memory.

I know you told Flanders orthopedic Doctor England that you found my personality change almost impossible to deal with, Maria but I can't voice what I want to say. Paper seems the only way. I pray this note will give you some understanding, because I don't understand either. I do know though, I love you, Maria.

Love forever,
*Alan*

In keeping with tradition, this intimate piece to my wife went straight to Yolanta, her mother. After consulting with Yolanta, Maria mouthed a smattering back to me but I did not fully hear her and asked for clarification. She loudly repeated the parts I said I had heard and then tapered off, leaving the parts that I said I had not heard, once again inaudible.

"You never acknowledged receipt of my letter."

"Yes, I read it."

"No, you didn't acknowledge it."

"I wanted to think about it first."

"So you shared it with your mother?"

"I needed to check with someone else."

"Check what? And why with an uncertified dental assistant?"

"She's my mother!"

"Master! You constantly complain to me about her and then go to her for any decisions or thinking. What else new have you shared with her about me?"

"Why should I share anything else?"

"Didn't answer the question."

"What question?"

"The one I just asked."

"O.K., so I needed to check how best to help you."

"So you went to her for direction. What did she say?"

"About what?"

"About what you said you checked."

"I don't remember exactly what she said. We talked about a lot of things."

In the hour that followed, I tried writing to a dear friend of mine, Manfred, a professor in Germany. I knew Manfred to be genuine and thought he would want to know.

Shortly, Manfred wrote back.

April 16, 1982

Dear Alan,

Mozart seemed able at a sitting to compose for 70-piece symphonies but Beethoven had to tug and yank out each of his notes. I think, Alan that you are now going to have to work for each note.

Alan, there is a probability that you have undergone a physically rewired personality change. You are now a different human being. Now comes the hard part. Alan, you are a supremely intelligent person with brain damage. You should experience cognitive improvement over the next 2 years but some of that damage may never change.

Alan, I believe our world needs you badly. You must undergo yet another personality change and that change rests on the impossible. You may have to undergo some exasperating experiences before reaching a new equilibrium.

Dieter, Regina and I met with experts and now feel you can do it. We believe in you, Alan.

Please, please stay in close touch.


Peace,
Manfred


Manfred was a loyal friend, even from a distance. Years later, I would try reaching him by phone and when he would call back days later, I would be unable to decipher in my black book, the cross-outs from 3 days earlier. Something else would happen with his 100-year-old grandmother getting my initial call, and I think he would blame me. From that moment, I would lose my close friend Manfred as I would lose over time, all others.


## Sex


For months, I had suspected a problem. Masturbating made it worse. My boss, Assistant Deputy Willy Cork had spent considerable time researching my brain damage and was confident he had seized on something.

Cork had long been trying sabotages of every sort and for a while it had been a game—while he had run around trying to destroy all involved, my dedicated secretary and I had planted decoys to ensure that the work would still get done. But as Cork's schizophrenia had become worse, his actions had become more desperate and far more personal. Cork had labeled my wife for all to hear a fat Pollack. Cork had also spread afar my supposed cavorting on the grounds of her reported ugliness. Cork's wife Anna was obese.

Before I recognized it as a certainty, Cork bellowed in front of my staff, "So, Cooper, we hear you can no longer get it up, ha, ha, ha."

He was testing my reaction and it was neither quick nor good. Cork was right and did not know it but my shocked face helped. I tried to hide my hurt but Willy Cork broke new ground for lowness. I could not get an erection and Cork wanted all to know.

## Alcohol and April of 1982

85% of us traumatic brain-injured (TBI) folk get into drinking problems within 12–24 months of the injury date. However, if we are motorcyclists, our probability is 96%. As a writer of this story, I am now supposed to footnote the Roth book *Alcohol and Alcoholism*, the year it was written, 1979 I think and the page reference. But Sir Roth, you are a famous psychiatrist and must understand that of which I speak—I cannot find the page; I cannot remember exactly where or how I read the book!

In growing exasperation and fear, I went out 4 times that April 1982 and got drunk. My reaction to alcohol, post-brain damage, was new. It took little to wreck my speech or gait, about 4 glasses of wine to snuff out coherence and about 6 drinks to lose it all. Never had I known such suddenness. Others commented on its newness but none knew why.

One day after work, I tried in vain, "But, most of all, he liked the fall. The yellow cottonwoods…I think that I have not yet synchronized with my destiny…All lawyers want to be poets and poets lawyers…Hemingway, Miller, Flaubert, Tropic of Capricorn, Madame Bovary."

"And Hemingway's book, pretentious Cooper?"

"Can't remember. The others are misquotes anyway."

Cork hung on the moment and started doing demagoguery on junior staff.

"The mighty Cooper is a drunken fraud, ha, ha!"

"The lowliest poet rests higher than the mightiest industrialist."

"Who said that?"

"I can't ..."

"Cooper's a drunk, ha ha!"

I paid as always for Cork and all. As I staggered out to leave, Cork provoked staff to laugh.

## Speech

"Maria, this book from the library. I'd like to try an exercise I've just read here. I have to take my tongue and put it behind my upper front teeth."

I was eager to start the exercise but waited for Maria to enter the living room from her kitchen. She snatched a tea towel along the way.

"Like this, Maria."

I tried the exercise again and exaggerated the movement, with mouth wide open in the hope that my wife would watch. She was standing about 6 feet away, with her arms folded and the tea towel drooping down like a warning flag. I took my tongue back.

"Now I'm supposed to use my tongue as a slingshot to trigger a few words off a consonant like 'D.' It says here to avoid 'L's and 'N's, especially when combined. Those are ones I can't do! I tried 'London' and 'familial' at work and I sounded drunk. I think people heard me."

Suddenly I remembered from childhood, seeing *The Music*

*Man* in New York and I recalled a speech-impaired child's singing "Gary, Indiana". I felt a moment's encouragement.

"Dirty, damn Cork. Dirty. Damn. Dam…n…e…d…that's much tougher."

"Good" was all she said, and then she swiveled her rear end to me and bulled her way back to the kitchen. I wanted to feel she cared and I raised my volume.

"The upper part of my tongue or perhaps its front seems lifeless, so my tongue has already been compensating. I have been trying to avoid certain consonant blends which have given me trouble."

"You mean when you've been drinking, according to Cork."

"No! That just makes it worse! I'm talking about always, now…What conversations have you had with Cork?"

"Well, I haven't heard it."

"That's because…"

The rest of my sentence I only felt, "… (you haven't listened!)".

## 2%

I never had the nerve to go to a lingerie shop in Toronto and had even looked over my shoulder before peeking in their windows. Suddenly I was on a trade mission to Brussels and found Belgians to be almost French, with lingerie as much a part of their life as chocolate. I tried to look married and very much in a hurry while on pressing business abroad, and bought a black camisole, mesh stockings and black garter belt. When I got back to Canada on that May 1982 Friday, the time was midnight and I faked fatigue.

Saturday morning proved different. Maria showered for what seemed an hour and spent an exasperating time trying on the lingerie. She strolled back into the bedroom, wearing high heels, mesh stockings, garter belt and open-door panties, and I started to get a hint of an erection. Maria took note, knelt down on the bed, straddled me and tried to put my penis into her vagina. My erection disappeared and tears formed in my eyes.

"Alan, you are not impotent!"

My post-injury need for numbers leaped to my tongue.

"2% potent is what a 90 year-old is."

"You don't know only 2%."

"True. It could be even double that! 4%!"

Maria got dressed and went shopping.

## Toronto and May of '82

That Saturday morning, the beginning of May, I shaved as I always had, with a bowl, brush and fresh blade but this time paused without my glasses on, to catch a look at my eyes. Their sense of being backlit was still gone. My post-accident pupils still appeared aloof and unaware. I showered as I had done daily since adolescence but now without much sense of smell. My post-accident want of a shower seemed to come solely from my desire to keep my body feeling scrubbed dry.

As a teenager in 1962, I had learned that polyester put red spots on my skin and in the 20 years since, I had worn only natural fabrics. My undershirt, underpants and socks were 100% cotton, and my winter socks all wool. My shoes, too, were of a natural fabric as were shirts and sweaters. I had a cotton jacket, cotton raincoat and wool overcoat for winter. What had also been true for those 20 years was my refusal to wear a logo, and no identifiers of any sort were allowed to adorn my clothes. Everything was always fresh but unpressed, my view of pressing being some sort of surrender to suburban values. Casual clothing pieces were always variations of green or brown and I remember answering "green and brown" in elementary school's first grade when others had fired off "red" as their favorite color. A neighbor, Mrs. Creighton, had told my mother that people who like green and brown were born in December and I had been born December 8th, 1947. I guess I would have first seen Canadian green at around 3 to 4 months of age.

Since backpacking through Europe in 1972, I had worn safari shirts, safari pants or shorts, and safari jacket, all with buttoned pockets. Now my pocket system was sanctified to minimize dependence on memory. My wallet went into the left buttoned front pants pocket, my keys and cardholder into the buttoned front right. A white 100% cotton handkerchief, un-pressed but fresh each day, went into the unbuttoned inner pocket on the right and any loose change into the left. A comb went into the unbuttoned left pocket at rear and a watch set to the exact time, went onto my left wrist and came off only for showering. If I were traveling out of Toronto, the pattern could expand to the 4 pockets of my safari jacket, to accommodate spare glasses, passport, Swiss army knife, facial tissue pack, heirloom compass or World War II binoculars. The system would never change and as I write this day, I am seated in safari clothes, with wallet, keys and cards safely buttoned, and inner pockets housing comb, coins and fresh un-pressed handkerchief.

After my morning rituals, I walked eastward over to the opulence of midtown Yonge Street and then south 5 miles to the corner of Yonge and College. On the last blocks south of Bloor Street, I hit the Yonge Street Strip and began sensing a film settling over me as if I were a TV evangelist whose pores oozed fried chicken. I opted to escape westward, along the north side of College Street, walking opposite Eaton's elegant 1930s midtown store. West of it was a new building, a silver-blue, soft-cornered monolith that was home to publisher Maclean Hunter. It was already being hit with rays of mid-morning sun and the building was beaming a blue hue over the old architecture all around it.

I crossed Bay Street and kept heading west, past the restored old Sick Children's Hospital and the variegated front of Toronto Hospital, gracefully scaled away from College Street. When I reached the wide and medianed University Avenue, I did not cross but chose instead to wind my way north around Queen's Park Circle, passing on my left the stiff Victorianism of Ontario's Parliament Buildings. Behind the Legislature, I slipped across the northbound lanes of Queen's Park Circle, plopped into Queen's Park and there I sat. I peered at Victoria College to my north, St. Mike's to my northeast, the faculty of Law to my northwest, beloved Hart House to my west and the old oaks all around me.

It was Saturday the beginning of May. Queen's Park's squirrels seemed somewhat baffled that morning—no nut givers were around. The University of Toronto's school year had just ended and the 1982 summer semester was yet to begin. But for me, that giant part of the Park which divided much of U. of T.'s campus was empty of human beings. Though the air was cool and moist, it felt bracing to a mind trying to heal.

It was rare to have 20 minutes free time before the university pool opened. Rarer still to be alone under a day's light in a big city's midtown park, experiencing it only with dozens of centuries-old oaks, hundreds of squirrels and one visible acorn, temporarily overlooked by those hundreds who had been fed until now on farmed peanuts.

I looked down at the acorn and then looked up at the oaks' branches, each of them working one with the other to assure room for all to absorb the sun, and all of them working together to form an organic superstructure of strength and harmony. This spring, the superstructure was re-creating baby green from within.

My eyes fell to the acorn. I feel that trees cannot necessarily unravel answers to the mystery of life but I do sense they can offer clues to the series of riddles related thereto.

My jacket's lower pocket held a book I had begun trying to

read post-injury—*The Holy Bible*. I was afraid to ask why "The", because I feared I knew the answer. But I was more afraid to ask why "Holy" because of the abuse of its allegories and cop-out of its writings as being divinely inspired.

Before studying the 2 Testaments of one of the many bibles of our planet's many religions, it certainly would have helped the clarity of communications, had I been fluent in Hebrew and Greek. It is difficult enough to read the writings of pseudonymous collators and interpreters of aged, word-of-mouth folklore, without having to worry further about the filtering and inevitable reinterpretation of message caused by linguistic translation. While trying to wade through schools of thinking found in both text and exegeses, one can feel an urge to get a pick and shovel. One can also begin to feel the size of loss in the burning down of the world's biggest library in Alexandria during the Western World's self-described biblical times.

Did not God give us brains and their intrinsic intellects and imaginations to question our beliefs forever, just as the same Creator recreates through all things forever? If $E = mc^2$, does not logic dictate that God is a verb, energy, the Big Bang behind the Big Bang, the reason the electron, indeed the big quark, behaves at random, in freedom? I fantasized.

Dear God,

Only a few feel, I feel, true you. I feel I as yet do not. Imperfect human beings too often want things to be finite and most often have simply labeled you "perfect". James, I feel, knew you as may have his brother Jesus. Göthe seemed to know of the importance of your creation nature as may have Mendelssohn and as did Chief Seattle. Nietzsche had enough penetration to see some light but was possibly clouded by hatred for so-called Saint Paul. Dostoevsky, I think I read somewhere in the last chapter of *The Brothers Karamazov*, seems to have understood the law of perfect liberty and a type of heaven-on-earth in helping others, and I feel knew of you. Church steeples point inward and are confining in their entropy. Trees like these oaks, branch outward. All animals apparently accept us human beings and do not harm or kill us for sport. You are, does it not follow, a loving God and you entered into a contract with us up front in totally good faith. You are thus true. I love you.

*Alan*


*Dear Reader,*

*Please come and look at Queen's Park's trees. Please then read at least the last chapter of* The Brothers Karamazov. *(Doctor Fisher assured me that Dostoevsky was not an anti-Semite). Please then read* The Bible's James *1:19-22 and 3:3-18. Whether or not James were Jesus' brother seems moot. James' words seem mushrooms amongst toadstools.*

*God brings forth life and good life. Left undisturbed, the better gene will be chosen. Only one of inestimable love could create such a world. The Creator—Energy—loves. The Creator loves us enough to give us freedom to enable us to make or break ourselves. God wants us to mature, to use our brains lovingly. When we do not, God weeps and tries again to help us. But God knows that the helping should not be so much as to cripple or retard us. The Creator gave us brains and thereafter is our catalyst if we seek God through good faith. God seems the source of the Big Bang and all big bangs before it. We human beings want to know where it all started. Our minds crave finite closures. Why should we assume that our Creator, Loving Energy, needs such closure, needs such a noun?*

*I think the old oak tree next to me knows of what I speak but I cannot speak oak. The oak is giving me protection from noise, ozone-broken sun and sometimes rain. It is giving me oxygen. It is giving a safe home to the squirrels and the many forms of new life within it. I feel it knows.*

*Alan*


People began entering Queen's Park and one old oak now had an owl sitting mid-height, watching all below. Tourists were dumbfounded by the tame squirrels who seemed to be asking "Where are my peanuts, person?" Children began playing, winos were quietly moving to remote benches, fountains looked ready to be turned on and flowers were sprouting. I healed more that day in May than I had done in 2 months.

Toronto in 1982. Safe, polite, clean. Tax-paid schools of excellence. Public transportation second to none. A city filled with trees. No U.S.-style crime and street people said "please." When refused, they said "Have a nice day." There was no SARS and people the Earth over saw Toronto as a model city for how urban life could work.


## Jobs


In New York, Toronto and elsewhere, Scope & Mack was ranked the top shop in advertising. Prior to the close of 1981, Scope had asked me to breakfast to woo me with the chance to co-direct Canada. I had accepted the breakfast, because of a threat by Cork for a fight-to-the-finish, but had felt the Scope offer unchallenging and had said a gracious "no." That was then. By early 1982, Scope was phoning me again and had no knowledge of my car accident. Soon, too, a national gifts company, Monarch, was offering me almost on my résumé alone, a general management position.

I was still on neurosurgeon Dr. Schwantz's timetable for a 100% recovery in 6 months and I repressed diffidence about being able to handle the Monarch Gifts job as re-entry into the private sector; moreover, Monarch had checked out my references and they also did not know of my brain injury. Based on the referenced reports, Monarch was talking about how impressed it was with Alan Cooper, and said it wanted me to take on a senior sister organization in 2 years, along the way to my becoming president of all 6 sister companies before I was 35. My outside reputation had not yet caught up with reality.

Things at the Ministry of Food were bad. I was promoted to Executive Director in April 1982, but that move had been in place since 1981, and my interfacings at all levels were unveiling my damaged brain. My speech had fallen in pitch to that of a deep baritone, because I had to shift voice projection from a dead front palate to the back of my mouth. People who knew my speech before, recognized the slow contrived delivery.

What little competence I did display was being set back by new brain mistakes each day and rumors so damning that I exhausted myself trying to defend what I did. The home economics section of my staff kept trying to reassure witnesses that I was to be 100% recovered in 6 months but these assurances came off as apologies, and Cork spread around the rumor that I'd had my staff coached.

Moment to moment, my days at the Ministry showed my bad memory, an inability to muster thoughts, slurred speech, a ghostly paleness and fatigue. Cork had the knife out and other fraudulent well-wishers were flinging backstabs as quickly as any semblance of fact could confirm them.

I sensed I had to leave and said "yes" to the flattering overtures of Monarch Gifts.

Days later I received a call from Connecticut, and a New York headhunter who had tried to lure me years earlier to London, England still had me on his favorite list. He wanted to talk to me about a vice presidential opportunity leading to president and he was talking U.S. dollars. It was with a Pepsi subsidiary, just 75 miles west of Toronto.

I heard again the marketing language I had known so well pre-accident, and I felt a comfort in retrieving long-term memory for a life that now seemed so long ago. The thought of moving to Kitchener-Waterloo 75 miles west of Toronto did not really sink in, and almost at the same time, a senior social work opportunity arose in that same little city. Maria was offered a job as was I. We both said yes.

# THE MONTHS LEADING UP
# TO THE ACCIDENT

It is now so long since the time of my pre-morbid state that I have difficulty grasping the life I led. Prior to the crash in late 1981, I had been acting as Assistant Deputy Minister and was to be promoted in early 1982 from Director of Marketing to Executive Director for multiple branches. I had been working in late '81 at a pitched pace, micro-managing my own branch, dealing with the Assistant Deputy mandate and spearheading a master strategy paper for the entire Ministry. Suppers had often been a granola bar and tea before my speed-walking 2 miles to a Mendelssohn Choir practice or 4 miles to a choral concert with the Toronto Symphony. Periods pre-breakfast had been at Hart House where I would do 1/2 a mile of the pool or 4 miles running, after 20 minutes in the weight and exercise rooms. Daytimes had been pockmarked with flying to Ottawa for a tussle with the feds, chairing in Niagara skirmishes between the wine council and grape growers, speaking to large groups of Ontarians on behalf of the Minister, being interviewed in the media or being in a Mendelssohn Board meeting. Photography had crept its way into things and in daily speed walks from place to place, I had begun carrying a Leica and fast lens, taking the odd close-up of spires, back alley lamps or the tender face of a bag lady. Late at night, I had completed a novel about Toronto and had begun scribbling down thoughts for a second book on the difference between spirituality and religiosity.

Home had been a midtown co-op kept immaculate by a cleaning lady, with little to do to keep it spotless. My wife had been doing her usual, getting home to our apartment 24 minutes after

5:00 p.m. and checking in with her mother. An hour or more later, I had been getting home for supper, after which time I would have done the dishes and if I had a Mendelssohn Choir practice, Maria would have gone food shopping. It had taken years to ease Maria into defying her parents and venturing the 200-yard distance for shopping in the evening alone. Occasionally, Maria would have practiced on the used baby grand that I had suggested her parents buy her as our wedding present, when I had encouraged Maria to resurrect childhood piano lessons. More frequently, Maria would have been going through her massive closet before undertaking an extended stay in the bathroom, and then preparing for her following morning's 30 minutes hair curling and renewed mulling about in her closet. Sometimes after my paying bills and with Maria busy in bathroom and closets, I would have taken off for squash and occasionally I had been in the U.S., Europe or Japan. Maria during those times would have had a chance to spend more time listening to her mother.

I had been invidious in those days, demanding extreme standards in each thing I tried. At work I had felt a need to get to the critical points of each issue and had often left others behind. If my probing were to have ruffled others, I would not want to believe that other people had been allowing insecurities to override their sense of intellectual integrity. But my talking could have been met with lies or a threatened face.

It was not that I had been insensitive to the needs of others, far from it. Instead I had been known to be a bleeding heart, generous to a fault and sympathetic beyond any level understood by almost anyone else. People had seemed to project their own views on me and assume from my outward worldliness, that I was not naïve. Often they could not have fitted me onto their scale for honesty and would have read what I had been saying in a less than charitable way. Their interpretation would have hurt.

Jealousy had also not occurred to me, though jealousy had run rampant. People had often been intimidated by my intellectual rigor and had mistaken thorough argumentation for bullying or pretending to be on stage. Some loyalists had tried to tell me but I think their euphemistic approach and wish not to hurt me had kept them from ever hammering home the fact that others had unfounded thoughts. One favorite thought started by Cork was that I was gay, because I had been a singer, writer and careful dresser, and according to Cork, was a womanizer to hide my homosexuality. It had been for him a thought that fit well into a pattern he could not understand.

Cork would have stopped at nothing to thwart my move up, but by late 1981, he had known my pending promotion to be only a holding pattern before becoming one of Canada's youngest Deputy Ministers. Willy Cork, as assistant Deputy, had still been my boss but for months I had been reporting straight through to Deputy Stewart MacCallum.

Throughout the autumn of 1981, I had watched Willy Cork grow paranoid, his desire to become Deputy ever-consuming as had been his alcohol. He had clandestinely met with the Ministry's ad agency to solicit support against me, after I had criticized its work in a confidential memo to Cork and asked for a related meeting with him. Twice my little sports sedan had been sabotaged in the Ministry parking lot and lying rumors had run rife about my fornicating female staff. Cork had bribed a drunken crony to report on my every direction. Just prior to Christmas, Cork had been shouting in my office an incorrect rumor that I had been bad-mouthing him—Cork had been going on in a rant, shaking the jelly in his Lou Costello body, pointing his fat finger up to my face and snapping that it would be a fight to the finish and he would win.

I had been Director of Marketing for only 2 years with the Ministry of Food but had brought about a doubling of Ontario's food exports, and had taken Foodland Ontario from its struggling infancy to an award winning multi-media program, popular on all fronts. Demands to speak had been frequent and Maria would be thrilled at banquets when cheers would have accompanied my being introduced.

I had moved 2 years earlier to government from the private sector, where I had enjoyed a career rapid in rise. At age 30, the marketing world had brandished praises and I had experienced multiple job offers. Pepsi had offered to send me to London and put me in charge of marketing management for Europe. Advertising agencies had heard of me in New York and I had been considered a future leader. Nonetheless, I had felt socially unredeemed and unmoved by money, and had said "no" to all the headhunters.

Now in the public sector, Capital Hill in Ottawa had witnessed my contributions to Ontario, and Alberta had a standing offer for me to move to western Canada. But in each job approach to me, I would have gone through turmoil, my wife not wanting to leave her mother and my feeling an insecurity which had bedeviled me since childhood.

One offer I had dismissed quickly after Cork had said it would finish my career. It had been for a one-year course given to the world's civil service élite at Canadian military headquarters in Kingston, 160 miles east of Toronto. The course had included my traveling around the world, seeing in depth how other governments worked and then entering into rigorous debate about the big issues facing the world. It had also included my being paid full salary for the year. My turning it down and not even studying the opportunity had been one of my life's biggest mistakes, pre-brain-damage.

# 10 YEARS BEFORE

In May 1982, I was in a situation where I had done the inconceivable and had said "yes" to 2 jobs, something I could not have fathomed ever doing pre-brain damage.

My confidence had needed to hear the adulations that senior people had flooded on me and their talk had thrown me back to the last 10 years. From a moment's crash, how things had changed.

Ten years prior in the late autumn of 1971, I had left my parents home, and with 2 other bachelors had been renting a dilapidated 3-storey house in midtown Toronto. Each of us had 2 rooms on a floor and I had re-done mine. I had converted the smaller storage area into a bedroom and I'd had my grandparents' brass bed re-lacquered. I had then used scrap materials and redone common areas in the entire house. Friends had been shocked at the design work and had coined me "Leonardo."

A month before the move-in, in October of 1971, I had gone for the first time to Europe on a 3-week vacation. In London I had met a German student named Rosi who had been doing graduate work back in Giessen. During my third week, I had gone abroad to visit her in Germany. I had agreed to help her with some work for her Master of English class and had reviewed *Understanding Media* by the University of Toronto's Marshall McLuhan. There in Giessen I had also met Manfred and Dieter, 2 professors who had escaped from East Germany. Manfred was to become, until my closed head injury, one of my dearest and most trusted friends.

By the spring of 1972, I had left an ill-fitting 2-year apprenticeship in chartered accountancy. An old undergraduate friend Brian Alexandra had graduated in United Church ministry. Brian had accepted my suggesting the 2 of us drive down the U.S. coast along highway #1. In South Carolina, I had picked up an old alcoholic Black man and driven him to his dream of seeing Charleston. When we had arrived, it had become apparent he had never been there. Until we stopped, Brian had not understood that I had wanted to drop him off with caregivers near a church in a Black area.

I had been driving the first of 5 successive German cars, an unadorned 1972 navy blue sedan bought in September 1971 at a price just over $3,000. It had been an all-manual piece of machinery with no options beyond a basic Blaupunkt AM-FM purchased later. I had succumbed to a radio, only because by then I had embarked on a practice judged pretentious or homosexual in my childhood home, that of listening to classical music.

Not long after Brian and I had returned from the U.S., I had been getting set to backpack again through Europe, this time for longer. I had been getting set to spend the summer doing what fellow graduates had done 3 years earlier, while I had toiled away 90 hour weeks in apprenticeship chartered accountancy. Before I had left, my mother had made sure to tell me she did not want me to go and had also made sure no-one else could have heard her comment. I had then vowed to break with the past.

When I had returned back to Canada, I had enrolled in business school at the University of Toronto and for the first time in 10 years, my marks had begun to soar with an A– average. Soon however, business school had become part-time, when at the end of the autumn 1972 term, I had landed a job as a Junior Account Executive at Maclaren Advertising. After a year at Maclaren, I had been promoted to packaged goods and had become Senior Account Executive on the Lever Brothers business. I had then begun making marketing decisions out of step with my superiors but lauded by the client, and thanks to the support of my Japanese boss, had kept winning the intellectual day. I had found myself working late into each night, comfortable in the knowledge that my boss would have supported me in my newfound confidence.

By year 2, the recruiters had heard of me and it wasn't long that, to my surprise I had been in demand. Without, however any recruiter, I had made the move to a full-blown Product Manager's job at Warner-Lambert and had been assigned Rolaids and a new brand Freshen-Up gum to launch. I'd had to work my way late into each night through every step of its marketing launch, but my secretary Marj had given me undying support. By the end of month one, I had been awarded an MBA assistant.

Soon I'd had the admiration and unknown envy of many. My brand had won packaging and merchandising awards, and had broken every sales record. Within 12 months to the day of hire, I had been promoted to New Products Manager, broken more records, won more awards and had then been promoted in another 12 months to Group Product Manager. GPM was a job that for those few who ever made it, normally took 7 years.

My reputation on the street had stunned me and I could not accept it. I had then turned down relentless job offers, reaching the late autumn of 1978 when a New York recruiter had led to my being offered Marketing Manager with Pepsi, to look after Europe from London. After 4 months vacillating and an enticing trip for my wife to London, we had said "no." Shortly thereafter in 1979, I had accepted the job as Director of Marketing with the Ministry of Food.

During those 10 years, my love life had gone through change. Break-up after 6 years with one girl, Jo-Anne, had finally come in 1971 after she had once again fornicated strangers. Monogamous I had then dared out into a world I had not known. The first lady I had dated had been Patricia Langlois, a beautiful girl of aristocratic breeding and one whom I had known in university. She had been younger than my 6-years girlfriend but still a full year older than I: I had been advanced in school and had never dated a girl younger.

Patricia and I would have gone out on the most proper of evenings and I think if I had ever leveled with her about my family, I could have felt some comfort. Such was not to be and an even richer Christy Judge was to have met the same fate. On my 24th birthday in December 1971, I finally had had sex with someone other than Jo-Anne.

By March 1972, I had begun a love affair with another virgin, "another" because I had felt myself the same, never having been able to evolve sexually at an unforced pace. Catherine McNaughton had also been the first girl I had ever dated younger than I. We had begun a sexless, but deep love affair in which we could not tolerate being away from each other. By August 1972, we had both been back from Europe and virgin Catherine had said "yes" to marriage. When she had changed her mind in the autumn, I had thought my new world had left me but within a month had met the girl I would marry.

Maria had been taking a Master of Social Work in the same U. of T. building where I had been studying graduate business and it had been suggested in the business school that we should invite social work students to our dance on that November 1972 Friday. I had worked up the nerve to ask some of them in a common elevator, when one of the social work females had responded with a glib sweep about the narrow-mindedness of business students. I had begun agreeing, when suddenly a haunting blonde had said she would come. I had lightly responded that I was from Missouri but had then realized she had not understood the expression. The misunderstanding had led to further conversation and before the elevator had opened, she had said "you'll see" with a soft voice, white teeth and sunbeam smile.

Friday evening had come and at 9 o'clock I was still at home. I had been thinking I might do what I had done for weeks and go to a movie but soon had struck on the idea she might be at the dance. I had put on my sexiest denim shirt, jeans and big leather belt, and darted in my car to the business school dance. There she sat, wearing a suede mini-skirt, at a table with other males.

No-one had known that I was shy and the haunting blonde had to feign 3 times going to the ladies room before making the move to my table. All it had then taken was my smiling and saying "You came!" for her to sit down. Within minutes, she had begun educating me on border collies, after she discovered I was a Wasp of mainly Scottish background. It seems that border collies are a mix between Scottish and Polish, and one of the brightest breeds. She had said we could produce the best of babies.

We had soon come to realize we both loved classical music and talk had worked its way around to Beethoven's 9th. This new blonde lady had already taken notice of my glimpsing at her big breasts, mini-skirt and long legs, and she had then dropped a bombshell by telling me that Beethoven's 9th was good for making love. Within a half-hour, we had been back at my place but soon she had been guiding my hand away, saying she was a virgin. I had sat up and started talking, assuming a position of presumed correctness and then had driven her home to her east European section of west Toronto and an orange garage door.

Sunday night I had telephoned her, with my memory still holding her surname and street address. She had expressed surprise at my wanting to see her again but had managed to enter into an hour's conversation. She had been intrigued that I had almost become a United Church minister. We had agreed to go out, the following Friday.

Later she would tell me during the interim period, she had bought new clothes to match the mood of the anticipated date. I had arrived looking considerably more Presbyterian than I had appeared in my denim. When her younger sister had answered the door, Maria had seized the moment to view me and alter her outfit accordingly. After a mandatory introduction to her mother, who had told Maria she had thought I was a very nice boy, we had been off to the El Mocambo to listen to some of the continent's best new music. It had not been long before Maria had stretched over, given me a full French kiss and had said "Hi." Then, after her telling me as she had the previous week, that the music we had been starting listening to was good for making love, we had been back again at my place. This time, when lying against my floor cushions and with my hand beginning to caress her legs, she had suddenly sat up.

"Why don't I just strip?"

I had pretended not to be stunned but soon had a blonde-haired, big-breasted, long legged, full beavered 22 year-old virgin with a honey smile, white teeth, cow brown eyes and long natural eyelashes, sitting on my used Iranian rug under the soft 25-watt lighting of my Japanese rice paper lamp. She had been the one who had spoken next.

"You'll have to show me what to do."

I have often been one who, when faced with an opportunity many of us would die for, has gone on to sabotage his good fortune. This time I had needed to stay cool and whatever happened, make this new Maria think that it was the thing to do.

"It's more comfortable in the bedroom."

My former girlfriend Catherine McNaughton's photo had been still on the bedroom dresser and her hand-done art on the wall, but Maria had not seemed to care and had started giving me what she had described as her great massage. Suddenly, with her sitting nude on her knees in the middle of my bed, her long blonde hair falling down over her face, her big breasts beaming out at me and her right hand masturbating my erect penis, she had thrust out her left hand to the ceiling and had declared for the old house to hear,

"Eat your heart out, James McGuire!"

I had started going soft and had pretended that I needed clarification. What had followed was a 20 minute history of each other's break-up and the fact we had both been on the rebound.

We then had had no further sex that night, and none at all beyond warm-ups until February 11, 1973, 2 months after we had agreed Maria should go on the pill. Maria had lost her virginity, and unbeknownst to her and the lies of her mother, she would have been the only person with whom I would have sexual intercourse.

That same February, I had been invited to cocktails at an old Forest Hill mansion and an unsure Maria had gone with me. Her surname had been mistaken for a famous Canadian, and after she had clarified the error, she had told me she had been exposed and would carry that social exposure for the rest of her life.

Beyond professional work in the 10 years leading up to the brain injury, my mind had begun blossoming after struggling against oppression for its first 24 years. I had resumed a university exercise regimen that, in post-brain injury modification, exists to this day. I had jogged, swum, lifted weights and practiced yoga. I had purchased a lightweight racing bicycle, played squash with executives, hockey with factory friends and baseball with all. Peers would have cheered at a grand slam out of the park or an end-to-end skate to score a goal. I had taken up downhill and Nordic skiing, and hiking in the Canadian wilds. I had bought a cedar-strip canoe and had used it on getaways to Ontario's lakes. Speed-walking had entered each day. I had looked athletic and my child-hurt ego had wanted me to stay that way.

I had purchased a sensitive stereo and had begun building a classical music library. I had taken singing lessons, rescued a post-pubescent singing voice and had passed audition into the world renowned Toronto Mendelssohn Choir. I had joined a writers' group and had found myself sketching little stories of things around me. By the end of the 1970s, I had completed a novel drawn around the lives of 3 young architects and their conflicting influences on a rapidly changing Toronto. I had enrolled in a creative design course and had co-taught the course. I had traveled to Europe 20 times on both business and leisure, and had gone to

Japan. I had been in the United States often and I had snorkeled in Bermuda, the Caribbean and parts of Mexico.

For a home, I had bought that one luxury bedroom co-op 2 months before marriage and had designed a cedar-paneled mini-office in the broom closet. For a car, I had kept buying the most basic of German sports sedans and the little things, still unadorned in those days, had kept going up in value as I had traded up 4 times.

# BACK TO THE PRESENT IN 1982

I had stalled my starting date with the 2 companies until late July 1982 and began agonizing over which job to take. The Ministry had not yet been notified and I was sitting in limbo while I waited for a 100% recovery, 6 months after the accident. I had marked the 100% recovery in my black book for midnight June 26th but the calendar pages kept turning and no neurological progress had been noticeable since winter. The Canadian economy had fallen into recession and the real estate market was in freefall.

I resigned my job and a day later said "no" to Monarch Gifts. Monarch seemed relieved, wondering how on earth it could possibly have matched up to what it said were my platinum credentials. I committed to taking the job with the Pepsi subsidiary and moving the 75 miles west of Toronto, and Maria secured her new job there too.

That same week, Cork took me to lunch, and I paid as always. He told me he had been surprised by my resignation from the safe civil service, as he and all others could see that I was not getting better. My biological parents were back from Florida. Both told me after I resigned that I was going to lose a fortune in selling my house, and that the economy was too terrifying for leaving such a soft government job.

Others followed suit, including the father-in-law of Maria's sister. In one of his drunken freefalls, he phoned me late at night. He said Canada was entering an economic depression, that I had left the civil service and would be out of work forever. By that time of 1982, Maria's sister's marriage was in trouble and her father-in-law wanted to level the playing field by damaging Maria's marriage.

That father-in-law then phoned Maria's mother and told a lie: he said that I was making Polish jokes about Maria's family.

All my life, I had been compassionate to the suffering of others, in part I think from my own pain. I also had a soft underbelly that I had learned to protect with intellectual quills. Some time in adulthood, I guess I had built up antibodies to most jabs against me, and I had rarely let people jealous of me see my sensitive side. But my brain damage killed much of that intellectual defense and left me like a burn victim, with skin wide open and immunities peeled back.

Discerning parts of the brain now sensed my exposure, though I still was not conscious of a changed personality. Maria had tried to communicate to medical experts, the new me and had gone with flailing arms to my orthopedic surgeon Doctor England. He had relayed to me her alarm over my changed personality but whether he had made any record of my new derangement, only his old files now know. Something radical had happened to my personality, an intricate re-circuiting of its entire self, but Dr. England, my clavicle doctor was the only Flanders practitioner who so much as touched on the issue.

## Unrelenting

There were so many manifestations of my multiply ripped and rewired brain that each week brought new ways in which my sensitivities and rearranged personality experienced them. My brain felt like a hamburger suspended in uneasy water, held to its basin by 6 strands of hair. If I were to turn my head at all, it would feel as if one of the strands had snapped away, with that burger adrift in threatening wind. That floating feeling remains to this day and if I make any kind of quick turn, things will come loose and I will feel woozy. My balance had improved from the sheer staggering, but I had learned by the spring of 1982 to compensate by walking bow-legged cowboy style.

Because of my brain's rewired circuits, getting an erection was almost impossible. Only once had there been the beginning of one. Problems, pressures and physical pain were arguably sexual inhibitors, but something more fundamental was electronically out of place. I still had the sexual desire and an undying attraction to Maria but regardless of what she did, my penis remained limp. When I sensed that my penis stayed soft, my rewired personality would further complicate the process and I would try to masturbate until I came without erection. A year later, an endocrinologist would tell me that my testosterone was below normal and my sexual release hormones sat at the bottom of the medical norm. All physical indicators would tell the endocrinologist that the accident had damaged my brain's hypothalamic inner nucleus. I would tell the endocrinologist of my prostatitis and occasional impotence as a young man, but she would dismiss both as irrelevant and not write them down. The endocrinologist would give me hormone shots for 4 months. For a while, my libido would seem to react to the chemical stimulant, but with no ultimate sexual ability, I would finally quit.

## Dr. Steve Jensen

To this day, it remains unproven how or if Doctor Steve Jensen took a bribe from the other legal side's #2 detective agency. If by chance, he deciphers from this story his real name and sues me, I would love it. But he won't. Regardless of whether he actually took a bribe from the facility Regal Insurance Company or the illegal cadre of CEO'S above it, by every code stated in medical ethics and by every principle of justice found in law, Dr. Steve Jensen should go to jail for a long time.

G. P. Dr. Jensen had been to see me when I had been in intensive care in Flanders and had said I should siphon off insurance money to fix my childhood-damaged cynical lip. On a later visit to Jensen in his doctor's office, I confided my impotence to him. He sarcastically asked if I got piss hards. I did not know the expression and he had to explain that it meant nocturnal erection, one experienced when waking up in the morning. I was about to confirm that I'd had none since the brain injury, when a loud Jensen interrupted with the jab that I was fine if I had to think about it.

During another appointment with Jensen, I expressed my new concern about alcohol. He interjected that I looked jaundiced and then bi-passed my telling him that I had looked jaundiced as had my mother since childhood. Instead, he lowered his brows and rammed a needle into my arm. Jensen said I was an alcoholic and that alcohol was the cause of my bad memory. When I refuted that I had drunk only 4 times, he mumbled something about denial and erroneously assumed Maria had forced me to come to him. He then asked a question odd to me and one I could not at first put in context, 'Were my finances in a total mess?' He seemed incredulous when I said my finances were all in order. Later, after all blood tests showed me normal and my not drinking for 2 months but still having the same bad memory, Jensen quipped that it was still the alcohol.

Maria made an appointment to see Jensen without me, to talk about my personality change. When Jensen asked her if Alan was "doing his homework", meaning sexual intercourse, Maria at first did not understand but then tried to shelve the issue with an "I wouldn't know about that." Jensen assumed Maria was shyly hiding sexual regularity and when Maria went on with her list of complaints, Jensen interjected with a shock, "Neurosurgeon Mark Schwantz hates Alan's guts."

At the end of his half-hour with Maria, Jensen fired another one, "Well, Napoleon had his Josephine."

Weeks later, I went for a follow-up visit with neurosurgeon Dr. Schwantz and asked him if he thought I was trying to do things to better my legal case. He blushed, said a credible "No!" and for the first time, I began to sense Jensen's distortions. The thought that G.P. Dr. Jensen was manipulating things was too unthinkable, and what would unravel in years to come, too unimaginable for anyone outside of Solzhenitsyn's Soviet Union to accept as happening. After Dr. Schwantz later wrote a summary report on the definitive damage done to my brain, G.P. Dr. Jensen heard of it and insisted on my immediately seeing another neurosurgeon, whom Jensen would prejudice ahead of time. Jensen would do this to Dr. Winter a neuropsychologist and every specialist I saw, right down to my dentist who told me he had a "lonnng conversation" with my doctor.

I had inherited Dr. Jensen from my old G. P. Dr. Brethren who had sold his practice to Jensen. David Brethren had been my child-hood next-door neighbor and had gone on to leave our middle class neighborhood. Along the way, David had married a prominent lady whom I had met in university and I think Jensen was under the impression that I was very wealthy, too. Jensen also thought I knew the vulgar-rich Peter Perry, from whom I had bought my home, and Jensen falsely assumed I had known Perry since birth. Dr. Jensen himself was from London, a little city west of Toronto with haughty roots of fallen English aristocracy. Jensen had tried to conquer Toronto's establishment by living in a Tudor mansion in lush Lawrence Park but despite Jensen's pretence, he had often grabbed the chance to tell me about Toronto's crass rich.

G.P. Dr. Steve Jensen did his best to make sure my qualifying for Ministry disability was out of the question. At one point, despite all the neurological tests and CT scan showing the damage, he said he doubted that the damage had not all healed. Jensen went on to insist I add bad hearing to my legal list, knowing of my imperfect hearing pre-accident.

What conversations Jensen had with my lawyer Gordon Dour, I would never know other than to hear after Jensen's irrevocable damage, that Dour had changed his understanding of Jensen to that of a horse's ass. Years later, when I had long stopped seeing G.P. Dr. Jensen, he telephoned me to say that his lawyer brother lived down the street from me and had been monitoring my goings-on for Dr. Jensen.

## 100% Recovery in 6 Months (?)

On June 26, 1982, 2 days after my farewell party, I lay awake at midnight, hoping at that magic 6-month point, I would undergo yet another "miraculous recovery" of the kind that a second Jensen-poisoned neurosurgeon would attribute to my first 9 days recovery. Somehow I expected the healing curve that had felt flat for 5 months to shoot into another upturn and at midnight lift me to the prognosticated 100% recovery. I eyed the second-hand on the tiny alarm clock and it ticked past 12:00. Nothing. Thoughts started to swell up that I was forever brain damaged and that I had taken a now impossible job, removed from my Toronto.

## Week 2 of Vacation

I never had so much spare time in my life as I did then in July of 1982, rotting my body on the beach with Maria. I had too much time to agonize over the misdirected brain decision to dive into new task territory, when that brain after 6 months had proven itself incapable. Although I was creative, that right lobe helped me realize I could no longer do the absorbing, collating or retrieving of new information. My left frontal lobe was damaged. Some of it was dead. Nothing, no further rewiring from the right could make up for a wild driver's having crushed much of my mind's library.

The right lobe saw disasters ahead and tried to warn my personality. My motor functions reacted by turning hyper-active, triggering acid blotches on my skin and diarrhea from my bum. The neurosurgeon had not known of my permanent brain damage.

## The Deputy Minister's Secretary

On the Monday of week 3 of vacation at 8:00 a.m., I telephoned The Ministry from which I had resigned In June. I asked to speak to my former boss' boss, Deputy Minister Stewart MacCallum. I asked his kind secretary Jane Briton if I could see Stewart and I began explaining that my job had turned sour. Stew was busy but Jane wedged me in at once.

Hollow cheeked and trembling, I went into the Deputy's office. Cork was ostensibly away on a trade mission in Britain but was actually on a secret junket to Ireland, visiting his parents and family. Deputy Stew MacCallum was a brilliant and dedicated servant to the public, a kind man with the sensitivity of a poet. Few knew that fact and people had branded him ruthless. In judging his lifestyle they had affixed "stewed" to Stewart".

"Coop! By now I thought you would have been slugging potato chips."

"No, Stewart, I wasn't scheduled to start until August 1st... Stew?"

He had been swirling around his desk, getting ready for a briefing, but caught my pause.

"Something's gone wrong, hasn't it, Alan?"

I felt a moment's relief and came as close to a lie as I could.

"Yes, Stew. The job is not turning out as I was led to envisage."

I could have said "situation" instead of "job" and have been distorting less. Stew, however, seemed ahead of me and his voice softened.

"How can I help, Alan?"

I felt a soothing on my inner chest as if a gentle paw were stroking it from the inside.

"Stewart, I was wondering if it would be possible for me to have my old job back."

I had said it and there was no ensuing silence. Stew re-entered the talk immediately; he seemed to know the purpose and direction of the whole meeting. His voice held mellow and his words were slow and deliberate.

"Oh yeah, Alan. There's no way I'll be able to get anyone of your caliber. We have some talented people but find ourselves missing the kind of zeal you inculcated into all who worked on your teams."

We both knew, I think, we were role-playing and I gasped the kind of sigh I would have had from front crawling a mile in the university's Hart House pool.

"Thank you, Stewart."

"When can you start, Coop? We need to get your pension reinstated."

"…Next Monday."

"Great! Oh, I'll check with the Minister and senior staff first, but I'm sure there's no problem. Just don't say no your employer, until we touch base."

That check made me a little nervous, but when Stewart phoned the following day to tell me everyone was ecstatic to have me back, I felt a small calmness. I phoned the company-to-be and it was gracious when I said I could not come. I canceled the sale of the house and undid all of the logistics that I had put into place in June. Maria was welcomed back with remarkable ease to her junior social work position but she never did tell me what explanation she gave. It was Friday and the one restful weekend to come in months, was one I needed.

A call came from a frantic Deputy. He had tracked down Cork in Ireland and had heard from him that "There were major Alan Cooper problems coming to the surface all over the Ministry and beyond." Stewart was wondering if I had said no yet to the new job. In an iced panic, I tried to undo the job turndown and made a fool of myself in trying. Maria started screaming and refused to try to get her new job back. I began to go catatonic.

Stewart's kind secretary Jane smelled the dirty Cork and appealed to the kindness she knew to be in Stew. Jane phoned me.

"Alan, we look forward to seeing you back on Monday."

"But Jane, the rumors…I had absolutely no idea."

"We checked with the other Assistant Deputies and they said they have never heard an unkind word about Alan."


## Back

Prior to my late July re-entry into the Ministry of Food, I saw G.P. Dr. Jensen and tried to raise the issue of depression. He immediately misread my words.

"Yep! There are 3 houses that have had forced sellings in Lawrence Park."

When he stopped promulgating, I had a chance to clarify that the depression was mine.

"How much alcohol are you drinking?"

"None for 2 months, since you last saw me."

"Well, I should check that with your wife."

With that sting, he prescribed 9 days of the antidepressant Amitriptylene to aid daytime functioning and Fluorazepam to ensure night-time sleep. The sleep drug hung over into late morning and exacerbated my slurred speech, and the Amitriptylene made an already deadened mouth dry.

When I returned to the Ministry of Food, I wasn't allowed to do my job. Cork spread rumors throughout the Ministry and beyond, and at every key point in my work, Cork sabotaged its doing. Cork tried first to prevent my pension being reinstated, then tried to stop both my public speaking and my meetings, then publicly questioned expenses. When I would announce to my secretary that I had a meeting with the Director of the Communications Branch, I would find in short minutes, the Director's office door rammed open by a quivering Cork.

Cork then tried to alienate all the workers from me, first within the Ministry and across the Government, and finally among my staff. Under false premises and without my knowledge, Cork promoted one of my underlings and gave her a 40% pay increase. The supporting document included a carefully constructed implication of my permanent brain damage, related incompetence and consequent need for the underling's promotion. Cork calculated that if I tried to undo the promotion, I would be seen as holding back my staff while trying to protect my fiefdom, and would also confirm the paranoia which he had rumored I possessed.

A former workaholic, I now spent days sitting with my office door closed. With each new hour, I would emerge to extinguish rumors of my brain deficits, all the while filling people with more knowledge that my brain damage was permanent.

I resolved to try fixing some problems on my own. My 9 days of drugs finished and on the evening of August 10th 1982, I began drinking 750 ml of 11% red wine before going to bed. I would drink no alcohol after 11:00 p.m. until the following day at 10:00 p.m. and would keep rigidly to this practice for 2 1/2 years until

January 1985. Each night, I would watch the news and taper off my day as I sat in the TV room, savoring each taste of a full bodied Rioja red.

Food appetite began to return, body weight grew back, a daily swim resumed and my complexion came back to a radiance not seen since the traumatic brain injury.

## Letter to Pravda

From the day I had met Maria 10 years earlier, never had a week gone by without Maria's complaining to me about how bad her mother was. From Yolanta's crippling of her son Constantine to the emasculation of her husband to her domineering personality, Maria spewed forth regularly on her mother's damage. Maria would also complain to her younger sister who confided not liking her mother's cooking. But it was always an aside—never was mother Yolanta to hear one word from either daughter. In front of the mighty mother Yola, Maria would turn back into the slave she had been since childhood. Her sentences would be completed by her mother as would all thoughts, and Yola's loudness would drown out the voice of anyone who dared venture to say anything.

Sixteen months prior to the accident, Maria had aged into her '30s and her mother had begun noises that it was time for Maria to have children. To this point, her mother had lied to extended family and neighbors about Maria's career, and Maria and I had put off having children because of her mother. Our fear had sat submerged under the comfort of Maria's young fertility but it was only a question of time before Yolanta swung around full force and gave the grandchildren issue its due.

Maria did not utter a thought that we should first see about recovery before considering children—the image-driven Maria stuck to my being 100% recovered in, now, 12 months. The realization that we had been unable to have sexual intercourse more than once in 8 months post-brain damage did not factor in, except in Maria saying 'We should practice no birth control if I could do it so seldom.' We both knew that Yolanta preached non-stop about being the world's best mother and that interference would come. A letter's writing to her mother asking her not to interfere fell to me and my wife agreed.

## The Autumn of 1982 and Early 1983

Four months passed. I hired a new Director to tackle the old job from which, de facto, I had been promoted pre-injury and was trying to give some time to teaching him. Graeme Pritchard lived west of Toronto as did Willy Cork, and Cork corralled Pritchard into buying Cork drinks along the way home. My drunken market researcher Sawchuk was enlisted to do work for Cork of an undefined kind—Cork deemed the work too confidential for Sawchuk to tell me, his boss, and Sawchuk began submitting mountainous bar bills above my head. Cork phoned my doctors' offices when I was there and later contracted a person solely to keep tabs on all my actions. When I was at meetings, Cork would pretend to try reaching me by phone, then lie and tell the Deputy I was playing hooky. It became impossible for me to leave my office or announce my business locations, without Cork and his henches following my every move and laying false reports. My poor secretary was going to quit so she wouldn't have to work in any organization that housed a Willy Cork.

The Mendelssohn Choir started again that September but this time with no annual audition—the Choir was scheduled to start in Toronto's new Roy Thompson concert hall and the conductor needed as little change as possible. After a 9-month absence since the brain injury, I re-joined the Choir and went through the motions in front of thousands in the audience, millions on television; I couldn't sing at all. Those singers around me kept mumbling they could not hear my voice. I was soon out of the Choir.

That same September brought my 8th wedding anniversary and on that September 20th 1982, Maria's mother began her attack. I was forced to be away at a conference but phoned Maria to wish her a happy anniversary. I was at the point of telling her about the dinner that I had planned for her, but discovered she was crying. Her mother Yolanta had received my letter in mid-August and had phoned Maria then to say Yola appreciated its understanding and agreed with Alan. It was only later that I heard from Maria's sister about the turmoil the letter had caused. Not only was Yolanta able to store her hate for 6 weeks but she also knew she could attack on Maria's anniversary when I was away. The mother's words were lies but that did not matter—it was her delivery of the poison that counted. The damage happened. From that night on when Maria was alone, Yolanta began a crusade to get Maria to procreate, and then alienate her egg fertilizer husband from every blood relative whom Maria had, and from the 2 later she would have.

# 1983

By the end of 12 months, I finished my part of recovering. My mind still hoped for further recovery but even my faithful home economics staff who had defended me—saying a 100% recovery in 3 months, then 6, then 12 months—now doubted aloud my ever healing. Neurosurgeon Mark Schwantz changed his guess on recovery from one to 2 years and added, possibly never. I continued trying to cope with the other sequelae, while G.P. Dr. Jensen balked at referring me to any specialist. Through Maria's work, she heard of the world famous psychiatrist Doctor Michael Fisher and I started to see him in October, 1982. There I talked about my childhood and only in passing, mentioned my bump on the head. I omitted telling him of the hematoma, because I had not then known I had incurred one or for that matter, what one was.

My worth at the Ministry was nil. In the outside world, the car crash news had not yet caught up to my pre-accident reputation and I stood in terror of the outside's finding out. Consultants to the Ministry suspected but they knew more about my bad Ministry situation. Without their fully understanding my deficits, they urged me to move back to the private sector ahead of any news, while my lawyer Dour goaded me, saying that I looked always to be a lowly civil servant.

Canadian marketing companies still seemed eager to grab what they perceived to be a one-of-a-kind find, and one such company began aggressively pursuing me. Perhaps I dreamt that a reversion to where I had shone, pre-accident would mean I could once again make a meaningful contribution.

The winter of 1983 saw me offered a new job, Vice President

Marketing for Blimiss Hope, a multinational headquartered in New York. Its Canadian President was Eugene Darling and he was good to me at the start. Darling had fired his former VP Marketing for reasons of personal chemistry and knew that any further people problems would raise questions about him, within both Blimiss Hope and the marketing community.

Within the resultant 1983 year long honeymoon at Blimiss Hope, I fell into a fantasy world, oblivious to people's jokes about my memory and never hearing staff refer to the car accident. I assumed they did not know of it and I worked hard with people whose names I would not later remember.

To hide the closed head injury, I became self-defensive in the extreme. One of my first acts was to buy a blazer with an eye-grabbing University of Toronto crest sewn on its front. It was in my possession by workday 5 and I began to wear it on day 8. I was insensitive to what the crest said about me and did not catch my new boss's winces. I told others that I was reading Joyce's *Ulysses* and Bronowski's *The Ascent of Man,* and I spent massive sums with Maria on weekends in places like Chicago to hear the symphony, Boston to see the schools and Montréal to see the people.

Within such hubris, I kept hearing Maria's want of children but gave little thought to not being able to copulate. I would try again and again but get no erection. At Dr. Fisher's urging, I bought a book by a Dr. Kaplan on sexual disorders but still nothing. One night in May 1983, Maria had been showering and I had been lying alone in bed, while masturbating with no erection. In a frenetic struggle to achieve orgasm, I was pulling and yanking a limp penis and finally squirted a soap-sized ejaculate. Maria caught the final scene from her entrance into the bedroom.

A week later at the end of May, a nude Maria began giving me fellatio. She then pulled my semi-erect penis from her mouth, embraced her right hand around its middle and wedged its tip into the outer parts of her vagina. My penis was there for about 4 seconds before full limpness set in, but limp and all, I came. For the third time in 18 months post-brain damage, we had sexual intercourse. Two more attempts were made in June, and one was a flop. The other resulted in a 4-second penetration, again with an orgasm. That month of June of '83 was the peak and it produced no more.

— • —

"Impossible!" was the thought that first came to me, but then followed a cautious elation. We were weekending in Montréal in the beginning of summer and were spending the afternoon hiking on Mount Royal, before taking the Sunday afternoon train back to Toronto. All she said in her climb up the mountain was, "If I didn't know any better, I'd say that I *am* pregnant."

She said nothing to my "Impossible" and I tried to remember if I had ever penetrated her at all. I may have had a moment's thought that someone else was the father, but if I did, the idea overwhelmed me and I suppressed it.

"Physically, we've had no intercourse."

Maria was programmed to wait for her mother to reply. She finally muttered, almost inaudibly out of fear of expressing a view without her mother's clarification. "W may have… (Maria may have ovulated late)."

Doctor Fisher had repeatedly emphasized that there is no relationship between one's ability to ejaculate and one's fertility, but the numbers still did not work for me. At any rate, we did not know she was pregnant.

The 5 hour train back to Toronto saw Maria in pain and when we got back, she had to be taken by ambulance to Women's University Hospital. After days of hospital incompetence, she was operated on to remove a giant ovarian cyst that had grown to be the size of a grapefruit, while being fed by hormones. Maria was pregnant.

Weeks later, in one of the daily walks I would put a pregnant Maria through, I blurted, "Maria, I have been a tyrant since that driver smashed my brain and I think I will be so on and off for many years to come. I hope not, because I truly love you, Maria."

## Winter's Tests

Flanders Hospital purportedly had one of the best neuropsychologists in the business in Dr. Gary Winter and when I first phoned him, he completely threw me off. Lawyer Dour had been pressing me for a year to have a battery of tests done on my cognitive abilities but G.P. Dr. Jensen kept delaying the tests. At first, Jensen had claimed it was too soon but then had started stalling, saying Dr. Winter could not yet see me. This tedium went back and forth for 10 months, while lawyer Dour hounded me on what was the hold-up. I had not known the reason but had repeatedly told Dour what Dr. Jensen had said to me.

In the spring of 1983, I finally got Dr. Winter on the phone after Jensen had told me Dr. Winter was reluctant to administer the battery of tests. From the second I mentioned my name, Dr. Winter was hostile to me, talked of my lawsuit and did his best to stop my taking his tests. When later his psychometrist performed the tests, she too was hostile and many more months passed, while Dour badgered me and said he had never experienced such delays in getting this type of testing. When the written results were finally presented, the content was sabotaged in such a way that neurosurgeon Dr. Mark Schwantz said it was portrayed to damage my credibility to the maximum. Among other things, the results made the lie that during my drunkenness post-accident, I had supposedly fallen down and incurred many head injuries.

I had no idea where this underlying hostility came from.

Months after the tests, and without my knowledge, neurosurgeon Dr. Schwantz in the autumn of 1983 sent an overriding report directly to Dour. The results confirmed both the severity of my brain injury and the permanency of its damage. I trustingly told G.P. Jensen that Dr. Schwantz had communicated directly with my lawyer, and Jensen immediately set me up to see Dr. Maul, another Flanders neurosurgeon. When the new Jensen-directed neurosurgeon saw me in early 1984, I was not in his office 10 minutes before he was commenting on my senior job position and how eloquent I sounded. Before he let me go, he told me that I'd had a miraculous recovery and it was obvious that except for my anxiety, I was fine now. He interpreted such anxiety to spring from my supposed zeal to maximize my lawsuit and told me that I should settle as soon as possible for the sake of my health. He communicated the same Jensen-initiated bias to the Flanders endocrinologist, whom I saw about my impotence. Later, G.P. Jensen repeated to me to take the first offer.

When the test results surfaced, despite all their distortions to render them unusable, they confirmed my cognitive impairments in now absorbing new information. Lawyer Dour nevertheless saw their poor usability and set me up to be seen by a second person.

The second neuropsychologist Kellerman asked me at the new hospital as to why on earth I would need testing again, if I had already had a full battery of tests done by the esteemed Gary Winter. I tried to talk of the sabotage but my words were misinterpreted. Kellerman repeated the now familiar word retrieval test but I still performed inadequately relative to areas of other testing. Without knowing, I also did disastrously on the personality tests, but Kellerman lied by telling me he could not find a thing wrong. He indicated with his hand to the air, that my intelligence was sky high, but then wrote to Dour a report that I was not to see, talking of my disordered personality and possible need for hospitalization.

Dr. Kellerman's diagnosis of normal cognition but deranged

personality, together with his distrust about why I had been unhappy with respected colleague Winter's tests, added to both Dour's disbelief and the damage set in place by the original source, G.P. Dr. Jensen.

---

## My Mother in 1983

By early 1983, psychiatrist Doctor Fisher and I had been seeing each other regularly. As may have been his Freudian bent, Dr. Fisher had included in our early discussions an exhaustive inventory of my childhood. I had mentioned my 100's in high school languages as well as scoring first in the Toronto school system on a series of Grade 8 Math tests. I had also talked about my history with music, being head choirboy, first desk on French horn and my current position in the Mendelssohn Choir. I had said I had been in track & field, hockey team captain and swimming instructor. I had stayed protective when discussing my family and it had taken some time for the kind, old Dr. Fisher to flush out problems.

Doctor Fisher did not suggest approaching my mother; instead it was she who said I should not keep things bottled up. My mother had come from her winter home in Florida in early 1983 and Maria had gone to bed for the evening. My mother at once mentioned a lecturing letter that I had sent her about love. She started by saying "not that other kind of love," her allusion to sex. I fell into a dissertation on the many meanings of love, but she claimed I was trying to hide things. Eventually, I began talking of my childhood when suddenly she shouted, "You're a liar!" then said it again and I stayed in shock. The things I talked about had "never happened, ever" and she furthered that I was a bit "tetched," her word for "crazy." The very foundation year difficulties that she had urged me to deal with were now being denied outright by her, right down to the minutest detail.

Before going to bed, she let fling that maybe I would appreciate her after she were dead, "like you now do Papa." Days later, after her visiting with my brothers, she flew back to Tampa and greeted my father with her rehearsed sad face and my purported cruelty.

## My Son James

Since December 27, 1981, few good things have happened. One of them is my son James and the other my son Robert. James was born February 29, 1984. Given my erectile dysfunction and near absence of sex, having a child amounted to something of a miracle. To my psychiatrist, I called James "The Miracle Baby."

Despite the obstetrician's telling Maria that I was obnoxious, the doctor mentioned problems on the Board of the Victorian Order of Nurses and I volunteered a marketing plan for it. Harnessing marketing to do good works made sense to me, and had motivated my refusals to be lured by headhunters and my move to the Ministry of Food.

I'd had a social conscience since childhood. I had done volunteer work with the kids in The Home for Incurable Children and had been active in philanthropic events around my church, Boy Scouts and the Y.M.C.A. As an adult, I had received letters of thanks from people whose careers and lives I had helped and was known as a person of ethics and social caring. Later I was a Sunday school teacher and Cub Scout leader, and would help my sons' school on trips and projects. Ecologically conscious, I was a member of the Temagami Wilderness Society and later member of the local residents association. I would play a lead role in making the Oriole Parkway safer for schoolchildren, push multi-faith representation on the Board of the King-Bay Chaplaincy and spend a year as student chaplain in Toronto's Don Jail. In our early married years, Maria had mocked me when I had cleaned up others' litter or declared at customs all goods that I had bought in the U.S. Later, I would intervene when Maria tried to hire an illegal nanny for cash.

With long-term memory still intact, I tried to help.

---

Dr. Heather Small
March 5, 1984 Women's University Hospital
76 Grandville St.
Toronto, Ontario M5S 1A2

Dear Dr. Small:

RE: EFFECTIVE MARKETING OF V.O.N.

BACKGROUND

I'm indebted to your delivering us James Cooper, February 29th, and would like to offer the following thoughts as a reciprocal gift, though it pales in comparison with yours.

SITUATION

I understand the Victorian Order of Nurses on whose Board you sit, to be presently running a cumulative deficit and the V.O.N. is attempting to offset it through supplemental fund raising. To that end, it has selected its public relations firm reportedly well, since the Wilson Group has been in business 25 years and has done work for such esteemed clients as Toronto's Baycrest. Such selection is important, since Toronto and Canada are evidently plagued with marginal performers in public relations work. That plague seems exacerbated by clients who have a dearth of knowledge in effective marketing communications; hence, well-meaning participants in philanthropic bodies seem to me often vulnerable to the seductive double-speak of slick but ineffectual marketers.

PRINCIPLES OF MARKETING

Regardless of what is being marketed, whether it be Tide, the Toronto Mendelssohn Choir or the Vatican, the 5 principles of marketing, the "5 P's," remain the same. They are:

1. PRODUCT
2. PACKAGE
3. PRICE
4. PHYSICAL DISTRIBUTION
5. PROMOTION

In V.O.N.'s case, the PRODUCT is an altruistically-based service, an ongoing concrete manifestation of love and caring for one's fellow person. The PACKAGE is V.O.N.'s shaping of the service in the form of nursing visitations. The PRICE has been laudably thought through and is based as I understand it, on a number of independent variables including Homecare (Ontario-subsidized hospitalization), Ontario's Ministry of Community and Social Services, private insurance plans, Workmen's Compensation and a sliding scale of cash payments varying directly with frequency of visits and income. PHYSICAL DIS-TRIBUTION is simply the logistics of placing visiting nurses in the home and should, I feel be carried out in a way that maximizes the speed and quality of patient service, while minimizing related costs. PROMOTION is the last of the 5 principles, though far from being the least important. It's in the PROMOTION area where V.O.N. has already perceived there to be opportunity for improvement in helping address the mounting deficit.

STRATEGIZING

The skeletal framework or superstructure for V.O.N.'s overall thrust can and should, I believe be shaped in the same disciplined manner used by say, Procter and Gamble. The mother strategy is the MARKETING STRATEGY from which all others flow. The eldest sibling strategy is the PRODUCT STRATEGY against which all other strategies must maintain a line of consistency.

MARKETING STRATEGY
- PRODUCT
- PRICE
- PACKAGE
- PHYSICAL DISTRIBUTION
- PROMOTION STRATEGY

As an outsider, I doubt I differ materially from many in having at best a vague understanding of V.O.N.'s raison d'être. There are 2 principal communication vehicles for executing a PROMOTION (COMMUNI-CATIONS) STRATEGY against us outsiders—ADVERTISING and CON-SUMER PROMOTION. The former, ADVERTISING, can be very effec-tive in reaching large numbers of outsiders (consumers). In reaching 1984's consumers, ADVERTISING uses 7 main media:

1. TELEVISION
2. RADIO
3. NEWSPAPERS
4. MAGAZINES
5. BILLBOARDS
6. PUBLIC TRANSIT
7. DIRECT MAIL

The first, TELEVISION, is high cost for both the medium's time and commercial production. It is suitable for relatively high-turnover items with frequent purchase cycles and mass appeal, such as laundry detergents. It also tends to be heavily skewed toward a lower-middle-class socio-economic viewer. Not a suitable medium, I would suggest for a philanthropic organization that is requesting financial donations.

The 2nd, RADIO, while socio-economically more upscale than TELEVISION, remains expensive and its message potential is too short-lived to motivate or induce one to make a financial contribution. The 3rd and 4th, NEWSPAPERS and MAGAZINES, afford more space and time to communicate a message but based on the guesstimated low average redemption rates on coupons at 1% and 12% respectively, are not cost-efficient vehicles for soliciting charitable donations. Of the 5th and 6th, BILLBOARDS and PUBLIC TRANSIT, the latter represents I feel, the better opportunity for getting a message understood, to the extent of being motivating in this instance. Again, however, the latter, PUBLIC TRANSIT, *tends* to be, (though it is far from being exclusively so), downscale socio-economically and thus not optimal for drawing huge numbers of donors. The 7th, DIRECT MAIL, can have a negative "junk mail" stigma attached to it and a corresponding annoyance factor. ADVERTISING, therefore, is not in my view the best route to go in realizing V.O.N.'s communications mandate.

CONSUMER PROMOTION, on the other hand, affords some interesting opportunities. The personal 2-way communications of telephone solicitation has proved successful for fund-raising drives, such as the University of Toronto's Varsity Fund and New York State's educational television station. Additionally, I suspect that a major corporation that markets drugs, medical or hospital supplies would be very interested in a tie-in promotion as has been done by other corporations with BIG BROTHERS or "CASH FOR KIDS." Door-to-door solicitation in selected upscale areas by volunteers has worked effectively in the past. Secondary schools could be approached through, say, Toronto's School Board, to perform such volunteer work on a group basis as part of a student's personal development and learning of responsibility. Ex-patients, that is the "converted," could also be approached (but not pressured) to assist in voluntary solicitation work.

The key, I believe is to zero in on targets which offer the potential for the kind of quantum leaps necessary to narrow V.O.N.'s deficit: corporations; prosperous areas of our urban environment; school boards. Once progress is made in narrowing the gap, V.O.N. can then pursue the third communications vehicle for executing a COMMUNICATIONS (PROMOTION) STRATEGY with a "TRADE" PROMOTION STRATEGY. The "TRADE," in V.O.N.'s case, consists of the governmental and charitable bodies on which V.O.N. relies heavily for funding. They can be reached either directly or indirectly, through the press with the proposition that the V.O.N. has underscored and substantiated its need by successfully soliciting private donations. The governmental and charitable bodies can then be fairly called upon to match such private donations.

SUMMARY

The Victorian Order of Nurses should attack the problem of its deficit through a focus on communicating its need for being. The need should then be carried further, such that private donations are motivated to help fund the V.O.N. The strategizing of such a V.O.N. thrust can and should be as disciplined as that of a sophisticated marketing organization. In executing such a communications thrust, CONSUMER PROMOTION, not ADVERTISING represents I believe, the optimal vehicle. The success of such CONSUMER PROMOTION can then be tied back to "TRADE" PROMOTION, to underscore V.O.N.'s need for being and consequent need for matched private/public sector incremental funding.

CLOSING COMMENT

I trust this paper is of some help, Dr. Small, in your role with the Victorian Order of Nurses. I hope so, for Maria and I love your gift to us.

Sincerely,
Alan J Cooper

## Legal Discoveries in 1984

It should have come as no surprise that my lawyer Dour had not bothered to obtain a copy of the accident report by the time of pre-trial Discoveries. The other side's lawyer clued into this at once and ensured that its cognitively impaired driver would not respond to Dour's asking whether this driver had been charged.

At one point during the interrogation, the opposing lawyer Gauze asked me about my speech and I explained how I now had to speak slowly and from the back of my mouth. Gauze interrupted me after each word of my explanation. He then asked me if I had always worn my hair the way I wore it now, to cover the accident's scar and broken blood vessel near my left temple. I mumbled "I guess," not stopping to think I had not always worn my hair that way, and Gauze proclaimed "Lucky!" When I went on to say that "lucky" was not a word I associated with myself post-accident, Gauze cut me off.

Weeks later, my lawyer Dour forwarded to me the Discoveries' transcripts and asked for my feedback on their fair representation. The entire part about my deliberately slow speech was missing as was talk of the scar and any discussion about my being now unable to sing fast words in the Mendelssohn choir. When I told Dour, he dismissed what he said I was suggesting, saying that Mr. Gauze was a respected lawyer from a firm that specialized in personal injuries. There was no way, Dour said that Mr. Gauze would have altered my testimony and what Dour claimed I was suggesting was a very serious charge. Furthermore, Dour had no memory of what I said was missing and my allegations threw further doubt on my damaged memory. Dour then added the stinging line I would hear often from him, that I should not be trying to run my life with lawsuits. The prejudicially and unlawfully altered Discoveries transcripts were allowed to stand.

<hr />

## Blimiss Hope

Before the end of month one in the new work environment, my weakened ability to absorb new information and poor recall showed. Vice President Personnel Don Slotherley asked about my problem with penetrating accuracy, "Are you still having difficulty absorbing new information?" President Gene Darling spoke to me about my "...terrible short-term memory." Countless times, my memory would interfere with my work and I tried to compensate once again by displaying how creative I was in the unbroken right side of my brain. Staff, associates and boss all saw through the compensation and joked openly about my bad memory. Subordinate Garth Good, to multiple snickers in an all-employee meeting, accused me of having none. Subordinate David Sun told me I had a "listing problem" i.e., an inconsistent, unpredictable memory, likening my mind to a pre-war Bentley—still of high quality but with weaknesses in the electrical system.

VP Sales Gary Brunswick, in fact all staff, joked about my black book, swamped with volumes of to-do's, follow-ups and details right down to the brushing of my shoes. Within months, Alan Cooper's memory was a joke among underlings, boss, peers and outsiders. By July 1983 and after 5 months work, I was formally told by an assistant to neuropsychologist Dr. Winter that I had an "absorption of new information" problem. I went straight to boss Darling and told of my weak short-term memory. He knew nothing about the neurological tests, and lawyer Dour and Dr. Fisher advised me not to elaborate.

Hour to hour, I tried to overcome my memory problems,

unable to confirm the injury out of danger of being "fired for cause" and made unemployable. I kept trying to draw issues back into the abstract where I could rely on a solid pre-accident understanding of marketing principles. To the growing annoyance of boss Darling who felt I did not care enough to "get into" the Blimiss Hope business. I also kept trying to draw on what I had learned pre-accident from Warner-Lambert, considered a first-rate Tier 1 company in the Canadian marketing community. To Gene Darling's chagrin because of Warner's turndown of Gene. Blimiss Hope was rated a nondescript Tier 3 firm; my blue chip Warner credentials should have allowed me to have enormous impact, but people saw my actions as brandishing those marketing credentials to the lowly practitioners at BH (Blismiss Hope) and as overcompensation for some memory deficit within.

I had bought that University of Toronto blazer with its crest to flaunt my graduation from a blue chip university and was seen as further self-centered when I repeatedly forgot the names of new staff or peers. I did not know that it is a predictable reaction for the brain-injured person to show off how intelligent he or she is or to become more self-focused in a way similar to the behavior of many people over the age of 90, knowing of their loss of faculties and wanting all to recall how contributing they had been. I had witnessed such behavior in another person, my pre-accident eye doctor Schulz. I had bumped into him post-accident at the University of Toronto where I had been buying the infamous blazer and he had begun telling me how important and accomplished a doctor he had been. Dr. Schulz had sustained a brain injury.

In the second 6 months at Blimiss Hope, staff felt increasingly free to mock my memory. A direct report employee Guy Vacks made fun in a skit of both my memory and Warner-Lambert analogies. Subordinate Rick Box joked in the open about my "memory impaired in a car accident," to the quick hushing by his peers and my posthumous pickup. Garth Good mocked me again in public, this time during a BH party, citing my bad memory and self-positioning as a creative Renaissance man. Drunken staff at an underling's send-off party, laughed about VP Marketing Alan Cooper, the has-been.

I was let off easily at the end of year one. My presentation to New York at the end of 1983 was stilted but rated a pass, with questions limited to 3 rehearsed points. Boss Darling assessed me in December as having good potential but indicated I relied too much on pre-Blimiss Hope information. It was time, he felt that I start demonstrating my lauded abilities in this new setting. He talked of my weak short-term memory but knew not its cause, and made reference to my bad memory perhaps being a function of narcissism.

By 1984, the honeymoon was over. Gene Darling realized he could not use personal chemistry as the reason for his growing Alan problem—the stigma of having fired the former VP still stuck. At the start of 1984, I steered out Guy Vacks, a direct report who had been like a son to Darling but now fell under Darling's disapproval. Gene then went on a wild swing from wanting Guy fired at any moment to hoping he would stay on. I got caught in the crossfire and when the start of year 2 saw me still struggling with new information, Darling put it down to my no longer being able to fall back on Vacks. Darling began a barrage of demoralizing digs against me, saying he had overestimated my abilities and indicated how lucky it was for me that Gene's boss liked me. Darling then fixated on the thought that I was spread too thin, and I was forced to abandon all extracurricular activities. I was working 11 hours a day and often nights and weekends, demonstrating a dedication far beyond that of any other Blimiss Hope employee. I knew things were going bad in a job that I could have done pre-accident with ease, but I saw no alternative other than working longer and harder.

My personal judgment, already cross-wired with a changed personality, reached a pressure point. Like a psychotic, I now had a knack for getting under another's skin and bringing out the worst in a person. I would overestimate people's rationality and liked to think myself helpful when pointing out another's key weakness. I seemed always to feel it necessary to clear the air. When departing employee Vacks asked me "When is someone going to tell Gene that *he* is the one who needs a psychiatrist?," I immediately relayed the bad news to Darling, not conscious of the self-damage that I, the sender, was doing. When I did a bold reorganization of my marketing department, I decided to show the plan first to market researcher Judi Jones, thinking her independent and thus objective. I was not mindful of her inability to understand much of the input or of her being Darling's cow. She deep throated her objections to Gene.

The worst was yet to come. By September 1984, I took what I considered high-road thinking to Vice President Personnel Don Slotherley and suggested I look for a Blimiss Hope transfer elsewhere. I did not give a thought to President Gene Darling's need not to be seen in New York as the source of Canadian management problems or Slotherley's reporting relationship. I assumed the VP Personnel would be neutral and did not see Gene Darling as his boss.

Darling took me to dinner. Over his usual cognacs at meal's end, alcoholic Gene began telling me of his failing Ontario's grade 13 but of having an I.Q. of 150. I kept looking at him, gently smiling and repeatedly feeding back "I know, I can read minds." Never in my wildest fantasies did I think Darling would take my tongue-in-cheek talk seriously or my kind smile for smugness.

The following day, I received a phone call from former employer Marty Rosen. Marty advised me that a detective was querying Maclaren Advertising's personnel department about Alan Cooper in a legal case relating to a car accident. Marty went on to say that the detective had been asking some provocative questions about Alan Cooper and Marty's personnel department had advised him to "watch out."

Here I was, a man trying his damnedest to pull himself up and do a marketing job in an area where he had always shone, trying to do with enormous new mental and physical deficits, in 11 hours or more per day, a job in which he had historically soared in normal hours. Here I was, still trying to contribute, to feel productive, to earn a living, and the opposing legal detective was trying to seek out negative information about Alan Cooper in Canada's tiny marketing village, despite an agreement between Mr. Dour and opposing lawyer Mr. Gauze at the time of Discoveries that such detective action by the other side would not be undertaken, since it could further hurt my career.

I telephoned my lawyer Dour, reached his assistant and told him that I had tried at all times to be as open, candid and fair as I could be with opposing Mr. Gauze. I also reminded Dour's assistant of Mr. Gauze's agreement at Discoveries not to make my job worse and added that "If Mr. Gauze wants to play hardball, I'm going after his shingle." Within hours, Dour's assistant phoned me back to say that Mr. Gauze too was upset by the detective's actions and in any event, the detective's investigation was now complete.

A day later, a second bomb dropped. Direct report David Sun, whom I was disciplining over a management issue, let me have it with, "Your memory was impaired in your car accident." I went numb and Sun saw it. I learned that all of my staff and many who had left for other firms, had long ago pieced together my "non-existent memory" and my car accident's brain injury. Sun went on to say that the headhunters, that is the contingency recruiters, all knew of it, too, and not just contingency headhunters but also Canada's prestigious Canton Group recruiting firm.

I phoned my lawyer Dour to say that both the workplace and marketplace knew. All the fooled Dour did was quip "...which you know isn't true."

I was caught in a hellish dilemma. Blimiss Hope, the recruiters and much of the Canadian marketing community already knew of

Alan Cooper's car accident and related bad memory. My own lawyer Dour was sitting in ignorance, duped by it all and believing in me nothing. Dour had even told me, "The other legal side could come back on me for malingering." My G.P. Dr. Steve Jensen had fed it to pivotal people that I was out to malinger for money and that my stress was a function of greed, when the truth was the opposite. I was doing whatever I could to offset the reality of my actual brain deficits. While all doors were closing around me, my exasperation with Dr. Jensen and his prejudiced people in pronouncing the opposite was making it impossible to function. The more I got stressed by my multiple brain damage, the more Jensen, lawyer Dour and pre-fed specialists thought greed was running away with me.

— • —

It was Friday and my broken brain's judgment was in one moment to do me worse. Boss Gene was in my office and wanted to know how my discipline session with David Sun had gone. Without mentioning Sun as the source, I began relaying Sun's desperate suck-up comments to me of a day earlier as if they were thoughts of my own. I asked if Darling had hired me because of my blue chip marketing and academic background along with culture and rounding, all the things that Gene was not. Darling emitted a quick "No," then paused, looked down at the floor, turned and charged back toward his office. He was unable to be found. An hour later, Gene was seen exiting the building, his face purple, his eyes to the ground, his lips spitting and his head shaking a continuous "No."

From that point on in September 1984, the pressure increased on me to perform at Blimiss Hope, to perform in Canada's tiny marketing community with all eyes upon me. Pathetically ironical, later in the autumn of 1987 was neuropsychologist Dr. Winter's second test feedback to me that typically an executive with such a brain injury still possesses post-accident, much of the former drive and high expectations of himself, and tries to compensate for his new brain deficiencies by working harder. By September of 1984, my 11 hour days changed to 12, then by October of 1984 to 14, then 16, then 18 hours a day of Blimiss Hope work. Subordinates, peers, expressed concern to me when they saw my exhausted appearance but I was determined not to let the car accident and brain injury beat me. I was averaging 18 hours work per day and proudly proclaiming to subordinates and boss Gene Darling that I was fine and "...could go on 4 hours sleep a day."

Mid-October, one Monday came and with it an invitation to Gene Darling's office. VP Personnel Don Slotherley was already there. Darling gave me the option of going or not going to a psychiatrist and if I decided in favor, going to the one of my choice. Darling expressed concern about my chronic bad memory, erratic behavior and mix-up of work priorities. In particular, he cited my comments to him about my blue chip, cultured background. I saw a setup but no option. Gene could not fire me for performance, because Blimiss Hope had been breaking record sales and profits. He couldn't fire me for people chemistry, because he'd used that reason for the previous VP. Insanity was his only way. I said "Yes" and chose Doctor Fisher, the one I had been seeing for almost 2 years. Blimiss Hope had not known about my seeing him and Dr. Fisher advised me not to communicate anything beyond my choosing him in response to Mr. Darling's urging.

Work got worse. The harder I tried at Blimiss Hope, the more reactive Darling got, and every decision I made was reduced to ridicule. Documents done by me were over-ruled and Darling began to make fun of my memory in front of hushed staff. Then my brain-skewed judgment got me again when I mentioned some marital problems to Darling—soon through his cow Jones, my marital problems were the news of the floor.

Next, Darling tried to stop me from going to New York for the annual plan presentation. He pretended concern about my being overtaxed work-wise and feigned fearing that New York would push me beyond the brink. He wanted to speak to my psychiatrist in front of Slotherley and me, and promised to keep the phone speaker open. He shut it off. Dr. Fisher confirmed I was fine for going to New York but when Darling hung up, he started off by saying Dr. Fisher couldn't comment upon Alan's "upsetting all staff."

Gene Darling got to his New York boss and cut off my line of communications to him. Darling then jockeyed plane flights to make it impossible for me to re-meet counterparts in New York and be part of the annual marketing plans rehearsals. Darling did not want me to be seen sane by anyone.

On the night before the New York presentation, President Gene Darling, VP Personnel Slotherley, VP Finance Tony Pudd and I met in Manhattan for dinner. I already had mistakenly told Don Slotherley that I was not going to stay for Gene's customary cognac blow-up. From the start, Darling stomped on my every comment, affixing "more of your bullshit" to each one of my points. I finally looked into his eyes and he stared back while asking, "McKenzie?" Then Darling nodded to me, mistook my straight stare for a counter-nod and in front of a silent Pudd and Slotherley, tongued out through his gritted teeth that he had used them too. He then began a piece-by-piece rip-up of my background, adding "bullshit" to each edict and then left before his forewarned cognacs. Gene Darling had timed all possibilities to push me over the brink in front of New York management.

I slept 2 broken hours. I tried in the morning to calm my nerves by speed-walking the 4 blocks to the presentation but was mistaken by VP Finance Pudd for being erratic. Gene's boss then pre-empted my presentation by talking of time pressures. Finally, I got to start. I stood up and made a jest of my pocket watch and compass in front of all world staff and Gene's boss shut me down. Then, with the meeting carrying on with other countries, Gene and his boss Dale Rogers met with me in Rogers' office. Rogers began by talking of my marital problems and how Blimiss Hope wanted to help me. I made the mistake of shielding Gene, not mentioning his hired "McKenzie" or the strategic timing of his acts and blow-up. Instead, I said I was under so much pressure that I might have a stroke. That was all it took, another misjudgment made by my broken brain.

I soon found myself with Darling and VP Personnel Slotherley at La Guardia airport, and Slotherley trying to reach Blimiss Hope's Canadian doctor by phone. I was unaware of how I had been interpreted or what I had done. Back in Toronto, I was checked by a medical G.P. and diagnosed as fine. But Darling was already starting the rest of his scheme to protect himself and see me fired. From the Toronto airport and doctor's office, he forced me that Friday, away from work and then, with Stalin-like censorship, cut me off from my trusted secretary and all of Blimiss Hope. I tried the following Monday to probe Darling about who was the "McKenzie" group he had referred in New York, but "End of conversation" was all he shouted, followed by a "Gotta go!" and a dial tone.

I was off work for the next 2 weeks of November 18 and November 25, 1984. On Monday of the first week, Darling had all my direct reports in his office and told them, "I guess Alan was under a lot more pressure than we knew." My direct reports were then told not to have any communications with me, without Gene's authorization. My staff already knew of my car accident, brain injury and "impaired memory," and speculation began to run wild within Blimiss Hope and the Canadian marketing community that Alan Cooper's bad memory post-car accident had finally caught up with him and that Alan had suffered a nervous breakdown.

That same Monday, November 18th 1984, Darling phoned Maria to assure her that Alan was not well, but she was not to worry, since Blimiss Hope would take care of him. Darling lied to Maria in saying I had been psychoanalyzing all my staff. Maria immediately relayed the lie as a truth to Dr. Fisher who was thus fooled by Maria into Darling's scheme.

I realized I was in deep trouble but also knew that my lawyer Dour had been duped into thinking I was malingering. The day after on November 19th, I resorted to an additional lawyer, along with his assistant Don Shin. Shin was to handle my possible dismissal case and I would find out only years later of his being fired for incompetence.

At the end of 2 weeks when I was scheduled to return to work, Gene Darling insisted on first meeting with me, Friday November 29th, off Blimiss Hope premises. He met me at the Blimiss Hope apartment and had with him VP Personnel Don Slotherley and VP Finance Tony Pudd. Slotherley and Pudd had both seen me at the New York presentation and had been with Gene and me the night before, for dinner and the Darling blow-up. Darling now said he wanted me to refrain from attending the Christmas Operations dinner for senior Blimiss Hope staff, scheduled for November 30th. Gene went on to say in front of the 4 of us that he did not trust my psychiatrist's judgment, which allowed me to go to New York on November 15th. Darling emphasized he had tried to prevent my going but had reluctantly agreed to it, only after talking to my Dr. Fisher.

Darling did not want me to return to work on Monday but instead to see Dr. Harry Hooker, a psychiatrist of his choosing. By now, I knew that all my staff were aware of the bad memory and car accident but did not know whether Darling, or VP Personnel Slotherley and VP Finance Pudd knew. I felt no choice but to agree to see any psychiatrist Gene chose, to prove I was still fit for work and my job.

The following week of December 2nd 1984, I began seeing psychiatrist Dr. Harry Hooker and visited him 4 times in all. My sessions with Darling's chosen Hooker were ugly from the outset. He started by saying he was in a difficult position, that he was to put nothing in writing and that his fees were to be paid in a special manner without any paperwork. Dr. Hooker went on to say that he held in high esteem the known-to-him Glib family who headed Blimiss Hope in New York. When I said the Glibs knew nothing of what was going on, he winced and for a moment displayed uncertainty but soon recovered. He flashed a copy of my résumé and said there were critical things missing from my curriculum vitae. He then began the first of 4 sessions of rants against me, shouting about my distraction, fragmentation and lack of single-mindedness. With rarely a question asked, psychiatrist Dr. Hooker said he had full and complete information, and went on about my lack of application and non-caring approach to the Blimiss Hope business. He talked of how my first and only performance appraisal by boss Gene Darling, done at the end of my first year, talked of my potential but with any conversion of that potential remaining a giant question mark. At one point, Hooker was interrupted by a phone call. When minutes later I said I did not remember our pre-phone conversation, he betrayed his lies of saying "nothing in writing" by starting to scribble frantically on a notepad.

Psychiatrist Hooker badgered me on what had so blatantly gone wrong with me in September of 1984. I told him nothing of the car accident and brain damage but my fears of his discovery grew. Perhaps I should have told this shrink Hooker but my chosen psychiatrist Dr. Fisher had advised me not to tell Dr. Hooker, and my car accident lawyer Dour still stuck to the thought that I was malingering.

Then came a battery of psychological tests by Dr. Hooker's assistant, psychologist Dr. Shalom Kulisky. After my first session in private with Kulisky, I told Hooker that I did not trust Dr. Kulisky, because he had looked at me through the corners of his eyes. Kulisky's final, written psychological report would go into detail about that "distrust and no direct eye contact" comment of mine, and included Dr. Kulisky's defense of himself.

The final series of tests by Kulisky were cognitive where I feared the brain damage would show. Before the cognitive tests' 5-hour completion, Dr. Kulisky shut them down and went downstairs to see Dr. Hooker, leaving me alone in his upstairs office. Maria was also downstairs but in a waiting room, and Dr. Hooker tried to get my wife Maria alone in his office to discuss me. Maria refused. Minutes later, without Dr. Kulisky's having analyzed the exhaustive series of tests and without Dr. Hooker's ever having seen them, Dr. Hooker yelled at me in front of my wife and Kulisky. Kulisky added to Maria that Dr. Kulisky did not need to analyze the results of the tests, because my "narcissistic, pre-psychotic nature" was self-evident. To my wife, Dr. Hooker yelled that Alan Cooper knew he was very sick and was using his intelligence to cover up his sickness. He yelled that the Dr. Fisher-prescribed Valium was doing me damage, and Hooker exaggerated 4-fold my recently given children's dosage. He shouted that I required immediate mind-altering, personality-changing drugs and probably emergency hospitalization by a qualified psychotherapist. Dr. Hooker then shouted that a pre-selected psychotherapist, Dr. Konrad Emin, was waiting in his office down the street to see me in a setup emergency appointment.

Dr. Emin saw me and after much delay, got Dr. Kulisky's notes. They included his defense of my not trusting him but I was not allowed to see the tests. Dr. Emin prescribed no drugs or hospitalization. It was now late December 1984 and I still had not been allowed to go back to work. Gene Darling would not allow it. I got wind of a wedding shower at a direct report's home on December 18th and there wished employees Garth Good and Guy Vacks well in their marriage-to-be. Other Blimiss Hope reports queried me as to when I would be returning to work and I said, "Soon," but also said I would be making a December 20th visit to my Marketing Department for the annual exchange of joke gifts.

Darling heard of my intentions and tried the intervening day to stop my visit. I insisted on coming and he acquiesced, provided

I did not remain past noon when the Blimiss Hope Christmas party was scheduled to begin. I went to my Marketing Department that morning December 20th and was still there at 11:00 a.m. Darling sent VP Personnel Slotherley to fetch me, and elbow-led by Slotherley, I reported to President Eugene Darling. Slotherley left. Darling said I had overstayed my allowed time and that he wanted me out of the building ahead of the noon start of the company-wide Christmas party. I said I would be gone. President Darling then told me that he would not accept my return to work at Blimiss Hope until Dr. Emin gave me a complete written bill-of-health. I then asked Gene Darling why days earlier, my German sports sedan dealer had been falsely told by a Blimiss Hope administrator that I Alan Cooper was very ill and had been in hospital, and that my order for a new car was to be canceled. I also asked why my car dealer had been told not to breathe a word of this directive to me and why I had to fight to get my car, through several phone calls to the VP Administration. Darling gave no answer other than I did get my car.

God, how I tried to get back to work that late December of 1984. I wanted to work, to function, to contribute. I had worked hard at Blimiss Hope for almost 2 years with enormous brain deficits. I had taken exhaustive pains to minimize those deficits to staff, Blimiss Hope and the marketing community. But Gene Darling insisted on first receiving a written bill of mental health on me from psychotherapist Emin and no other doctor, despite my protesting that my chosen psychotherapist had been and was still, Dr. Michael Fisher.

A grim Christmas of 1984 passed. An attempt at a Bermuda vacation before New Year's came and went, one in which I tried rekindling feelings when my wife and I had been there pre-accident. My mind was elsewhere and I sensed I was finished at Blimiss Hope. One bit of light had occurred during my December 20th meeting with Darling—he had talked of a mid-winter 1985 presentation to

U.S. management, planned for Canada and I had assumed that by Gene's telling me, I was to be part of the presentation. January, however, crossed over, I was not back at work, my secretary was phoning me in tears to talk of her frustration and I was still being forced to see psychotherapist Emin.

Dr. Emin by now was confronting me with bills. When I said that Blimiss Hope was covering those bills, Dr. Emin advised me that he had checked with Blimiss Hope and the bills were all to be paid by me. When I then protested by phone to VP Personnel Don Slotherley, he replied that psychotherapist Emin was my chosen doctor and I was to pay his bills. When I said that Dr. Emin was not at all my psychiatrist of choice but Dr. Michael Fisher was, Don Slotherley told me that Blimiss Hope doubted Dr. Michael Fisher's competence, up-to-datedness and accessibility to emergency hospitalization, and Gene Darling would not accept a written clean bill-of-health on me from any psychiatrist other than Dr. Emin. He also said I was free to choose whatever psychiatrist I wanted and that Dr. Emin had been my choice, so I had to pay Emin's bills out of my own pocket. I protested to Darling but he said Hooker was their guy and Emin was my guy and I, therefore had to pay.

About the same time, I told dismissal lawyer Don Shin about my brain injury in a car accident. Shin looked askance at me and said, "Well, Alan, so you really *are* paranoid." I tried to protest that paranoia had never been at issue but my credibility with my dismissal lawyer from that moment on, ceased.

On Monday, January 6, 1985 I saw psychiatrist Dr. Konrad Emin in a morning session. I told Emin of a recruiter phoning me and making queries as to my health, saying that my staff wondered why I was not back at work. Dr. Emin told me he could understand my source of anxiety and phoned in my presence, boss Gene Darling. A meeting was set up for me to see my boss Darling that afternoon at Blimiss Hope.

I arrived at 4:30 p.m. to be greeted at the front door by VP Personnel Don Slotherley and escorted directly to Darling. President Gene Darling sat behind his desk and Slotherley sat down beside him. Both looked at me seated, some 20 feet away. Darling told me that a written clean bill-of-health was no longer necessary. I was fired. VP Personnel Don Slotherley orally supported the firing. Darling took the opportunity to throw 2 hurtful jabs: 1. he did not respect my judgment, citing a decision for a price increase which in reality was made by a group; 2. I presented myself well on hiring but was poor in decline, stating that I blamed others. Slotherley saw me to the door, and then thinking nothing of his role in my insanity setup, curled his finger to my face and lectured that between a president and vice president, "There has to be that chemistry."

Blimiss Hope was anxious to settle my severance and I had not yet pieced together the damage already done to my reputation. True, subordinate David Sun had confirmed to me in September that the contingency headhunters had known of my injury and memory impairment since the time of my accident. I had even heard the story in October from former Warner employee Kasia. As would prove ironical later, Kasia had also asked me if I, Alan Cooper, were still the same health and physical fitness buff I had been during my many years at Warner-Lambert. But I still did not understand that the gossipy headhunters and much of Canada's marketing village had linked together my car accident, memory impairment, 2 months absence and firing from Blimiss Hope.

Darling did not seem to know the entire story but did realize it was in his interests that all believe that I had been fired for reasons other than personal chemistry. Darling also knew he had made a disastrous ass of himself in thinking I had hired a detective to research his background. His hiring a detective and front-end loading a shrink to pronounce me crazy, looked to me to be some low point for professional behavior. Then.

In despair, I agreed to a damning 1-pager as to why I had left. My lawyer Don Shin told me he was impressed with the nice-guyism of Blimiss Hope's lawyer O'Hara, who offered to let me go off severance and onto disability payments for as long as 6 months if I relapsed into my "illness." I refused, saying I wanted not to malinger, but to work. My dismissal lawyer Shin also joked with my accident lawyer Dour about my skill in Trivial Pursuit, and both failed to note that such trivia was pre-accident knowledge.

References for any new job were virtually impossible to obtain. Subordinate Steve Pince went out of his way to say that Alan Cooper was only half the man he had been before the car accident. Another Blimiss Hope direct report Paulette Montreuse, one I would have been promoting without her knowledge in my pro-posed reorganization, refused to give me any reference at all. It was January 10, 1985 when I began to appreciate the full extent of the damage and to realize I was unemployable.

# 1985

I had been fired because I was brain injured and the market knew more than I thought.

I sought out the executive recruiter who had hired me into Blimiss Hope and he referred me to outplacement counseling. John Bridge was to be my counselor, and from the week in January when I met him, he began probing about my car accident, memory impairment and need for neurological help. Bridge was reporting back to Blimiss Hope as part of my settlement and I was again advised not to disclose anything.

My first job interview in mid-January was for a more junior marketing assignment than the ones I'd had at Blimiss Hope or Warner-Lambert but it was for a position leading to general management. Contingency headhunter Richard Fast secured the interview and my agreeing to go marked the only time I had ever come close to finding work through a headhunter. Before my going, Fast told me he had been "... a big member of the Alan Cooper fan club" but followed with "How's your health?" I replied, "O.K.", not yet fully appreciating how damaged my reputation was. Fast then remarked on my black book.

Before the interview, I researched the job and company thoroughly, interviewed well as I had done pre- and post-accident, and earned a second interview with the general manager. I then received a phone call from Fast, indicating that my reference Steve Pince had told the company the "half the man since his car accident" story about Alan Cooper. I had actually mentioned to Steve Pince that I wanted to hire him into the new place under me, but he had gone after the job for which I was applying. The opportunity was dead.

Alarmed by Steve Pince's blackening reference, I sought out another Blimiss Hope direct report David Sun for a face-to-face meeting. Sun told me that VP Personnel Don Slotherley had told my staff that Blimiss Hope had to keep changing my supposed return to ensure that I was responding well to my prescribed "drug treatment." I had been taking none in the period other than the occasional use of a children's dosage of Valium prescribed by Dr. Fisher.

I was then set up for an interview with a small ad agency. During my interview, the president tried to check my memory and I gave no reply. I did not get the job. In another interview for a job as Vice President Marketing of Toronto's famed Roy Thompson Concert Hall, I was told that a reference check had revealed my brain injury.

Two other recruiters fed back to an old Warner-Lambert peer how difficult it was going to be for black-balled Alan Cooper to get another job. In one case, the prospective company phoned former Blimiss Hope direct report Guy Vacks to ask if Alan Cooper had actually had a nervous breakdown. A headhunter Bloomfield, who had been shunned by me, phoned Vacks for the same news. Bloomfield then wrote me off as a prospect and phoned me to say that he was going to hunt me down and make sure all staff knew, no matter where I was. When I confronted Vacks face-to-face, he told me how he had "...heard from everybody, in and out of Blimiss Hope, of Alan Cooper's cracking up."

Creative Toys President Samuel Doner was looking for a VP Marketing and interviewed me as a candidate. He queried me about my recall and viewed my explanation as defensive behavior.

My reputation was shot, my ability to get another job all but impossible.

## Unemployment

I seemed permanently out of work. The ability to provide was gone. I am sexist enough to believe that built into each father is a need to care and provide for his family. When that ability is taken away, I feel the father falls down further than any father would want known. I felt I could not provide what a father must, and had failed my family. I was brain deranged and unemployable, and no pivotal person was listening.

Maria and I had bought our English Tudor house, 9 months before the December 1981 accident and had planned in due course to have 2 children. Our mortgage was huge but money from double incomes had always been running in. During his first year, James had been colicky and Maria had taken the maximum leave allowed, then had gone back to work in September of 1984, leaving James to the daytime care of a nanny. Now Maria dropped a surprise. Our sexual intercourse had been nil for 9 months but it seems I shoot with live bullets. In our 8 days in Bermuda, we had managed sex for seconds, twice, and neither of us had imagined her conceiving. Maria was due in September 1985.

I applied for countless jobs, composed 200 faxes and interviewed as often as 3 times per day. But my references no longer checked out, news of my brain damage flourished and all who saw me said I was spent. Old Warner employees tried to warn me but only added to an anxiety already there and soon wounded confidence was added to the list. As people's suspicions grew with my overcompensating, my confidence worsened and a kind of bloodlust poured forth disguised as concern. People who had once seen themselves as less exalted, now relished the downfall of one they had perceived so high.

Maria fed all to her mother and I had no one to talk to. I tried to write myself a letter.

January, 1985
Dear Alan,

Worry will not increase your help to others one bit. I will not help you overcompensate for your brain damage but do ask you to reflect on your remaining powers of love, reason and the potential for help to others. Inasmuch as you can still strive for love, justice, truth and their realizations, try to consider your life valuable.

You have experienced autonomy and initiative, and have proven your industry and competence. You have repeatedly demonstrated integrity and compassion for others, and have shown some glimpse of life's meaning.

I think you need to know your newly restricted condition and not be overwhelmed by it. I think you need self-acceptance.

Sincerely,
*Alan*

I completed another battery of tests for my outplacement counselor's psychologist, this time not on cognition but on vocational preferences. To my counselor's shock and contrary to everything he had heard from Darling and company, the vocational results revealed that I was a person of ethics and social responsibility, and was a helper, healer, social worker, minister, philanthropist and altruist.

## To the Desert

Near the end of January 1985, I broke my 30 months of 750 ml nightly water and wine, and switched to straight vodka. I did not want to see real day. Hopelessness had ground down the soreness of my unhealed clavicle and I felt the future black.

Not only was I able to knock myself out for 6 hours after midnight but when daylight came, I could face it with 2 more shots of vodka. The odor on my breath was not at first decipherable and I could still shave and shower with discipline. For the 9-minute walk to the liquor store and 9 minutes back, I could stash into my safari pockets, 2 little 2-ounce "ponies" of vodka and then could walk along swigging and faking a cough, finishing 4 ounces on the round trip.

I don't know how many days went by with my doing such drinking, except to say that I did at all times pay the bills, keep the house neat and take out the garbage. I could be 3 horses dead but would still hang up my clothes, shower and take out the garbage. Neatness and cleanliness seemed to give me some symmetry missing in all my other life. Perhaps I was overly anal, perhaps just a severely brain-injured person whose idiosyncrasies pre-accident were now greatly magnified.

On a Tuesday in February, late in the day, I was on my way to the liquor store when I took note of a pub I had passed for years. I heard through its front door, laughter and a hint of British accents. I went in.

Many folks from Glasgow, I have now learned, rank among Earth's best. Rough, agile, articulate but most of all, kind. The Duchess pub taught me so. What one working-class Scot said to me there on a February Tuesday was that modern science was founded against both the necessary capriciousness of free will and the human need to satisfy a sense of unfulfilled purpose, the result being a construed reality of orderliness rather than spontaneity. After his 4th drink, he continued by telling me that to be vital, people should risk madness or else life is left with no flavor. He saw a person's job as needing Scotch, not herbal tea, to turn one's vision of life inside out.

I listened dumbfounded as working-class Scots switched from prose to poetry, English to Gaelic and back again. These Scots accepted me and were very kind. Using philosophical espousing I had not witnessed since my sophomore days, they tried to help me out of my pit.

"Alan, new friend, sorrow can find a voice when supposed happiness is saying nothing. A sincere lad respects honesty and the person who suffers for it." Big Scottish Jamie put his hand down on my shoulder and I felt tears come to my eyes.

"Thank you, Jamie. You're a good person."

"Thank you, Alan but..." He swept his long arm around the pub. "...There is many a good person right here. Is that not true, Drew?"

"Aye, Jamie. Alan, the devil was invented to avoid the shame of suffering. But what shame? It's bullshit, lad. Not truth but imagery at its worst. Ah, but freedom of choice and conscience often take great suffering, since one has no scapegoat devil to blame ...Take sin."

"Sin?"

"Mediaeval Christian chiefs, the only ones then allowed to be educated, knew they had only to make a good man feel sinful in order to redeem him. Am I sinning right now as I drink? Not I believe, if I hurt no one. Alan, you are an educated man and a true one. We do not have your formal learning but we've seen many an honorable lad like you hoaxed like a trusting dog."

"Alan!"

"Jamie?"

"I agree with Drew on sin and freedom of conscience. God gave us desires, hormones and instincts. Your life is down right now, so I don't think you can see it but as you come back up, and we'll help you, we hope you'll see that instincts, following those instincts without hurting others and happiness, all hang together."

"You're a creatician, Alan and right now show the feelings of a tragic artist. Unleash, Alan as you must have done before, the freedom to express. Have no fear in the face of the fearsome and questionable people who want you to copy life and not express it."

Jamie and Drew and their fellow Scots asked me on the following night, to put on a jacket and tie. The group of newly met Scots then took me out to a full-course dinner, back to the Duchess pub and home. In later years, I would be dismissed from the Duchess for making a textbook brain injury remark but for now, noble working-class Scots with their knowledge of poetry, prose and so much more, humbled me into understanding again that acts of love and acceptance can make up for much.

It was not the Guinness of the British pub that did me in but the vodka before and after. During my second week of the ritual, I began realizing my body could not take it. Each straight vodka triggered revulsion and the revulsions built to vomit. I had to stop.

I fetched an empty milk jug and poured into it 4 ounces of vodka. I filled the rest with water, took the milk jug in hand and started a slog though the winter's night, the 3 miles to Flanders Hospital. Along the way and as necessary to counter any shakes, I sipped bits of the vodka-water mix. At Flanders, I misdiagnosed myself as having delirium tremens but did not have it; nevertheless, the intern recorded my DT's misdiagnosis as his own.

Of the 8,800 hours in 1985, I was overdosed on alcohol for about 1% of them. Alcohol was not the cause but the effect of the brain injury, the personality displacement, the firings. Many of the characteristics I displayed as closed head injured could be easily misconstrued as caused by alcohol, especially by the ignorant layperson

and those pimp-like experts who were willing to prey on the ignorant. My binges were done out of rage, indignation and the extreme
dilemma of my situation, but they were short lived and all post-accident. No-one freed himself or herself, of prejudice to hear me.

## James

I sobered up that second week of February and took again to
writing, mostly job applications and the positioning of myself for
hire. I kept to the unfinished basement, not to drink but to work
on top of a tiny table. I put off interviews and seeing again the outside world for another week. As I had done when Maria was pregnant with James, I spent evenings helping her get as much exercise
as possible with our Robert-to-be.

One bright February, as the daylight hours grew longer and a
stronger sun radiated off the white snow, I took my son James to
the park. James was now almost one year old and had been trying
to talk for weeks. The playground was cushioned with snow, and
James and his dad first tackled the jungle gym. James was at his best
that day and seemed to revel in his time alone with his daddy.
James loved me unconditionally and I had the feeling that if I had
told him I was brain damaged or out of work, he would have loved
me just the same. From these moments of fun came an inner
freedom over me as I listened to James' bird speak and looked at
his gleeful face.

One of the biggest mistakes I then made was to keep applying
for jobs instead of being with James and later Robert. As things
stood, I did give them much, but I missed this opportunity to be a
stay-at-home father and give my sons a childhood richer than anything some people deemed possible.

## Biological Mother

Pre-brain injury, I had taken my mother to concerts, arranged an elaborate 65th birthday party, written her massive letters and had bought her a subscription to the *Harvard Medical Journal*. I had grossly overestimated not only her abilities but also her goodness.

Before my brain damage, I had not in my adult years felt vulnerable to my mother's venom. I was not fully aware of it, thinking such a thing unthinkable. My younger brother's wife had made mention of my mother's jealousy and Maria had mentioned my mother's denigrations, but I had given their comments the swift dismissal that I felt they deserved. I had not conceived of my mother seeking out a soft spot for her poisoned tip. Most likely in the last 10 years leading up to the accident, I had built up antibodies to my mother. That had been a time when I had left home, the career had soared and my Mendelssohn Choir, creative writing, philanthropy, cultural Board memberships and world travel had contributed much to the growth of myself and others.

My mother and I had stopped communicating after her liar accusation of 2 years earlier, but she had tried in the interim to milk the guilt in Maria, under the guise of healing.

Perhaps indicative of some induced need I had to be downtrodden, in 1985 I visited my parents alone. With no way of my escaping and no person around, other than my father focused on himself, my mother lashed out at her brain-injured and unemployed son, "You deserved to be fired. You're absolutely spoiled rotten. You're no good at all. What you need is a good swat."

## Cross-wired Thinking of a Car-crashed Brain

As I write this story, more that 2 decades after my medically categorized "severe" brain injury of late 1981, I find it impossible to describe or even depict parts of my physically shattered personality. I am stuck forever trying to describe the way things were, using as my main instrument a brain so changed that it can no more describe the way things were than can a dead person describe her life before death.

There is no-one else who can help. As befits left lobe injury people, all close friends are now gone. My wife was never there, my father was never there, my brothers don't know me and my mother stays stuck in her own world of self.

I can perhaps shed some light by divulging some writings that I began in 1985. Those writings were done in that unfinished basement, in a damp cellar room on a late grandparents' wicker table, away from Maria. A neurologist, Doctor Day, would later say that the stories were a classic manifestation of a left frontal lobe injury.

Maybe one test for demonstrating to you, dear reader, the broken-brained "soured symphony" effect on my personality and perceptions of reality, can be done through comparing some of these 1985 stories with stories written pre-brain damage. I cannot help you with this exercise beyond my giving you the stories and saying what I have already said.

Here are the stories and if they don't help you with further neurological understanding, maybe you will find a bit of yourself in them.

# PRE-BRAIN DAMAGE

## A Toronto Saturday Morning Writing Class

Dear Ed,

As a new member to your Group, I was made at once to feel at home. The informal setting and relaxed atmosphere you set up front eased us all into a new environment. Thank you.

Given your interest in people of rich character, I thought I would pass on to you my first dealings with a carpenter. Forced to go through the Yellow Pages and fearing financial rape, I decided to obtain estimates from three separate contractors. The first two companies were large and have long since drifted from my memory. The third was a self-employed carpenter, Pat Smith. Mr. Smith's quotation was the lowest— the other two quoted $1,100 and $1,400 but Mr. Smith was $220.

Who was this Pat Smith who could guess the dollar amount to be 1/5th that of the next estimate? Would Mr. Smith stick to his quotation? What sort of job would he do?

Pat Smith arrived punctually on the agreed upon starting date. He was short, five feet two at most and in his early fifties. He had white curly hair and old-fashioned wire rim glasses. His face was multi-colored-purple in the cheeks, red in the nose with many broken blood vessels and grayish overall. He was slightly hunched over, exaggerating his smallness. With his little box of tools, denim overalls and tattered working boots, his impression was that of a cartoon character. As a carpenter, he did not look expensive and appeared incapable of charging more than $220 for anything.

Pat was a Scottish immigrant from the slums of Glasgow, and his nineteen years in Toronto had done little to soften an accent that one could cut with a knife. His speech was riddled with Scottish expressions—instead of the mini-study I described, Pat was going to build a "wee den"; he was going to use "wee" strips of cedar, "wee" copper nails and construct "wee" shelves; during our conversation, he excused himself to go to the "kybo" to take a "wee" wee.

Pat labored in my little apartment for three days, cutting, hammering, singing and cursing. The songs were sometimes in English—"And he loved a lady, a fine young lass..."—sometimes in Gaelic. The curses were gentle while he was in my wife's presence—"Lord love a duck" when he hit his thumb with the hammer. The curses were less gentle and more spontaneous when they were out of earshot, most referring to the sexual habits of ducks and bears. One had the impression that a fiery temper lurked beneath the otherwise jocular manner of this tiny Scotsman. For all his idiosyncrasies, Pat was a man who loved his work and performed it with supreme skill, a seemingly Scottish version of a little Austrian toymaker.

When Pat had completed his work, he said to me that in addition to his contracted work, he had "cut" six doors and put on extra shelving. I was ready for it. Here it came—no $220 now...No, Pat had upped his finished cost to $230. Two hundred and thirty dollars, for a paneled den, bookshelves, racks and six cut doors. With my hand slightly shaking, I gave Pat Smith the $230 in exchange for his "Thank you."

Three years later, I was again in need of a carpenter and had no doubt whom I would phone. I still had his number in my date diary. A woman answered and was surprised to hear my request for a Mr. Smith. When I finished my embellished

request for Pat's services, the woman quietly replied that Pat
had died six months earlier.

I haven't yet found a replacement for Pat Smith.

Alan J Cooper
January 1979


## STORY # 1

### I Declare You Beautiful

Seven p.m. Back to work after supper. I glance through the
cold rain at the little German sports sedan and sense its
glancing back. Lonely in the dark corner of the night, waiting.

I veer south, winding through the streets of Rosedale. I
bloop over potholes in taut comfort. Then the car and I enter
the turn onto the Parkway, sucked to the road's slippery surface. My hands cling to the wheel at 3 and 9 o'clock, my
arms stretched out, seat tilted back. Northeast to the steppes
of Scarborough. When we reach the car dealers of the
"Golden Mile," the glitz seems muted by a welcome rain. We
stop at an office parking lot.

I get out and look back at the unadorned piece of engineering. I walk into my office and choose for a moment not
to do brand planning but start instead this little story.
Somewhere in it, I am supposed to say "I declare you beautiful." I'll do that later in tribute to my little all-manual driving
machine, but now I must go back to brand plans.


## STORY # 2

### The Elms of Childhood

I think I will never feel anything as lovely as those elms. Four,
with forty years of rise to majesty. Birds sang in them, squirrels homed in them, fresh air came from them. And unending

coolness. All summers cooled to sleep with windows wide open under those mothering elms.

Dutch elm disease. Hacked down in forty minutes.

No squirrels. No early morning birds. Stark, hot, no air, our house naked.

Our mother elms gone.

Alan J Cooper
January, 1979

## STORY # 3
### The Heavy First Date

I was to pick up Dawn Kellet at 1:30 for Saturday's matinée. The critical link to a successful quest was to take control. Quickly. I couldn't let my anxiety show. I couldn't allow myself to be overwhelmed by the magnetism of our school's most popular blonde.

As I edged my way across Davisville Park to her Millwood Road home, my eye returned the glare of Davisville's young bloods. As per ritual, they were gathered in a circle near the old clubhouse, smoking Buckinghams non-filtered and carving obscenities into a weary picnic table. Their heads were fixed on my total movements—my aloof strut, the windbreaker with collar raised, my shirt-tail out, the faded blue jeans, the ultra-thin, silver belt with buckle at the side, white bucks with pink shoelaces, and a double-curled haircut, slicked with Brylcreem to mirrored perfection.

"Where ya' goin', Cooper?"

"Got a date with Kellet."

My calculated histrionics had won me the first battle— the other bloods were stunned into a suppressed silence, envious of my social adroitness.

Dawn's mother answered the door. Glamorous! Red lip-stick, tight skirt and two big ones pushing out of a Banlon sweater. As I sputtered out my rehearsed "How do you do?" the lady pivoted in front of me and twisted down the hallway to the staircase bottom, where she belted out, "Dawn honey, your guy's here." Then as I ogled her, Mrs. Kellet sambaed into the adjoining living room and slouched into the sofa in front of a *True Confession* magazine...Why couldn't all mothers be like her?

Dawn ambled down from the top of the stairs. With each step, her golden locks sprung softly from her head. She was smiling coyly and whispering something that my bewildered mind couldn't grasp...I was to make it with the renowned blue-eyed blonde.

We strolled up the west side of Mount Pleasant Road; I remembered to walk on the street side. Some Davisville Park studs spotted us and were following fifty yards behind. No time for cowardice—I took Dawn's hand in mine.

The first landmark on our half-mile promenade was "Pop" Moray's Cigar Store. Pop returned my customary wave. Next, Parkmount Cleaners where Ben, the old Jewish tailor stopped with arms on waist, shook his head and winked at me. Near Manor Road, we passed the Fish 'n Chips store where several more of the cool set peered out the front window at the dandy duet jaunting up Mount Pleasant, sporting the latest in 1956 fashions. At Manor, we cut across to the east side, to ensure our passing the ice cream parlor. Mr. Fung's Ice Cream was doing a booming business that warm October and several of my fellow warriors were in there, trying to hustle two aspiring flames. What fortune! Eat your hearts out, also-rans.

For the final block northward to the Mount Pleasant Theater destination, the trailing throng had grown to a dozen. Once we arrived, my 55¢ budget went fast—50¢ for our admission, 5¢ for Pink Elephant popcorn. As I marched pompously down the aisle, Dawn in tow, the train followed. Only the royal box would be good enough for this occasion—

front row center. The crowd of admirers settled into lesser seats. Battle number two had been won. The final battle—making it with Dawn—would decide the total quest.

As the onlookers focused on the two front heads silhouetted against the screen, I did it. I reached over and put my left arm around Dawn for all to see, with my right hand's slyly slipping into the popcorn box.

I had made it. On my first ever date. With no less a prize than Dawn Kellet. And the prize a full year older than I. Dawn was nine.

Alan J Cooper,
January, 1979


## STORY # 4
### Watson

David Watson had called me a "suck" once too often. Until then, I had avoided returning from school via Mount Pleasant Road so as not to confront Watson and his gang. But avoiding them was becoming more difficult week to week until by November 1963, it was virtually impossible to leave home without being in danger. Faced with a choice of continued humiliation or confrontation, I chose the latter—walking home past the gang's Mount Pleasant hangout.

Watson had singled me out months earlier, though the sociological schism had started 3 years prior. I too had been a roughneck while at Hodgson Elementary School, partially for survival, partially out of ignorance of other ways of life. Unlike the vast majority of Hodgson's 1960 graduating class who had later entered technical and commercial courses at Northern Vocational School, I had entered North Toronto Collegiate. The reason—I lived on the west side of Mount Pleasant Road, on the periphery of Hodgson's district.

Watson and company had become harder during their

first year at Northern, concentrating on cigarettes, street fights and loose teenage girls. By contrast, I had come up against a radically new environment—gray flannels, blue blazers, orchestras and a group of highly motivated upper middle class students.

I could still be seen by the old crowd, marching home with my newly worn glasses and braces, a pile of books under my right arm and a French horn case held by my left. I would pass former friends, I in gray wool slacks, black oxfords and dress shirt, they in blue denim jeans, greasy T-shirts and sharply pointed shoes. Early on, I was received with curiosity and jokes, later with a low-key nod of the head and finally with increasing contempt as the split became more crystallized in the gang's minds. The contempt's first outward signs were confined to insults, the most frequent being "suck." Later, the verbal darts were accompanied by flicked cigarette butts.

My new prep friends were aghast to hear about these episodes, their travels being through the safer areas of Lawrence Park and Chaplin Estates. They advised me to take an elaborate detour through their areas, do my homework in their homes after school and sneak home when it became darker. Sneak home? I had lived in the area for all of my 15 years. Was I then to accept a life of fear?

I told no one in advance of my intended walk directly past Watson's gang headquarters. I merely set out, books and French horn in hand, and heart in stomach. Watson saw me from a greasy spoon and though betraying surprise, quickly composed himself long enough to get out the "suck." I returned the barb and there was a moment of silence as I walked onwards. He had to save face in front of his goons.

Watson bolted out of the restaurant and attacked me from behind, kicking my music case open and sending the French horn into the gutter. I dropped my books and started to windmill my fists, trembling too much to land one stroke. Watson ripped off my glasses to blur my vision and then landed a direct hit against my mouth. My braces cut into my top lip and I spouted out blood. The blood temporarily made Watson back off but then his gang emptied out of the greasy spoon, encircled us and edged him on.

My luck had bottomed out. I was surrounded by Watson and his thugs, was spitting out a steady stream of blood and could expect more of the same. Strange at this point, the only thought in my mind was my not being able to play French horn in the upcoming Ontario-wide Kiwanis competition, because of my mutilated lip. I was angry. I had toiled long and hard in the first-desk orchestra position.

With my fear turning to anger and little left to lose, I was the one who became the aggressor. Not expecting me to rally, Watson was forced to change strategy, keeping me at bay by resorting to boots. He landed his pointed shoe in my left ribs, with a second shot bruising my right thigh, narrowly missing the genitals target. The third shot went for the ribs again. This time I managed to grab his shoe and without thinking, lifted his leg high into the air, flipping Watson backwards. The small of his back landed on top of a fire hydrant and he let out an excruciating groan, before slumping to the sidewalk.

Watson fallen! I thumped on his chest and began pounding blows to his face and upper chest as he desperately tried to return the blows and wriggle free. Finally, with Watson's screaming "Stop, stop!" his comrades pulled me off. Then, expecting a ganging up, I tried to out-psyche the thugs by standing firm and yelling "Who's next?" The reply that came from the second-in-command was quiet—"The fight's over. Get lost."

I went to sleep that night in pain and a confused state as to the rightness of my actions. Word spread throughout the local teenage gangland that, "Cooper had kicked the shit out of Watson." I was scolded by my prep friends for the foolish and dangerous solution I had undertaken, and their unanimous opinion was that reprisals would be forthcoming.

Reprisals never came. I walked Mount Pleasant past the tough crowd for the rest of high school and invariably, one or more of the group would nod his head and greet me, using my first name as his sole salutation. I continued in my direction, they in theirs.

Alan J Cooper
February 1979


## STORY # 5
### Canadians Have Always Known Their Duty

The train to Rome had been an impulse decision. I leapt on board at the stroke of 4:00 p.m., just as the express rolled out of Munich for the 14-hour trip. First class as usual was almost empty and I wandered down the corridor, peering into the lush seating compartments, searching for a passenger who wouldn't find my safari jacket and knapsack out of character with the sumptuous surroundings. Near the back of the car, I found a young blonde sitting alone in one of the posh 6-seater booths. I tried to appear unassuming as I slid open the glass door and asked in stumbling German if any of the seats were free. She replied in fluent German, they were all free.

"Sprechen sie Englisch?" I politely inquired.

"I sure enough do," replied the lady, in a deep southern drawl. My fraulein was a Texan.

"My name's Alan. I'm from Canada."

"Howdy, Alan. My name's Cheryl."

We sank into a comfortable conversation about her exchange studies, when the glass door slammed open and two obese, middle-aged Italians, husband and wife, plopped themselves down on either side of us, with their bags monopolizing floor and rack space. We exchanged nods but soon discovered there was no other means of dialogue. All conversation halted and our new neighbors spent the next hours stuffing themselves with bread and sausages. Cheryl went back to reading Göthe, I the *Paris Herald Tribune*, every damn word of its meager 26 pages. It was going to be a long 14 hours.

By 10:00 p.m., lights were being turned off in anticipation of an early sleep before the 6:00 a.m. arrival. The space was cramped and stuffy, and our four sleeping positions were awkward, each one being more or less a slumped seating posture. Once my Italian friends appeared sound asleep, I slid their leather bags across the floor to use them as a leg rest. Cheryl who sat opposite, was tempted to follow suit but stayed inhibited until she too stretched across, fatigue finally overcoming any fear of presumptuousness.

The night passed in pain. Once into Italy, the train rocked on uneven tracks, banging heads against walls and rubbing legs against suitcase buckles. The plump Italian woman remained sprawled in a position that confirmed to me once and for all that obscenity in absolute terms does exist. With the booth's glass door locked tight, the booth became mustier and I couldn't sleep for lack of oxygen, but I feared opening the window, since the other three occupants were already bundled up against the night's cold. The squatty husband slept with his mouth open and snored incessantly, and whenever the train made an abrupt, lateral shift, his snore would break into a grunt. The low point in the evening came when an acute, sideways jerk bumped the husband against the wall and he emitted a slow, relaxed fart straight in my direction. It was a long 14 hours.

Rome came. I wanted out and so did Cheryl. Fighting the washed-out feeling that comes from broken sleep, we scurried over the strewn bags and pushed our way to the train car exit. As Cheryl's foot hit the last step to the platform, she was fondled by a male passer-by. Ah yes, we were in Rome.

"Guess the next job is to find a place to stay," I said, eyeing the hotel booking kiosk.

"Yes we must," replied Cheryl.

I looked at her with slight surprise, thinking for some reason that her final destination had long been determined before her taking the train. The hotel referral center sent us both to the same pensione.

"Guess we have similar budgets," I said.

We strolled together the eight blocks to the pensione, our conversation non-existent in deference to fatigue and the overwhelming din of car horns. Finally, we saw a sign "Pensione Maria" and a small building, gilded with wrought iron.

The foyer was in-your-face ornate, and one almost expected a Madame to take one's coat and murmur "Good evening, sir, Sofia is waiting in room number four." There was in fact no Madame, just a short, friendly concierge and his chambermaid wife.

I stepped forward to the pensione counter to explain my arrival but was interrupted. The concierge had already been phoned by the booking center.

"We have your room made up, sir!" he proudly proclaimed in broken English.

Cheryl appeared nervous, so I attempted to do her booking too.

"Oh yes, signore, we have her room as well."

On cue, the wife grabbed our bags to take us to our rooms when Cheryl looked at me with a blank expression.

"Why do we need two rooms, Alan?"

I started. The concierge started. The chambermaid started. They looked at me for a reply.

"Well uh, Cheryl, I didn't know you wanted us to, uh... sleep together."

"Well, we already slept one night together on the train."

"Yes, yes, so we did."

The little concierge was beaming from ear to ear, rubbing

his hands and gleaming at me. The wife scowled at Cheryl in disgust. Seconds passed, with the four of us standing in a circle, waiting for someone to assume leadership. Finally, Cheryl spoke.

"Don't misunderstand me, Alan. I'm no floozy, far from it. In fact I'm a virgin."

The wife smiled a blessing at her.

"Of course, right!" I spat out. "Economics. We save money by doubling up."

This seemed to satisfy the wife but the concierge winked.

"Not exactly. I'm 20 years old, figure long overdue in losing my virginity and this seems as good a place as any."

By now, the concierge was giggling and drumming his fingers on the registration desk. The wife let go of our bags, hurled the word "Puttana" at Cheryl and departed.

My move. "Fine," I said.

The concierge smirked, "Yes, fine, fine." He took over the chambermaid role and helped us up to our room with the bags. He was still smiling as he closed our door behind us.

We stayed in Rome seven days. Each morning when we came down to breakfast, the concierge would glow a radiant smile and pat me on the back. His wife never spoke.

On the eighth day, Cheryl departed for Munich, I to Switzerland.

Alan J Cooper
March, 1979


## STORY # 6
### Chicanery

I spent Sunday morning alone, deep in thought—how would I seek revenge for the previous evening? How to come up with the perfect coup?

There was no excuse for what Café Güte had done. The

young lady and I had been enjoying a quiet tête-à-tête across a small table for two. Over the long course of the evening, we had sipped several Irish coffees in deference to the January cold outside. Long after the check had been paid, we sat, eyes glued to each other through the soft candlelight, my left hand stretched across the red tablecloth and clasped in her right palm. We both could feel that this our third date, would determine whether the relationship would blossom or fall off into obscurity. The mood augured well.

My right hand had been subconsciously playing with a swizzle stick, lazily poking it against the thick white candle in the table middle, when suddenly a woman's arm reached between us and snatched the candle. My startled glance upward was met with the scowl of a middle-aged matron who was scolding, "We don't treat our candles that way." Snickers and chuckles emanated from the surrounding tables. I was mortified.

After several minutes attempting to regain some composure, I arose from the table with my lady to leave the now dark corner. At the exit foyer, I stopped to ask for the manager, my sense of justice demanding an explanation. The same matron—the manageress—appeared. Behind her hulked an obese chef with a meat cutter clutched in his right paw. Instead of an apology, I received a reprimand for not being able to hold my liquor. I was fuming but had not yet burst and my lady was entreating me to leave quietly. I struggled with a civil response to the matron, when the white-coated ape belched, "Out."

Outrage! A quiet evening; a few drinks; a generous tip and then an unceremonious stripping of the colors and laughter from those around me.

By noon Sunday, I had the plan. Oh, sweet revenge! It would require an accomplice and one or two props. Nothing more...except chutzpah.

The following Thursday, my comrade and I entered the

Café during the heavily populated dinner hour, my friend in normal dress, I in dark glasses and carrying a cane wrapped in white adhesive tape. I saw my first target in the middle of the dining room, a recently abandoned table for four, complete with dirty dishes and relish tray.

With the aid of my partner, I labored forward. While passing the large center table, I stumbled and reached out to grab the tablecloth to prevent my fall. To the floor I crashed, tablecloth in hand as the dishes, old coffee and relish splattered over an area six feet in diameter.

Patrons reached to help me and the manageress beckoned her hulk from the kitchen. The massive white-coated pork leaned over to help me up and I struggled to my feet, feigning an injured knee. The knee gave out and I half-fell again, my cane's accidentally crashing across the hulk's nose.

Finally arisen, I was helped to—poetic justice—the same quiet table for two. My comrade and I quickly gulped our cappuccinos, our emotions pitched with pent-up laughter. My partner then left first, paying the bill at the cash register next to the front door. The manageress gave him change. No tip today! My comrade then pivoted in my direction and hollered for me to come. The matron and other customers looked at him, then at me in disbelief—how was I to negotiate a solo trip through the tables, over fifty feet to the exit door? But negotiate I did with flair, finesse, and speed.

Once out the door, my friend and I bee-lined across the adjoining courtyard in clear view of the Café dwellers, as they looked on through the floor-to-ceiling glass. We disappeared into the St. Clair Avenue crowd.

Alan J Cooper
March, 1979

# POST-BRAIN DAMAGE

## The Autumn of '48

Television in Canada was still 4 years away but American CBS had turned on to channel 4 and Buffalo's signal could be picked up with a towering antenna. Before I was one year of age, a massive, walnut-casketed television set would arrive at my childhood home. My father was still wealthy from his patronage job under his own retired father, and at a time when the average annual wage was just $2,000, my father had put out half that sum to be the first on a dozen blocks to sport an aerial soaring atop his roof.

The giant set landed on the front side of our living room, across from a recessed 3-seater chesterfield. To the left of anyone seated on that chesterfield was a large, cloth-upholstered chair turned to the hulking TV. In fact, with the exception of an upright piano wedged against a wall on the far side, all furniture was positioned so as to make the center of all attention, the television set.

The big wooden unit was to become an altar. Neighborhood children on our front porch drew lots to decide who would be allowed inside that day to lie on the rug and watch TV. When their parents would arrive at dinnertime to take the children home, my family would shift to the dining room but the set would not be shut off. At most, its volume would be turned down and the sound would never cease to reach every corner of our 2-storey house.

Mealtime would be quick, with dinner conversation limited to logistics and each eater putting up with my mother's cooking only for so long as it took to fill up. Then each person would bolt back to the living room, to plop down again in front of the TV.

And so began 2 decades of my living in a home where television reigned over all attitudes, actions, decisions and thought. Books, apart from school texts glanced at amidst noise in later years, were just not read. The TV even managed to keep my father home from the horse races, and he had to find a bookie nearby where he bought his cigarettes. Our family values were shaped by Mickey Mouse, Milton Berle, Friday night boxing and Gunsmoke. Weekends were built on cartoons, The Three Stooges and Hockey Night in Canada.

Time doing things constructive, especially creative, was minimized. My piano playing ran into conflict almost from the moment it started. Later, French horn playing was condemned to the cellar. Homework was done in a din; studying was never tried.

Late in the evening while children tried to sleep, the television would rage on until my father took his cigarettes and *Racing Forum* to bed. Then the TV set would be left to cool.

## The Winter of '49

"Ryooraha, uhooah, uhooah..."

I could keep the bellow going for almost 5 minutes. At 13 months of age, I had begun imitating one of the most compelling noises I had ever heard. It was the noise from the mouth, voice box, throat and lungs of my father, shortly after he arose each morning. It was his innards-heaving smoker's cough.

Four packs a day, non-filter, of the strongest brand then and now known to our world, a cigarette some said had killed more American G.I.'s in World War II than had bullets. Eighty, countem', 80 a day. In the non-sleeping 16 hours of each 24, that meant he puffed one every 12 minutes. Except that my father did not sleep 8 hours—he would awaken at 2:00 a.m. and realize he was out of cigarettes, then drive 2 miles to and from Fran's all-night restaurant to buy 4 more packs.

For the 9 months I was a fetus, he had smoked 4 packs a day. For my first 13 months of life, I did not see him without a cigarette. He smoked while he ate, bathed and shaved. He smoked late at night in bed, while he studied the horse races. He smoked while watching TV and smoked while he continually paced the floor, up and around our house.

In years to come, at those times when my father would be affixed to the TV, I would walk the 12 minutes round trip to Pop Moray's Smoke 'n News shop to purchase 2 packs of the world's most powerful. I was never questioned by the storeowner, because I had a letter from my parents. In my father's car, I would be nauseous in the back seat as he puffed away in the front but be told not to complain, with my nausea dismissed as neighbors' quackery.

When my father reached age 62, after smoking for 50 years, a doctor told him "Quit now or we'll have to cut your legs off." He then switched to cigars and built to 16 stogies a day.

I don't think any time was spent assessing the financial drain from my father's smoking. What it did to suffocate the minds of my father's children, I also cannot say.

## The Spring of '49

As an infant, I was medically ordered to sleep in the winter, under a thin blanket with the window wide open. My body needed fresh air, lots of it and I gave off carbon dioxide in equal amounts. In the countryside, I was to become a mosquito's best prey.

Overheating from my parents' house had left me sapped and along with cigarette smoke, dust and TV, I knew little freshness. The bedroom was noisy and next to a street stop sign, and when my younger brother was born, the tiny room had its window shut to keep in the heat. The bed I tried to sleep in sagged in the middle and creaked from weak springs.

Overheated, in a din, confined and with little air. That's how my mind now thinks of it.

---

## The Christmas of '49

I vowed to obey her training. The shame not to was gnawing and always there. I had to remain clean but could I do so with my fantasies blooming?

She and I had been close, very close for 2 years. I did not want to disappoint her but could I perform, could I reach those standards set by her? I feared I could not.

It was Christmas and the bulge in my pants could not remain hidden. Could the many guests detect the bulge?

Shyness, sensitivity, self-doubt exiled me to the bedroom where I remained until the guests dispersed. Would she then climb the stairs to my solitude? She did.

The bulge grew more pronounced when I heard her deliberate pounding on the stairs to my second floor retreat. She swung the door open and stood in full frame, her eyes locked on mine. Her gaze shifted to my pants where the bulge was now big and overt.

She grabbed my arm and flung me onto the bed, pulling off my lumpy trousers. She tore off my underpants and yanked me out of the room to another, then pressed me to my knees where she pinned me. With her hands clutching the 2 sides of my head, she held me. Her commands were passionate and unbending. There I knelt, shivering as she took total charge. There I knelt beside the toilet.

"Put those underpants in there!"

I sank the bulge's source into the toilet's clear water and it turned murky from the stools left in my underpants.

"Scrub them against the bowl!"

I did so while she flushed. My hands were covered in excrement, and it splashed my face and arms as I fought the suction of the flush and tried to hold onto my underpants. I was forced to look down on my dirt with horror, and as I reared back my head from it, her hand met the back of my head and pushed my face down again into the toilet and my own filth.

"Scrub them in your hands! Clean it all out!"

I scrubbed and she flushed. Waste splashed. I held the underpants. I scrubbed and she flushed. Waste splashed. I held the underpants. I scrubbed and she flushed. Waste splashed. I held the underpants. Tears spilled onto my excrement.

The water cleared. My hands and arms were chilled but the pants stayed held. The waste was gone, but for my hands. It clung to my fingers and stuck under my nails.

I felt filthy. I had failed my love of 2 years. I had worshipped her. She was tall and strong of body, emotion and voice. I had not met her demands. I was unclean, untrained.

In the weeks ahead, if she sniffed any odor, she would threaten my having to scrub my dirt again. I would try with all I could to earn her love but would fail. I would earn only "proud".

It was Christmas of 1949 and I had just turned 2.

## The Winter of '50

"Don't be looking in the mirror! You're so vaaaiiinnn!" The hard "a" of her long "vain" grated, while her tongue stayed arched to retain the grate. One time of many she caught me glancing at myself when passing the hallway mirror.

No doubt her criticism had started long before that winter when I had just reached 2, but I now tend to think I was not aware of such stings, for I had not heard much else. It did not matter what I did or did not do. If I talked, I was chastised. If I walked, I was told my bum wiggled. If I stood, I was told my bum stuck out. If I sighed, I was told I was trying to make people feel sorry for me. If I breathed, I was told I was doing so too heavily and trying to attract attention. Every word I spoke, every facial expression, every move I made was met with vicious criticism. In later years when I made my grooming impeccable, I was told I was trying to be too particular about myself. If I laughed, I was told I was trying to be smart-alecky. If I smiled, I was told I was smirking. If I looked sad, I was told I was wallowing in self pity. When I tried to do my best in everything I did and my academic, athletic and music marks soared, I was attacked for feeling superior. When my grandfather gave me attention, I was criticized for causing favoritism. There was not a waking period of 15 minutes when my mother did not have something to say to crush my self-esteem.

If my mother critiqued me in public, her tone and words would be re-configured so as to present herself in a kind light. But in private, she would conclude with her right hand raised, my talk having been stopped and her declaring, "I'm absolutely disgusted with you!," "You're spoiled rotten!," "What you need is a good swat!," "Shame, shame on you!," "You're no good!," and finally, "You're just a dirty rotter, absolutely rotten to the core!"

## The Spring of '50

The ordeal of eating in my parents' home was made worse by the onslaught of visitors from extended family. Judgmental acts would be the order of the day.

I remember one Sunday when a large contingent of Roman Catholic relatives had arrived all the way from Montréal. At the beginning of their arrival, people had fussed over a sweet, old greataunt with them. I knew what the word "great" meant and certainly the word "aunt," but I'm not sure the concept of "greataunt" was grasped.

At any rate, the fussing dissipated as the time for eating drew near. My greataunt was abandoned lying down on the living room chesterfield when the professed well-wishers adjourned, and eleven people sat down at a stretched dining room table. I was allowed to be propped up on 2 telephone books and sit with the more mature people, provided that 2 year-old I minded my manners and did not act up.

After the food had been passed around, my mother muttered to her plate a sentence that I had heard her say only once before, about a year earlier in front of guests then too: "You may begin." The Protestant hosts of the family dug in, while the Montréal Catholics began lifting their right hands up and down, then back and forth, mumbling words that sounded like "cheeses", "are" and "lowered". Soon thereafter, the Montréal Catholics caught up to the Toronto Protestants, and everyone's self-centeredness cross-fed into a clamor of voices, clanging of cutlery and dish banging, all fighting to dominate the dining room air.

Nobody seemed to care about my sick greataunt, lying alone in the living room. No one seemed to be thinking about her needs.

I quietly took an extra plate from the table and started stacking it with different kinds of food. People close by helped me, not pausing for a moment to see my own plate full. Then without saying a word, I took my untouched glass of milk, lowered myself off the phone books, lifted the plate off the table and left for the living room.

"How are you feeling, Greataunt Agnes?"

As I entered the living room, a feeble and prostrate lady turned her eyes from the ceiling to me. Her voice at first sounded feeble but suddenly gained in strength, "Oh not to w'…My! What is that you have, dear?"

"I brought you some food. I thought you might be hungry."

Just then, my mother appeared and grabbed the plate that was wobbling in my right hand.

"You're acting up and you promised not to! How many times do I have to tell you, you're not to carry food into the living room!?"

She then clutched the glass I was carrying and its milk spilled over the rim, onto the rug.

"There! You spilled it!"

The sick old lady managed to prop herself up on her elbow and she smiled at me. "That little boy of yours was bringing food for me."

"No, he was just bringing his own food to eat in front of the television. He knows he is not allowed to, but he was trying to sneak it in, while the rest of us were eating."

The sweet old lady tried to rush to my defense.

"That boy should be a doctor! Or a bishop! A doctor and a bishop. He's so kind…"

"It's nice of you to…There! Now have poor Aunt Agnes trying to cover up for you."

Aunt Agnes then looked blankly into some space in the air and her eyes turned ghostlike. She struggled again to have her words heard.

"A doctor and a bishop." My greataunt's elbow lost strength and she sagged into the chesterfield. Her face once again turned to the pale ceiling and her eyes gave off a wilting hope.

I was harangued back to the dining room but not before I managed first to get over to Aunt Agnes and squeeze her drooping hand.

"Thank you, Greataunt Agnes."

Her despair looked to lessen. Through frailty and pain, her lips turned up and she grinned.

---

## The Summer of '50

I was 2 in the summer of 1950 and my elder brother had just turned 6. We were in my father's car, en route from Toronto to my grandfather's cottage, an arduous trip in those days and my parents chose to stop 80 miles north, in Orillia at a famous Chinese restaurant. The town of Orillia was not far from both my father's boyhood village and a known insane asylum on the town's edge. As my family entered the outskirts, we began driving by the asylum and my mother labeled it "The Crazy House." She tried to stop her children's peering at the hospital, claiming she did not want to hurt the patients' feelings. My elder brother Murray said she had told him that if he looked in, he too would go crazy. I looked, and the images of walls, giant gate and long driveway welded onto my mind.

When our family arrived at the Chinese restaurant, my elder brother began putting his hands on the sides of his eyes, trying to imitate the appearance of a Chinese person. I watched him, laughed and tried to do the same. Murray continued against parental attempts to hush us and he sang, "Aran is a clazy, vely, vely clazy. Come from Olillia, that too bad." I repeated the song to my elder brother, substituting "Mullay" for my name Alan.

Two days later, my father returned us to Toronto from my grandfather's cottage. The following morning, I went visiting 2 doors away at the Macdonalds' house. The Macdonalds wanted to know all about our trip and Orillia in some way, worked its way into the talk. To the Macdonalds' delight, I told of the Chinese restaurant.

Within hours, my mother was castigating me for making fun of "Murray's craziness" around the neighborhood. She said that my mocking had been made the worse, because Murray had to wear eyeglasses for astigmatism and was sensitive to impersonations done by others. My mother used the words "stupid" and "crazy" interchangeably and behind my back, made my elder brother feel I was mocking his intelligence.

Murray and I would never appreciate what my mother had done. We would not talk to each other and the silence would continue for 20 years under a manipulative mother who saw it in her best interests to have us resent each other, such that she could keep the peace. She would be our sole go-between, passing herself off as diplomat and healer but secretly making her every move a manifestation of her own sibling hate. She had been the eldest girl in her childhood family and was jealous of any second child.

## The Late Summer of '50

I was terrified when I was 2, of going to the outhouse at night. Waking up in the small hours, and then having to plop down over a deep, black hole wide enough for me to fall through to the guck below! The trail to the outhouse was gucky too and my mother always forced me to go the final part of it myself. On any wet night, the walk was worsened by rainwater running under the rotten leaves sticking to my feet.

One drizzly night in August, I must have felt I could not take the last 30 feet, and rather than try to pitter-patter atop the last gooey part, I froze and clung to my mother. She started complaining of my interrupting her sleep and goaded me to overcome what she broadcast to the dark was my cowardice. When I wouldn't move, she began cajoling and offering me her treasured flashlight.

I crept my way forward, opened the door and shone the flashlight into the big hole. Then I inched my way forward to the baby step for elevating toddlers to the moldy seats, lowered my pajama bottoms and began easing my little buttocks around to the hole. Suddenly I was shaken by my mother's distant yell.

"Don't drop the flashlight in the hole! It's Papa's and very expensive."

I rested the flashlight down on the moldy platform and tried with both hands to suspend myself in mid-air above the swallowing hole. As I pressed to work out a bowel movement, my urine ran forward and soaked my pajamas.

It was at that moment that I looked to the right of the door and saw the giant shadow of a hairy spider. I tore out the door, with my anus still carrying a half-out poop. My mother saw my lunge to freedom and moved to lash down at me.

"There was a big spider."

"Get the flashlight! Hurry!"

"But..."

"Gwan!"

Her right arm rose as if to strike. Petrified, I retrieved the flashlight and returned.

In nights to come, I would pretend going all the way to the outhouse and would let slam its cracked front door. But I would pee and poop to the side, my wanting nothing to do with the mold, odor, spiders or hole of the dark outhouse, back in the woods.

## The Autumn of '50

When there were no witnesses and I as a toddler acted in a way not suited to my mother's temperament, she often dropped 2 words on me. I understood the first one but not the second. During the early autumn of 1950, a neighbor's daughter from my mother's village came to stay for 2 weeks. Diane West was to take a course in typing and from the moment Diane arrived, my mother altered her expression—the second word became different. She called me a "beggar" and I became confused. When I asked Diane what a beggar was, she told me that he was someone who wanted something for nothing, but I thought I was giving my mother as much as I could.

One afternoon, a half dozen women were present in my mother's home, appearing to be not giving much either. Perhaps, I thought they would know the meaning of the second word, the one whose sound upon Diane's arrival, had been altered. I decided to give it a try.

"Do you know what my mother sometimes calls me?"

Three women paused in their chatter and looked down.

I carried on. "She calls me a little bugger."

A gasp followed but little more, and then the women resumed their talking.

I tried again. "A lit...tle... bug...ger!"

Eyes opened wide, jaws dropped and all women stayed silent but for Diane West.

"Now, Alan. I have been here 2 weeks and have not heard your mother use that word once."

"But she changed..."

"Hush! Diane said you're ly...fibbing. You must have heard that word at nursery school."

"But I just started nursery school and I heard the word from you before."

With tears of frustration forming, I listened to my mother's and others' loud laughter. I did not know then that I was experiencing revisionist history.

## The Christmas of '50

School concerts are a big deal to most children when they are growing up, and before nursery school's Christmas Concert of 1950, I had just turned 3.

The nursery school teachers began assigning the instruments one-by-one to our school orchestra, while the group of 30 or more of us children was seated in a semi-circle on a stone floor in the church games room. Two teachers were standing at the front of our semi-circle and appeared from my lowly vantage point, to be over 6 feet tall. In front of them were 2 long wooden tables, with each table displaying an array of drums, bells, horns, whistles, shakers, rattles, cymbals and even recorders.

The larger teacher was a distinguished lady who was evidently a musical specialist for the greater Toronto region. She Mrs. Rumpton began officiously reading off children's names from a prepared master list. Through her drooping bifocals, she read both the first and last names of each child and the correspondingly designated instrument, and each child then marched to the front, retrieved his or her instrument from our regular teacher Miss Thedford and then returned to his or her seated position, with legs punctiliously folded.

There was little noise, apart from some excited whisper—all children appeared rigid, with eyes locked on ladies Rumpton and Thedford. The teachers were obviously working from some previous consultation and I seem to recall at the start of the autumn, we children having been allowed to choose and experiment with any instrument we had wanted. I remember I had tried bongo drums, snares, 5 different kinds of shakers and 2 horns. I also recall I had been steered clear of recorders by students older and professedly more accomplished. Most everyone was older.

I sat glued to the front in a cross-legged seating position on the musically bright-sounding floor. As each child got up and went forward to receive his or her instrument from Miss Thedford, a massive Mrs. Rumpton looked on over her bi-focals. The rest of us on the floor watched the number of instruments on the big tables dwindle, until those children who remained without instruments were beginning to look tense. As the number of noisemakers dwindled down further, the remaining children's looks gave way to fear.

The last 3 instruments left the long tables and I alone was left without one.

My name was then read out. I was asked to come forward but saw no instruments. I then looked up at my teacher Miss Thedford who smiled and said nothing. She looked up and over to the mighty Mrs. Rumpton who opened her big purse and pulled out a baton.

A week later, my mother came with others for our nursery school concert. I tried to hold in tempo the allegros, subdue the adagios and hold intact the playing of my 30 fellow students. To my peers, I was forgiving; with myself I was ruthless. The concert was heralded by all present.

During the performance, another mother had turned to mine and said the little boy conducting had more rhythm and music in him than the rest of the children combined. My mother had been angry and had stayed so, not from what the other woman had said but about my not announcing the concert.

"Alan hadn't peeped a word."

## The Spring of '51

My nursery school rested next to a church atop a hill on its own city block. It was the highest point of land in non-suburban Toronto and from the south of the playground, one could see tall buildings 5 miles to the south and the streets in between, covered by Toronto's trees.

My favorite house was across the road from the southwestern rim of the grounds at the bottom of the church hill. That house was on a corner at the top of a boulevard that ran down a slope to a sort of traffic delta shared with 2 bigger streets. The boulevard had a driving surface that was narrow and left to neglect, to deter traffic. Between the paved part and east-west sidewalks were grassed medians that made the route feel pastoral, somewhat protected, and rarely would one see a car taking this route. One could sometimes wonder whether anyone lived in any of the boulevard's character homes.

That favorite house of mine was not much more than a bungalow. Its tiny second floor had 2 leaded windows that faced the church park and playground. The house was stucco and its doors, windows and corner walls were outlined by a mosaic of roughened bricks, with colors mixed and dark. The tile roof was within easy eye angle from the playground and from an uphill position, one could see the roof's long runoff over the sides. The chimney looked to have 8 rectilinear smoke spouts cut into it, 4 long and 2 abreast. The corner lot's yard was hedged so as to make it invisible to any passing pedestrian but from the hill, one could see a curving, red-bricked walkway that made its way from the house through the yard and past a flower-filled well to a brown wooden gate going to a garage of like design.

For reasons I still cannot explain, the house looked to 3 year-old me, Dutch.

In those days of the early 1950s, regulations for children's safety were not, I suppose, what they are now and that part of the playground's southern fence behind the equipment clubhouse was rusted and curled up at the bottom. Any risk-taking child could crawl low enough to wriggle his way to freedom.

It was a sunny day in late April and I paused, as I had done many times since September, to look down at the house and the individualistic others running downhill away from it. The boulevard had become by that 5th week of spring, resplendent with trees that had begun to bud and the day seemed ideal I thought, for a walk.

When our teacher Miss Thedford temporarily abandoned us 3 and 4 year-olds in the fenced-in playground for her to go I guess to the bathroom, I made the suggestion to Big Brian and several others that I give them a guided tour of some of the finer architectural contributions of our North Toronto neighborhood. I was the first to slide under the upturned fence behind the equipment clubhouse and then I turned around and held up the rusted fence for 6 more children—4 boys and 2 girls—to follow. Big Brian bullied his way up to second-in-line but as he tried to drag his fatness under the jagged fence, the backside of his trousers caught on a rusty barb and his pants ripped open, while the sharp barb scraped through to his bum. Big Brian let out a yelp that drew the rest of the 30 toddlers to our place of escape. Still, no teacher was in the playground. After a girl and I pried Big Brian loose, the 5 remaining escapees made it through under the fence, while the other nursery school children looked on, in some blend of fascination and fear of the taboo.

The 7 of us sauntered down the slow hill to the sidewalk, then stopped, somewhat stunned by the appearance of a road in front of us. No one had ever crossed a road without an adult before and we did not even know how to do it. Sheila St. Vincent was the eldest among us and said that we should first look all 4 ways, but there were only 3 ways to look. No cars were coming from anywhere, so one by one, we followed Sheila across the road.

Once on the other side, I began to regain the confidence I'd had in escaping the playground. Our group stood in front of the Dutch house and I looked for the first time at its front. The veranda must have been 15 feet wide and was recessed into the house some 10 feet or more. Sitting on the porch's tiled floor was a 2-seater sofa of plain wicker.

We started our walk down Wilfrid Avenue, my taking the lead and commenting on the different designs of each structure, including one that had been built—I did not know the word "financed"—by my grandfather. The day was cool, the scents were fresh and the greenery was young. Except for us, the boulevard had no people.

We made it to the bottom of Wilfrid to a rounded corner shared with Belsize Boulevard, and stood opposite a freshly flowered Belsize Park. Behind where we stood was a gracious old home that sprawled across a huge corner lawn, lined with trees. Were it not for its harmony with its own space and endless greenery, the house would have overwhelmed the more modest surroundings of middle-class North Toronto. Like my Dutch house, this one, too was stucco but its color was charcoal and it looked to be keeper-of-the-flock. On either side of its chandeliered entrance were long, small-squared windows that stretched from near the ground to a height some 20 feet or more above the lawn. "French," I thought.

Along with my 6 elders, I was about to continue our architectural tour, with a stroll back eastward along Belsize and parallel to the pretty park. Suddenly, a piercing scream of the kind that stabbed women make in grownup movies, came from Wilfrid Avenue. We turned and saw Miss Thedford scrambling down the sidewalk, with her arms flailing and her words impossible to decipher amidst her high-pitched squeals.

Neighborhood doors opened, even the front doors of the designated French mansion and a woman in uniform barged out to stand and stare. Soon, adults were outnumbering us and as they closed in, a mad chatter seemed to be flying everywhere above our heads. No one really seemed interested in communicating with any of us and we had to wonder what all the fuss was about.

We found out. It seems we had "gone missing" from the school for almost 6 minutes and within this frenzy, someone had called the police. Then, when a police car arrived, the finger pointing began.

"How could the toddlers have escaped? Who was responsible?"

At no time did anyone stop to ask if the remaining 24 children in the nursery playground were at that moment being left unsupervised. The adults were far more interested in assigning blame for children's circumstances or in just acting out the drama of the moment. Then, without so much as a query as to our safety or welfare, Miss Thedford tore into us, her questions firing out like slow World War I machine-gun fire.

"Who let you out? How did you get down here?"

"Alan did. He started it."

True to form, Big Brian tattled on me.

"No he didn't! Alan is only 3. He's the smallest. Big Brian is just trying to bully one of the younger kids again." Sheila St. Vincent came to my defense, for whatever reason, I did not know.

No matter, since the police looked at little me and immediately bought into her argument. Miss Thedford then adjusted her theatrics to make sure her thinking was onside that of the police.

"Brian, you're a bully! You started this, sneaking these little children away right from under my sight. We're going to have a talk with you and your parents," she said.

The acting drew to a close and we children were all packed into the police car. For some reason, Miss Thedford charged back up Wilfrid Avenue by herself and by the time the 2 policemen had filled out a report, several minutes had passed. When their car finally did arrive back at the church hill and nursery school, a puffing Miss Thedford was already in the fenced-in playground with the 24 remaining children, and the question of who had looked after those 3 and 4 year-olds for the previous 10 minutes was never asked.

The rusted old fence behind the equipment clubhouse was never mended but it became an absolute no-no for any child to go back there or even close to the area. I do not know what happened to Big Brian but any time after that when he tried to bug me, Sheila St. Vincent would intervene on my behalf. She seemed an honorable person, rather attractive too. But not as attractive as my Dutch house.

---

## The Summer of '51

I was curious during my youngest years and an act at age 3 bore that out. One day, I was standing at the edge of the park opposite my home, watching from atop a small hill a group of older boys playing a game I had seen before. One boy was swinging what was called a bat. Behind him, a second boy crouched in a position I more or less knew from my having done it, but I had never done it while playing whatever game the older boys were playing.

Down the hill I traipsed and no one took note of me as I wedged my way in front of the second boy and behind the batter. The bat came around, struck me on the left side of my mouth and sent my body flying.

I was dazed but managed to get up. I felt a wetness on my mouth but still no fright until 2 things happened. The first was wild yelling by the boys who had been playing baseball. In a moment they were gone. The second involved my elder brother who saw me bleeding and charged homeward in hysterics, "They killed my brother!"

I gave out the best cry I could, and with face covered in blood, made my way across the northwestern section of the park toward home. By the time I arrived at the park's corner opposite my house, my mother was being dragged down the house steps by an hysterical brother. At that moment, it was plain he still loved me.

Pediatrician Dr. Gleasome used little care in pulling out my stitches, and I was left with both a line scar and a ball of skin emanating from my left upper lip. The doctor downplayed her error and told me to strengthen my lips by playing the trumpet.

Ten years later, I did play the trumpet and played the similarly mouth-pieced French horn. My lips did strengthen but the ball on my lip remained, as did the sarcastic distortion in the shape of my mouth. From the age of 3 years, I spent the rest of my life having a "cynical lip," one that made me look in a scowl or in contempt when I was not. In later life, comments of mine could often be met with a look of cynicism or doubt. I will never know nor ever be able to gauge, the effect of my unfairly misinterpreted "cynical lip."

## The Autumn of '51

I was not yet 4 but did love touring the neighborhood and visiting anyone whom I felt to be lonely. Neighbor Mrs. Brethren had called me the Good Samaritan, the area's evangelist who cared for all, eager to seek out and help those less able.

Mrs. Macintosh's house was always a delight. She was a sweet old lady who had long outlived her "Darling husband." My visits would never be announced but the lonely woman loved to see me. I would sit in her parlor and listen to her playing the piano, while buns warmed 2 rooms away. Then we would share a half-hour's conversation, talking about what I can't remember. At some point after that, I would finish my milk, try my most gracious "Thank you," and depart to my awaiting tricycle.

One day, my mother saw my leaving Mrs. Macintosh's house and caught me before I reached my trike. I was severely chastised for "bothering poor old Mrs. Macintosh" and "taking advantage of her good nature to get shortbreads and treats." My visits were terminated. Nobody told Mrs. Macintosh why.

## The Spring of '52

My first exposure to evangelical fundamentalism occurred when I was 4. I was in Davisville Park, across the street from where I lived. It was a Sunday evening when I heard music and wandered over in its direction. The music was coming from about 100 yards away in the baseball diamond, and what looked to be hundreds of people were gathered in its open stands to listen to a preacher talking into a loudspeaker at the catcher's mound.

In my rough-and-tumble clothes, I ventured into the free seats, sat and sought to listen. No sooner had I sat down than a small man who had the look of a sick Eddie Cantor appeared. With Bible in one hand and proselytizing literature in the other, he climbed up through the stands to my remote location, then stopped and stood over me and lowered his head to mine. For a moment, I thought he was going to give me a welcome and offer a question as to where my parents were. Instead, his bilious, bug-eyed face gave me a dead person's look and he commanded, "Get out."

Indignation shot through me at the man who appeared particular about the decorum of his church's clientele. I was hurt, but moved out of the stands along the rusted-out fence behind the withered seats, leaving these shiny-suited Christians to themselves.

The little man then shifted to the stand's center. I caught note of his absence and sat down again, this time on rotting boards near the end of the first row, yards away from any churchgoer. The music resumed and a fat woman at the catcher's mound started warbling in a sound that seemed to me a mix of Kate Smith and screeching streetcar wheels. I was entranced and sat unaware of the goings-on around me when without warning, again appeared the little man. Like a nasty teacher, he snarled, "I thought I told you to get out."

Get out I did. But not without thinking as I wandered off, about the lack of substance in this small man and his fellow parishioners. With their park permit for worshipping and practicing the teachings of Jesus, were they right to refuse a child's entrance to their gathering? Could they see their religious issues on any level of love? I thought about what Jesus would think, when people of bent intent got together to worship whatever, under the rubric of his name. That was my first exposure to evangelical fundamentalism.

## The Christmas of '52

I thought it odd that TV grownups gave each other long lasting kisses. My mother would curse such things and her words would eke out between curled lips atop a Mussolini chin, "A Holllyyywood kiss." Each time she made the pronouncement, her right hand would leave its position covering up her mouth and would fall away in a kind of judo chop to underscore the incontestability of her decree.

People hugged on television, too. Funny, around our house we never did that. I had just turned 5 years of age and had little idea what a hug felt like. I had tried at times to give my mother a hug but had been confronted with her arms, struck out and quivering.

Enough. It was our kindergarten's Christmas party, classmate Mary Moray looked like Lana Turner and we pre-schoolers were gathered in a large circle. To the delight of peers, I strutted 40 feet across the circle, embraced Mary, swayed her back, gave her a long warm kiss, set her upright again, and then walked back across the floor to my station.

The kindergarten teacher reported me to my outraged mother but did pass compliment on my taste.

## The Winter of '52–53

I do not know when, if ever, before my broken brain, I saw a cause of gloominess. Recognizing it would have been difficult, for there was nothing with which to compare—there was no other family where I had lived. There was, however, one thing about the gloominess I do now feel—that it self-renewed.

The cause was the litany of things about which one could feel sad at any given moment, the objective being to overwhelm, such that my mother could make public her empathy. It was my mother who would have built the litany in the first place, her crippling all dependents around her, thus keeping her in power and drawing attention to her as she pretended to be concerned and share in our pain. People would see how much she was suffering and therefore, how saintly she was.

She was excellent at it. Her face would be cast in a caring but poor-me look, her eyes would water and her voice break. Then her children would feed in their own litanies. The whole process—recital, ensuing mood and final pitying of my mother—would be sealed in a wrap-up by her.

I lived that way and knew of no other. I was 5 years old in the winter of 1953 and my mother's methods had by then been going on since at least the time of my babyhood. Whenever guilt or shame was interjected into the cause of gloom, the emotion could make me feel apologetic for ever having been.

I cannot think of a time when the cloud of bad news was not over my head, ever reminding me to feel badly about my circumstances and my role in their making.

## The Spring of '53

I did not appreciate my threat. She was taller than I, older too, and she seemed a monolith of wisdom, absolute in all she said. For me she had been truth, but I began to see flaws. At first, I was dumbfounded she could have weaknesses and was certain she would thank me for my attempts to plug the leaks in her seamlessness. She did not thank me.

During my first 5 years under her, my knowledge of language, math and music had soared. She had shown little concern about that expansion, her seeming to sense some purity in the exactitude and concreteness of such subjects. It was rather in the gray areas, and within them, my growth, that caused her distress. She could not suffer grayness. She feared and destroyed different perspectives or evolution of thought. When that other point of view came from me, her adorer for half a decade, the destruction was absolute. She took each of my questions as an attack, each of my doubts as a challenge to her worth.

Her position would be bedrock. Swats to my head, face and ears. Less painful though than the threat of such swats. "Yit!" "Cut!" A sharp clip of one's words, enough sometimes to pry her husband away from the TV long enough for him to yell, cuff me and leave.

To speak, to utter, to open one's mouth, only to see the raising of a mighty arm is to recognize the plight of any who are treated unfairly under authority's sanction.

One time I tried to appease with a gift and a note, both done in secret. The gift brought guilt but the note brought mockery and a straightening out of my misunderstanding. Some 35 years later, that writing would be seized upon, blown up and said to have been done "always." It would be one courtroom concoction about my purportedly troubled childhood.

## The Early Summer of '53

There are some things in my childhood I would rather not talk about. Hookers have often been abused in their childhoods; others have been violated, only for the hurt to show later.

My mother's private lashings and public praises had one common outcome—both cemented dependency. It was as if I needed her in-home stabs and outside adulations.

I do not know when it was that she started sleeping with me. Whether she had started before the birth of my brother 4 years younger, I cannot be sure. At some point after his infancy, I found myself lying many nights in my parents' double bed, alongside my mother's big warm body. A ritual became engrained whereby my mind in the middle of the night was trained to wake up, go to my parents' room and answer questions from an always awake mother.

"Can't you sleep? Are you hearing noises?"

The second question always mentioned "noises" and would be a variation on a theme. She would tap into my fear and I would succumb. Then as if by script, she would nudge her snoring husband and say, "Alan can't sleep." She would ask me if I would feel "safer" if I slept "there," and on cue, I was made to feel shame.

After my admitting "Yes," my father would move to my room and my mother's sleeping with her son would be realized, once again.

There was never anything physical in the sense of my biological mother touching. But her presence would be a real one from the heat of her body, inches away.

## The Autumn of '53

When John Muller and I began Grade 1, most schoolmates thought we were twins. Our eyes seemed to beam an inner radiance, making them look backlit. In our own ceremony, the two of us became blood brothers.

Both John and I were missing 2 teeth at the front. John's dentist, a professor from the University of Toronto, told John's mom that his teeth configuration was a rare sign of extreme intelligence. John would prove Dr. Evans correct.

One day, my mother told me what the dental professor had said about John Muller's teeth. She added a word that across my childhood, she held in such contempt as to be almost unable to say it. That word was "genius."

"It's a fine line between genius and crazy," she said. In later years, she would add another sentence. "It's not so much how intelligent you are as what you do with it that counts!"

What counted was all she said and did.

## The Summer of '54

By the time I was 6 years of age in the summer of 1954, my mother had made sure that my elder brother had not spoken to me for 4 years. My second brother was 4 years younger and seemed most of the time to be sick. Thus, summer life at my grandfather's cottage was lonely. When I was not swimming alone—my elder brother's visiting a similar-aged friend and my younger brother's staying with his mother—I often wandered in the woods, trying to communicate with the trees and small animals.

One day, a farm dog found his way down the long, curving cottage driveway and ended up right in front of our large front porch. I had been behind the cottage in an off-limits woodshed, exploring pots, sickle and abandoned junk, when the dog's bark to the other side of the house sounded like a call to announce his visit.

I did not recognize the bark. It was not that of the neighbors' cocker spaniel Skippy—by that time of day, he would have been beyond the back hill, on the gravel road to the village, waiting for the next car to chase.

I ran around to the front and there stood a collie. He had a mix of black and white hair, wagging tail and kind face. Knowing nothing about dogs other than not being allowed to have one, I lunged forward and gave the border collie an embrace. "Lassie," I said.

The fact that the collie was male or the thought that he already had another name did not seem to matter. As far as I was concerned, Lassie had dropped out of the sky to be with me. He began licking my face, we rolled around on the ground and together dashed down to the lake to get him a drink of water. I shook his paws, rode on his back and together we danced. We looked for a long time into each other's eyes and I felt he knew "Lassie" to be my name for him. We played until supper, and when I was coaxed into the cottage, he stayed and stared. I tried to look back but was hauled off to the cottage rear. I shoveled down my food and dashed back to the front to see Lassie but could not find him. Lassie was gone.

I was not really interested in getting up out of bed on cottage mornings and the following day was no exception. I more or less found my way to the breakfast's Rice Krispies and sour milk, and then strolled away from the dining nook through the living room to the front door, to see what the dull day had in mind for the long hours ahead.

Lassie was there, waiting for me for who knows how long. I hugged him with all I could and held his head next to mine.

We romped together for 4 days. I did not seem to care where his home was, only that he was there every morning when I jumped out of bed.

Without announcement one day, a red pickup came bouncing down the cottage driveway. Don Scarsdale was a farmer from the other side of the lake and twice monthly delivered our ice. Lassie it turned out was his dog, Shepherd, and Shepherd had been neglecting farm chores "…for the better part of a week." Mr. Scarsdale took him by the collar and as the pickup turned and departed, Lassie's eyes stayed on mine.

## The Autumn of '55

He had been pushed out of the nest too soon, had bought his father's house, had a bi-sexual brother and perhaps because of that brother, had clung to a macho manhood. At age 51, my father had a smoker's skinniness but still looked big to 8 year-old me. He could command his version of respect by hitting me at bedtime, then later giving me candies in bed during TV breaks.

One Saturday, he started on my elder brother. Murray had been loath to go to the YMCA, because the boys swam naked and my father was swatting him for his perceived perversion. I prayed for my brother as I heard his yelps but then came my turn. My father kicked open my bedroom door and demanded to know why I had argued with my mother.

I began to respond and he began hitting, until I screamed blue murder and he backed off. He stood at the foot of the bed, silhouetted against the hallway and for a moment, seemed off-balance. Then came his move. While I lay screaming, he pointed his index finger down at me and did a make-fun-of-me laugh, worse than any I had experienced from a school bully. My screaming grew louder and he curled back his finger, scoffed and then turned to go back downstairs.

Next commercial, my father brought candies.

## The Spring of '56

"Fuck off!"

The only words I could think of to wrench him away from the television set long enough to hear my point of view. At other times I would have received a yell, a hand or demand for respect from one much more powerful.

I had not understood why childhood had to mean having no freedom to express, why wisdom automatically followed age. Could not elders err? If their views were flawless, why the need to crush questions? I found it almost flattering to be threatened, because such retribution was a kind of compliment that my questions held validity.

Yes, the "Fuck off" had wrung my father's attention away from the TV and I had his attention at last. But not attention for hearing my point. The hand that struck me was closed and I repeatedly pleaded, "I'm sorry" as I rolled around the living room with the man pounding my shoulders, back and neck.

"Get to bed!"

Intensely religious by age 8, I never swore, never a "Damn," "Hell" or even "Gee Whiz." When others had done so, I had prayed for their forgiveness. From where, therefore the "Fuck off" had come, I do not know. Even I had been stunned before the "off" was out.

In bed, I prayed in deep repentance, but also began in some strange way to feel a different hurt, a kind of indignation.

My father clomped up the stairs at 9 o'clock when his TV program was over. He had hurt me but I waited for his intrusion with light anticipation—always when he had punished me, he had later brought me treats. The door thrust open.

"How do you feel?"

I thought he felt for my pain.

"A little better, thank you."

"No, I mean about what you did?"

"I have been praying for forgiveness."

He dragged me from the bed to the bathroom, propped me up against the sink and rammed a bar of soap into my mouth. I tried to cough it out but some of the soap went down my throat. Again and again, he washed the soap around the insides of my mouth.

"Have you had enough?"

I was crying. "Yes, Dad."

I was allowed back into bed, with my mouth unrinsed. As I lay there whimpering, I could hear downstairs, the TV.

## The Summer of '56

I could not appreciate the dangers of hitchhiking. I was 8 years old. I probably would have taken free rides anyway, even had I known. I was desperate to escape the flat loneliness of our summer cottage.

South River, population 1,000, was 8 miles of dust away. Gravel trucks and the odd American tourist seemed the regular fare. I particularly liked pickups where I could catapult into the rear, then while the truck rattled along, bounce over the road's stones in open air.

It did not seem to matter to drivers that I actually lived in Toronto, 200 miles to the south. I looked and smelled like a farm boy, and my language by early August was well-schooled in the voice of Northern Ontario's vernacular.

I would usually trip into the village with one of 2 older boys, usually villagers on a day's outing to Eagle Lake. One veteran, Chuck West, and a tough kid, Davey Baker, had taught me the intricacies of forcing drivers to stop, and I rarely had to wait 20 minutes for the second car.

Once in the village, I would trail behind my local elders, downing a Hires root beer at Happy Landing truck stop, and then visiting the railway sidings to climb onto old box cars and play daredevil on the river dam's wobbly top. Rain would not dampen the 4 hours of independence, just move it indoors to the 5¢ juke box in the clapboarded rear of time-worn Murphy's hotel. It mattered not that the hotel's 78 rpm records were near death from scratches. The sounds were still soothing—"Hound Dog," "Don't be Cruel," "Keep-a-Knocking," "Whole Lotta Shakin' Goin' On."

One particular "trip to town" became different. It was to be my first solo and I had a mission—to find and visit the grave of my dead brother.

I had never known him and my mother would answer nothing about him. My dad would answer only with a twisted lower mouth and a mumbled voice that it was a good thing he had died. I did not even know whether he had been stillborn or as someone else had uttered to me, had lived 2 days. One recurring mumble seemed the most constant—he had been large and "not normal." I was certain of 3 facts about my dead brother: he would have been about 1 1/2 years my elder; no one had ever visited his grave and I wanted to visit the resting place of a sibling I would never see.

A truck was coming and I could hear it from over a mile away. It sounded heavier than a pickup and it seemed to be coming quickly. I promptly yanked the shirttail out of my jeans, threw my hair forward over my face and rolled up my pant legs, 4 inches above my ankles. "A Northern boy on a day's swim at the lake." As the truck made the last hairpin turn before coming into view, I began my sad grin to underscore my plea for help.

It worked. Dust swept over my grin and body as the big truck slid to a stop. A tattooed driver yelled from his seat through the doorless hole on the passenger side of the cab, "Get on." There was no second seat, so I scrambled onto the sideless and empty back.

Before I could find anything to hold onto, the 10-ton charged off over the gravel, the movement hurling me down onto the truck's flat rear. I tried to get up but the truck began rolling around another hairpin, and I clung to nothing as my torso bounced help-lessly, while dirt and chips of wood leapt over me. Finally, I crawled to the rear of the cabin, grasped a thin bar and pulled myself to my feet as the 10-ton bulled its way along the dusty road. Once on my feet, I peered into the cabin to view a 250-pound man, guzzling a bottle of beer with his left hand, and his right hand on the wheel. The beer was the only hint of moisture in a cabin which like the man, appeared to have grown out of the dust.

Surprisingly, the speedometer worked and the needle was passing 70 mph. The road's rocks were blurred but seemed precariously close to a truck without sides. The truck's long flat rear jumped over the close gravel, each time the truck tossed around a jagged turn and I kept expecting its clumsy weight to roll over the entire chassis. My fingers were white from clutching the steel bar on the cabin's rear and my feet were spread apart for stability but not enough to fight off the sideways force towing at me on the jagged turns.

We finally hit asphalt as we entered the last mile before the village. The truck then sped up and hit 80 mph in a 30 mph zone. A quick pitch into a pothole sprung my hands loose from the cabin and I fell again onto the flat back. Then the driver suddenly braked for the village's only stop sign and before the truck could stop, I was tossed over its steel side onto a mercifully soft shoulder. The driver looked back long enough to see me, struggling from my fallen position and then he barreled left through the stop sign and off into the village.

My limbs were torn but nothing seemed broken as I crawled back to the road through the soft sand. I thought I felt like one of the surrounding tall weeds, irreverently smothered in gravel along the road's sides and I wondered if they hurt like me.

I pulled myself to a standing position. Bruised, scraped and thirsty, I felt not at all like a city boy. I felt like a "Naho" child, one of the Finnish family of 15 poverty-stricken children who rode the trucks daily from their shack to the village school, where they were beaten by the local boys and teachers.

The South River cemetery was not in the village but a mile to my right. I began the walk.

I had never been to the cemetery; I knew no one who had. The mile seemed long. After stumbling down a homeless road, then up a steep hill, I saw a tiny house of tired wood. Daisies and 2 large sunflowers draped its broken, iron gate. Someone lived there.

I had my 8¢ and was ready to buy a Hires root beer or a glass of water from anyone inside. A worn woman pulled open the door and gawked at me, saying nothing. She thought I was a Naho and would not let me in. Her look was then of astonishment when I pulled out a nickel and 3 pennies for a glass of water.

She took the 8¢ and slammed the door shut. Several minutes passed while I waited and then I kicked the door. It opened again and a large, unshaven man with overalls and an eaten wool shirt looked down at me.

"You a Naho?"

"No, sir. I'm a Cooper. From Toronto."

"You Nahos is not to come here for your food. Where'd you get the money?"

"It's yours now, sir, for some water."

A filthy paw lunged forward with a smudged glass of well water and I grabbed it. "Thank you, sir. I'm leaving."

Up the hill farther west and south to my left, I could see gravestones. I was at the cemetery. Inside it were stones from the '50s, '40s, '30s, even '20s. The cemetery looked to be mainly a between-the-wars one, though one gray slab did don a Royal Air Force emblem. The names seemed stunningly familiar—Woods, Baumgartner, Elliot, Sohms, names of people from the village. Why, then, was this burial place so forgotten? The grass was long and wild and I pushed through it slowly, peeling it back to read the flat, green stones.

An hour passed. Nothing. My brother, I guessed had no stone. I sat down on a gravestone and pondered my plight. I had to find my brother.

I noticed to the right some 20 feet away in an open stretch, 3 flat squares, each about 4 inches in size, each clinging to the earth. The second one read COOPER. Nothing else...I knew I had found my brother. The marker was mossy from age and chipped in the upper, left hand corner. But it was unhidden, free to see the sun and it said COOPER. My brother.

So different from Toronto, so different from Mount Pleasant

Cemetery and its lush greens, manicured foliage, labeled trees and majestic stones. This was not a cemetery. It was a graveyard for forgotten, dead people. Strange, I thought, the sun was beaming and the sky was blue and cloudless. There were no trees but the long grass seemed healthy as it swayed wistfully in the afternoon breeze.

I tried to find the piece that had chipped off the marker's left corner but it was lost. Some moss did come off the top and the soil was easy to pull away but the stone itself was embedded. I let it be.

I wasn't sure what to do. I had never been to any cemetery by myself. Papa, my grandfather had always knelt down in Toronto's Mount Pleasant, so I did the same. My brother's grave seemed to stretch out past the marker 2 feet to the south and one to the east. I eyed it carefully along each imagined side and then I eyed the tiny stone.

Alone, I knelt with my dead brother. For 5 minutes, maybe 10. I looked at it all, the little grave, the stone, the grass, the earth. An 8 year-old boy with his brother, alone in the sun's silence. I felt I had to do something else. My eyes fixed on the grave's head.

"Please don't be lonely. I'm your brother. Your younger brother. You have an elder one, too. You have 3. We love you." I don't know why I started to cry. "You'll never be lonely again. I know you're here. Do you know?"

No sound but for the grass. Nothing. But I felt he knew I was there.

I don't remember the ride back to the lake. It was a car. A local.

I've been back to the gravesite only once in 40 years. Go through the fence to the left of the gate, go forward 30 feet, go right just over 20 feet and you'll find 3 small stones, about 4 inches square. Please don't step on the second one. It's the grave of my brother.

## The Spring of '57

"Business isn't worth a nickel. You see this car?" I looked at the 2-tone Cadillac. "We don't own it. We don't own the house. It's not paid for. We may have to move to the slums before too long...Not a nickel."

For that I can never forgive him. For the 4 daily packages of non-filter cigarettes, yes. For the incessant pacing of the floor, yes. For the constant complaints of being diarrheic, yes. For the 100 mph or more every time he took to the highway, yes. For my car sickness when in his cigarette-smoked car, I think so. For his making fun of my car sickness, I think not. For his poker games, yes. For his nightly vigil to the horse races or bookies, I don't know. For his rednecky and macho attitudes, I think not. For his relentless bragging and know-it-all attitude, yes. For his hitting of helpless children, I don't know. For his giving those children candies and treats after the beatings, perhaps not. For his pointing and laughing at me when as a 7-year-old, I had cried hysterically, no. For his religious devotion to the TV, yes. For his never attending any academic, musical or speaking performance of mine, I'm afraid not. For his mockery of my fondness for classical music, poetry, drama, no. For his never listening and constantly interrupting, I'm afraid not. For his claiming loudly as he paced the floor that he was a good listener, I think not.

But for telling a 5-year-old, then a 6, a 7, an 8 and then a 9 year-old "We may have to move to the slums," never. I did what I could with paper routes, with usher jobs. I paid my way and asked for nothing. I topped the school academically but never dreamt of university. Instead I dreaded poverty, slums, insecurity. A young child lying awake at night worrying about our home, our clothes, our warmth. "Not a nickel...the slums." Not forgiven.

## The Summer of '57

My father bought a budgie bird from a breeder and the budgie still had his neck stripes when he joined our household. The breeder said such stripes showed the bird's young age and young age was key to their ability to learn.

The budgie was dubbed "Roscoe" in homage to a comical character on television's *77 Sunset Strip*, and from the day Roscoe came into our home, he displayed a comfort and confidence that few small pets ever have. The breeder's words rang true—Roscoe learned quickly. His cage door was kept open and he loved finding hidden perches in all corners of the house. One of his favorite activities was to sit Long-John-Silver style on a person's shoulder, or perch on a person's pen while he tried to do his homework.

He loved joining the family dinner and thought nothing of bouncing around the dining table, pecking away at greens. One Sunday morning at a golden bread breakfast, Roscoe tried to come in for a landing on my younger brother's plate and slid right across the syrupy surface. At other times, Roscoe could be discreet and sense from where his bread was buttered—he would not poop on people.

My mother was not vindictive in her normal talking of Roscoe, though she did object to her having to clean his cage—"It's the dirtiest job alive." What she thought of Roscoe's daily defecating onto her jewelry box while he jumped up and down in front of her mirror, she did not say.

One of the few rules the family had about Roscoe was making sure the bird was away from any outside door before one opened it. An additional, instinctive rule was that each person would call "Roscoe," upon entering the house. Usually, that call meant one would hear Roscoe chirp from a distant room before zooming to one's finger. Just witnessing the process could amuse anyone who had never seen such closeness from a little animal.

— • —

Late in the summer of 1957, my mother and her children were as always at my grandfather Papa's cottage and Roscoe's cage had been parked in the cottage's living room. There was little fear of his getting out of the house, since the living room's front door was kept closed and in any event led to a large screened porch which itself was self-contained. There had been a fright once when Roscoe had managed to make it to the front porch but he had been rescued and returned to the cottage living room.

One afternoon that August, Papa and my mother's children were gone from the cottage and I was with Cousin Brenda, my mother's niece from the local village. We were on the lake's other side, looking for souvenir stones and did not arrive back at the cottage until late afternoon. I remember then being shocked when I saw Roscoe's cage set out on the front porch. My mother heard our arrival and she charged out of the living room.

"Oh! I'm glad you're back! Roscoe escaped up into the trees and I need help rescuing him!"

My chest went tight.

"Rosc..out!?...How could that possibly be? You would have had to have both inside and outside porch doors open at the same time, and they're too far apart!"

My mother sounded rehearsed. "Don't talk about that, now! Don't you care about what's happening to our little Roscoe? The other birds may be hurting him!"

No one had actually seen Roscoe escape. My mother would later explain that she had brought Roscoe's cage out onto the screened porch to keep him company as she kept doing "...all the cottage work." She added that Roscoe, once outside of the porch, flew straight up to the very tops of the tall birch trees. There were inconsistencies in her story.

Toward suppertime when my grandfather, brothers and cousin were all present, I started to cry but tried to do so alone, to be at greater ease with myself. My mother's eye caught my display of feelings and she began making fun of me, saying that even my female cousin Brenda and younger brother Don were not displaying such weakness.

My 81-year-old grandfather, who had been silent throughout the transpiring turmoil, took it upon himself both that evening and at dawn the next morning to venture out with birdcage in hand and chirp up at the forest, in an attempt to lure our beloved budgie back.

At breakfast next morning, nothing was said. After cereal, Cousin Brenda coaxed me back again to search for rare rocks, and hours later while returning home for lunch, Brenda and I stopped at the summer store to get 2 glasses of water. It was there we learned that news of the missing Roscoe had hit the area—my mother had been to the store to inform the owners, in order, she said, to help with Roscoe's rescue.

As Cousin Brenda and I left the store, a soft-spoken man with a European-sounding accent stopped us and asked if we were the ones who'd had a little "bud gey bird" go missing. I sputtered back an excited "Yes!" and the gentle man's eyes watered. Roscoe was dead on the beach.

Brenda and I tore down to the lake's public beach and there found Roscoe, lying 15 feet from the water's edge in dry, white sand. He was bone dry, feathers unruffled and his body showed no signs of blood. In fact, there was no evidence of attack or torture anywhere. His eyes were closed and he seemed at rest.

I buried him in front of the cottage and Brenda made a gravestone.

My mother commenced her story of Roscoe's being found

washed up on the wet shore after having drowned. She would tolerate no other version.

Summer passed and with the coming of September, my father made a purchase. To my mother's horror, it was another budgie. We named him "Roscoe."

## Entering the Autumn of '57

I went into an enrichment class after accelerating a grade and was suddenly 9 years old in Grade 6. It was rammed into me that I was in a special class and I was told without end that I had come first in a piano competition against older grades, had won a school music test and was lead choir boy at church.

Now I won public speaking contests, was interviewed on Canada's biggest radio station and plopped onto TV, 4 times. I started a neighborhood newspaper and neighbor Mrs. Brethren praised my work. But at home, my mother spied on my writing, saw the word "sex" and told me she had once thought I had some writing ability but now was sure I had not.

In visual arts, I saw girls using elaborate materials and I took toothpicks to put together a design that won school praise. At neighbors' homes, I designed ranches at the Cliftons and farms at the Brethrens. Both Mrs. Clifton and Mrs. Brethren talked of my architectural gifts. I suggested to my mother that I wanted to be an architect.

"No. Architects have to be *creative* and you don't draw."

Designs all halted.

Drama class was such a no-no that it was coded "effeminate." Secretly, I slipped in.

## The Autumn of '57

Mr. Green seemed the hardest man I had known. A bulbous head with a lightning fork creviced down his brow and a barrel of a body whose aping shoulders arched over all of us boys. Over me the more, since I was smaller.

Green's manual workshop was held not in our school but a half-hour walk up the streets of North Toronto. The walk was liberating at first, since it showed me fresh shades of the city, but the walk soon came to be lonely—our grade 6 took the class with grades 7 and 8, and most boys aged 11 to 14 years, kept only to themselves.

I was 2 years ahead of where I should have been and afraid of the once-a-week workshop. The power saws were almost as loud as Green and the older boys exaggerated their toughness when it came time for "Manual Training."

Early in the fall of 1957, workshop students were given a chance to design and make a Christmas present. I chose to do a product that steered clear of my needing to use either "the jig" or the villain power saws. I had to keep closed-mouthed about what my present was, since its concept would have earned me ridicule— it was to be a gift for my mother's December 1st birthday, a perfume atomizer and there was such a stigma against working on this type of object that the 2 pieces of raw materials were neither readily available for workshop nor for that matter, free. One part was a crystal-like cube for whose design I needed to make blueprints and then I had to heat, cut, mold, buff and drill the part, readying it for the second piece, a more delicate one. The second was a glass cylinder with a spray-pump top and it alone cost 3 weeks' allowance—2 dollars!

Time was nearing the end of September and the 4th workshop,

when Green bellowed across the floor for me to come to his office. When I went through his doorless entrance, the shop din muted and I instantly craved for noise to soften Mr. Green's growl. I stood in front of him and his old desk, thinking I was going to get yelled at for taking too long in my design work or for forcing him to order such socially unacceptable parts. He stayed seated, so that his massive face held level with mine, and he sent a piercing sternness straight at me.

"Cooper, I've got the parts for your…atomic thing. Here is the first." He handed me a 3-inch cube and then lowered his head to his desk drawer. "Now the second one." Green opened his desk drawer and brought out a blue, velvet bag. He couched it in his work-tough hand and then he ceremoniously rose to his feet and towered over me. "Don't break it, Cooper. I don't want you to think there are more of these."

I took the soft bag in hand and eased out the spray-pump trigger.

"(Elegant, bought on my own, to be in a creation of my own!)", I thought.

I sensed my mother would be thrilled.

During the 2 months that followed, I tried crafting with all the care I could. My hands caressed the work in what became for me a labor of love. The atomizer's housing was shaped and reshaped, buffed and buffed again. To aggressive questions as to what I was doing, I stayed vague, but occasionally when no-one was looking, I would go back to my work station, pull the purchased part out of its hidden bag, feel heart-warmed by my mother's anticipated reaction, then place it back into safety.

In the final week leading up to my mother's December birthday, I bought a card, draining my assets to 6 cents.

"(No matter, for I did not need money to buy her a present. I had made one!)", I mused.

I told my mother that I was making her something but only Green and I knew what I had been up to for 12 weeks.

I was going overboard during week 13 at November's end, trying to hand-buff the shaped holder into some sort of finished craft, when the buffer accidentally nudged against 2 books that concealed the felt bag. It fell to the floor and with an almost inaudible tinkle, its cylinder shattered.

I was stricken at first with shock, then with a flash of fears, then with a grip in my chest. My pulse raced, my breath was in short quick pants and I stared into blankness. I began to cry. I rushed for the cloakroom and once inside away from all others, pulled frantically at my winter coat pockets, doing I know not what but trying to stifle tears and a recurring peep. If my upset were made known, the older boys would laugh and call me a suck. I stared at nothing, except the coat and wall in front of me, and it was becoming harder and harder to quell the cry. Then I heard floorboards creak near the cloakroom entrance. Green was coming around. I buried my head in my hung-up coat but his giant hand came down on my left shoulder. With tears on my cheeks and gasps of air coming from my mouth, I turned and looked up to see his massive face. His eyes were on mine and his brow was wrinkled. His eyes were full of compassion, his mouth beginning a grin.

I fastened on his face in bewilderment, still gasping from lost breath. His eyes never left mine as he pulled from his brown tweed jacket another blue, felt bag. Another one. I looked down from his face and stared at the felt bag.

"I never order one of anything, Alan, in case I make a mistake or have an accident. This one is free of charge to you, courtesy of the school."

He called me "Alan." My eyes went back up to his and I stared in awe at the man over me.

No-one found out about the breakage. The bag had been removed from the floor next to my work station and the rest of the class saw only the finished product.

"It's for my mother, for her birthday!"

ALAN J COOPER

There were no scoffs.

Mr. Green seemed the kindest man I'd known.

---

## The Early Summer of '58

I was 10 and did not know enough about the cause, but I knew my mother hated my hanging around Danny Weinstock. She had been particularly heated about an earlier Jewish friend, Stephen Korn. Stephen was what she labeled "effeminate," was into drama and "abhorred violence" as my mother liked to mock. Some 30 years later, she rang victorious when "Stephen Korn died after a pro-lonnnged illness." Stephen died of AIDS.

Danny Weinstock was the start of a number of Jewish friends where the surname could not hide their Jewishness. Michael Crumpton had been a Jew too, but his name as my mother had said, "hid it" and he did not get beaten up the way Danny did. Moreover, Danny looked Jewish and his clothes were flashy, the way she said "Jews like." The Weinstock home was next to our church and my mother instructed that no one at church was to know.

The Weinstocks had a cottage 40 miles from my grandfather's, and despite motherly attempts to sabotage, they invited me for 3 days. Danny was to come back later to Papa's.

Before being driven south to the Weinstock cottage, I was taken aside. The Weinstocks car would be passing through the village of Burk's Falls, my mother's place of birth and the birthplace story had been recited each time our family had passed the village on the way to Papa's cottage. This time, though, my mother let her 10 year-old know that under no circumstances was I to mention that Burk's Falls was the place where she had been born.

I feared probing but her answer came anyway.

"Jews are city people."

## The Late Summer of '58

Even to have been selected to go was an honor. The "chosen few" among Canada's choir boys, the people at church told me and I had been picked to share their experience.

I had never taken a lesson. I was lead choir boy in my church but my Anglican church seemed a trifle when matched against St. James Cathedral, St. Paul's on Bloor or the Anglican castles of other parts of Canada. I had no idea what Port Hope's posh private Trinity School would be like—I had never heard of it.

August of 1958 took me there. As I slunk out the bus door, Trinity stood massive before me, majestic, "Gothic" I think some boy said. Its green grass sprawled across playing fields, the scale of which dwarfed my Davisville Park, and the fields themselves were built for sports I had never seen. The driveway overwhelmed me— longer than any street lane I had ever seen and lined with soaring maples, all standing at attention. Trinity's front door or entrance or whatever it was stood high at the driveway's end and appeared steeped in self-importance. The grounds, the buildings, the scene were not of my world. Mine was 10 years of television, chocolate bars, comic books and questionable food manners. Suddenly I would be expected to dine with elders, sing with choristers and worse, wear shorts.

As I ascended the stone stairs to the entrance, cool air hit me. Two older boys in shorts and knee-length socks scurried out the door like élite officers leaving a regal ship. They paused long enough to look down at me and my threadbare suitcase.

"Fix that hair, junior! Fabian haircuts are not allowed. We are gentlemen, not hard rocks."

The one older boy, 4 inches taller than I, flicked a roll of my hair. "Not allowed, junior."

They giggled and scampered off.

I entered the giant building and heard the echo of my new shoes' heels on the stone floor. Thirty feet in front of me and stretched lengthwise down a hallway was a long oak table, where 6 important men were processing boys. There was one ahead of me.

Suddenly, a grown man's voice barreled out as I stood alone in the grand entrance.

"Name?"

"Alan."

"First?"

"First. I'm new..."

"No. First name!"

I remained solo in the huge hallway with 12 adult eyes on me.

"Alan."

The 12 eyes stuck, with uniform scorn.

"Alan, what!"

"Alan Cooper."

"Alan, sir!"

"Right."

"Wrong! Last name?"

"Cooper."

"Cooper, what?"

"Just Cooper."

"Cooper, sir!"

"Right."

"Wrong! Come here, Cooper."

I slid across the floor, fearful of my shoes' making a noise on the stone floor.

"Where from, Cooper?"

"Toronto."

"Toronto, sir!"

"Right."

The 12 eyes stayed on me.

"You're rude, Cooper, impudent. Where are your manners?"

I was confused. "I use a knife and fork."

A gasp came from man #5 and he leaned forward, while the others sat erect. Then the #1 man, who had been shouting at me, slammed his right hand down on the long table and the slam reverberated down the hollow hall, like a gun shot through a canyon.

"Tuck in your shirt, Cooper!"

I put down my bag and stuffed my shirt in under the belt. The man got up, leaned across the table over me and his eyes rode down my jacket, shirt and trousers.

"Your shoes are white, Cooper."

"Thanks, they're new."

Another gasp from the row of men.

"You're a saucy brat, Cooper."

I knew those words—I'd had them drilled into me often.

"Cooper, you're now B3. Take this to Brennan House."

The man thrust a single sheet of paper at me.

"Where?"

Another gasp. The man murmured.

"Where, what?"

"Where is this house?"

"You're a brat, Cooper! Off!"

I looked around and there were now 4 other boys behind me at the doorway, all staring. The 6 men stared too. Finally a kind voice emerged from the silence.

"It's that way, Cooper."

I caught the man's soothing tone and I smiled. I then turned to the hollow hallway and departed, with all ears on my every step.

— • —

I had never been away from home and Trinity was new to me but old and cold. Cold floors, cold walls, cold people. Rich people. Cold, rich people. I was poor, a brat. I was scared.

As each day passed, I lay at night in my dorm bed with its wool blanket itching, looking at the high, pealing ceiling and from time to time, listening to spits of rain on my window. I was poor, different, "a brat," they told me. I was 10 years old.

In the days ahead, my hands were slapped, my face slapped, my bum slapped, first with a strap, then steel brush, then while swats echoed down the halls, with the cricket-paddle.

— • —

Something unexpected did happen to me near the end of week 2— I was pulled from class and given a note.

"Cooper, you're wanted in the infirmary."

The infirmary! I wasn't sick. Were they going to give me a needle? Where was the infirmary? From across the mile of playing fields, the infirmary, the "sick place," looked like a tuberculosis hospital, sitting by itself in a long white house of wood. I entered with my note.

"Cooper? Oh, yes, follow me."

I followed a white-coated man down a hallway, past the cries and groans of ailing children. The coat stopped at the door.

"Millworth sent for you, Cooper."

Millworth? The boys' favorite Millworth? I entered the room to find white walls, a white sink, a white bed and Millworth. He looked sick as he turned his head to me.

"Cooper? Come in."

"Millworth...John."

His face softened but he could not hide his pain. His eyes turned to the ceiling and his language held stiff. "I sent for you, Cooper. Sit down."

I sat down on the room's single white chair next to the bed.

"Did they teach you how to write where you come from, Cooper?"

"I have had A's in handwriting, Millworth…John."

"No, Cooper! I mean to write! Can you write anything?"

"You mean a note?"

His face pained. "A note, a letter. Can you write a letter? Did they teach you that where you come from?"

"No, but I can sort of write a letter."

His face softened again, though his eyes held fixed on the ceiling. "I want you to write a letter to my parents. I'll sign it. I want you to do it now."

"What will I say?"

"Anything you want." He turned his eyes to mine and his were full of tears. "Anything, Cooper…Alan. Only you…Please do it for me."

"Why me?"

He cried and stretched out his long, athletic arm. "Please, Cooper. Please, Alan."

Write I did for 15 minutes and then handed what I had done to the mighty Millworth. He read my letter, signed it and turned his head back to me. His language again turned stiff.

"Thank you, Cooper. You're a good man."

I returned across the green playing fields to class.

— • —

Another week of Trinity pressed on by. Singing, singing and more singing. In the chapel, in the dining room before eating, in private, in tests.

Trinity drew to a close and the final evening was a gala, with hundreds of privileged young boys gathered in the Great Hall for awards night. Near evening's end came the result of the boys' own voting, the vote for Trinity's most all-around boy.

I pondered, "(Cranston? Possibly the mighty Millworth? Undoubtedly, since his name sat on the lips of all. Pendleton? Knight?)"

The hundreds sat waiting.

"To the man most respected and heralded by the rest of the troops...Alan Cooper."

I sat still in my chair, with hundreds of eyes, friendly eyes, turning to look upon me. Cheers rang across the Great Hall.

Morning checkout included a final meeting with the Headmaster. Each boy took his turn for 1–2 minutes and then came out of the closed office with a smile. I felt a moment of rest.

"Cooper?"

The office was massive, masculine, old. The Headmaster was massive, masculine, old. I stood while he sat. Between us was the high desk where I had received my first strap. His face looked down on me.

"Cooper, we want you to take lessons."

My heart sank. No 2 minutes for me. Had I failed all the singing tests?

"Cooper, you have perfect pitch. Your melodic line is impeccable. Your harmony is immoveable. Your tonality is clear, round and full. Your resonance is pure. Your diction precise. Your rhythm exact. Your ear is extr...Cooper?" His face warmed. "You should start lessons at once with the Royal Conservatory."

— • —

I don't remember the bus ride back to Toronto, only ending up home. I entered the door with my trophy and the television was blaring, the house full of cigarette smoke. My family was watching wrestling, eating doughnuts and drinking golden amber ginger ale.

"Alan's back from camp!"

No one at first got up from his spot. All eyes were locked on midget wrestlers.

My mother came to the door and I beamed up at her.

"I have perfect pitch."

"No, good pitch. Perfect pitch is extremely rare."

I put down my trophy, dropped my bag and peered at my family. I pulled out my shirt, mussed up my hair, went back outside and got a Pepsi.

---

## The Winter of '59

Four-letter words were a no-no in my home, even "Damn" and "Hell" and whenever I heard either word uttered around the neighborhood, I prayed for the user a quiet wish for forgiveness. "Shit" was a bad word but "shit" did not carry the sexual overtones that some words had. One 4-letter word was the worst in my mother's lexicon—"Fuck." It had earned for me a person who never swore, a washing out of my mouth 3 years earlier. "Cunt" was a word so foreign that I am not sure I knew its meaning.

One 4-letter word was so unutterable that it had not been used in my house. Any attempt to say it would make my mother's face turn jaundiced, and her tongue would get stuck behind her upper front teeth. That 4-letter word was "love." When my mother tried to describe her feelings about me or a sibling, it would be in terms of how proud she was of us. If she wanted to underscore how much love she felt, she would begin by shaking her head, then tilting it back and proclaiming she "thought the worrrld" of that person.

She could not get out the word "love."

## The Spring of '59

"Lord, to thee..."

Hanging onto high F, an octave and a half above middle C. No vibrato, only the solo sound coming from a boy soprano.

Coming from me to him. Hundreds listening but only one who counted. My grandfather, "Papa", his eyes fastened on mine.

Uncanny how much I was like he. Sunday mornings, I would listen to the classical music coming from his little radio in the far off bedroom, the sounds struggling to be heard through a crackly speaker and the tumult that was our house. I would hunger for the harmony.

God, he was honest, immovably so. Didn't cheat either. I remember watching him play shuffleboard with his son, my father. My father would cheat and Papa would know it, and my father would win but Papa alone would know he had won.

Papa was generous. We were in Florida, he and I, back in the 1960s when Blacks still lowered their heads to Whites, and a Black lady in front at the cash register was 52¢ short. Papa slipped her the coins, so that no one could see and she showed her surprise to us, "Oh, thank you, sir!"

Loud, I remember, but Papa was unembarrassed. He smiled benignly and lowered his head.

Papa's car was manual, his son's automatic; Papa's doors were 4, his son's 2; Papa's tires were black, his son's whitewall. His son's elongated car had a flashy radio, Papa's upright car none. His son's was a treasury of trinkets, Papa's a means of transport with lumbar cushion and car robe. His son had a whining speed boat, Papa a rowboat. Papa hand-carved the turkey, his son used batteries.

On any point where I used my mind to think, my values seemed invariably like his. Hiroshima, capital punishment, help for

Ontario's Ojibwas—I would arrive at a conclusion on my own but it would always match his. Funny, in early years, neither of us said much about this similarity and we both listened silently as opposite thoughts flung around us.

Papa took me fishing. He showed me mint leaves and their magic smell. He showed me reservoirs, big parks and places to buy flowers. With his son at the horse races, Papa took me on little adventures.

He took me to his wife's grave in Mount Pleasant Cemetery, always a time of reverence for a grandmother I had never known. But his most reverent time was his most secret—his time by himself at night before sleep. On his knees beside his bed, his head held deep in aging hands, here a once powerful Victorian businessman knelt down in prayer before a God he had seemingly always known.

A man at peace with himself. Self-righteous, I suppose. Even guilty, I guess for co-creating a non-listener, one generation between us. But I can't be objective about that…

Papa. I was his favorite and he mine.

## The Spring of '60

I was graduating that spring of 1960 from grade 8 in elementary school and year 3 of a gifted class. I had participated in a series of city-wide aptitude tests for graduating students and was told by teacher Mrs. Hill that I had come perfect in Math and first in Toronto. Grade 8 capped 7 years of elementary school in which I had accelerated a grade, topped music, been singled out for studies in Russian, elected Red Cross representative and had spearheaded volunteer help to the Home for Incurable Children. I was branded with crests on my windbreaker and medals on my blazer.

In public, my mother displayed her pride, and I was repeatedly photographed with my medals on me and her at my side. In private, she would quip, "You think you're better than the rest of us, don't you?" and would seize each chance to make my elder brother jealous. Then she would do the reverse with me—she would whisper "Who's this Susskind guy anyway?" mimicking my brother's mock of the Toronto Symphony conductor.

My father did not think much of my musical, artistic or poetic achievements. They simply did not constitute for him the right things for an aspiring man. My father and mother did not even know of my first love, drama.

Sports constituted acceptability. I had thus begun to run races and come first. I had played baseball and hit home runs. I had entered bicycle rodeos and won on TV. I had swum past all. I had skated and no one could catch me. I had become captain of hockey teams.

On one hockey game at the YMCA, the team had won 5–1 and I had scored 4 goals and one assist. My father had bragged aloud in our house and for a night I had felt accepted.

## The Autumn of '60

I was 12 years old, trying to open a thick front door. The most demanding high school in Ontario, perhaps in Canada, North Toronto Collegiate. For 48 years, a paragon of musical, artistic, academic and athletic excellence and I a graduate from Hodgson, the "hood" school. Not from Blythwood, Brown, Oriole or John Ross Robertson, schools whose grade 8 graduates aspired to be judges, neurosurgeons, professors, composers, otolaryngologists. No, Hodgson. Garage mechanics, secretaries or no aspirations at all when asked. Almost all had gone on to Northern Vocational but I had been sent to North Toronto. I worked.

Christmas and the marks came. Latin, French, Math, Physical Education. Firsts. Then came music. Despite others' private lessons, first. The "Hodgson hoodlum" typecast was crushed but soon came another isolator—"The brain."

## 1961

As 9th grade drew to a close in the late spring of 1961, I found myself at the top in music and was given use of the famed Alexander French horn. I started to be groomed for solo desk in the year-to-come Ontario Kiwanis competition, and school pressure began at once for me to start private lessons at the Royal Conservatory and to play publicly.

I began trucking the Alexander 2 miles to and from my house each day and trying to practice the French horn in my parents' home. Almost at once, I was forced to play in the cellar but soon discovered there, too that my playing interrupted the upstairs TV. I moved my practice back to the Collegiate and played in a rear stairwell.

By June of first year high school, I had been urged by North Toronto Collegiate to take the Alexander full-time for the summer and I took the $1,200 instrument to my grandfather's cottage. During the first week, the music stayed untouched until my father drove up again at week's end. Early that July evening, he took me aback by expressing interest in hearing the French horn. He said he wanted to hear a "number" he had heard me play in Toronto. Within minutes, he convinced me both to go with him in a rowboat to the lake's middle and to tow in hand nothing less than the famed Alexander.

Once in the middle, he began singing "Down in the Cornfield, dee da dee da" and I acquiesced to play a few bars of his Mozart "tune." I was soon accompanied by his noisy voice and it did not matter to him that his melody was out-of-sync. Cottage lights turned on around the lake.

"Try another number!" he urged, but I expressed fear of dropping the $1,200 French horn overboard. We left the lake.

I did not get my private lessons. "Too expensive" I was told. "Besides," my parents said "...you don't want to be a musician." Both parents affirmed that musicians were sissies and my father decreed, "Musicians starve." Nor did I get the Bach mouthpiece that the school had been pushing me to purchase, at least not at first. My parents could not comprehend spending 10 dollars for a thing like that and when I asked on my birthday for nothing other than the mouthpiece, my parents said they could not locate the store. They gave me instead the $10 and pressed me to reconsider. I got the Bach.

Starting that September, I played first desk, concerts and a solo passage in the Ontario Kiwanis competition. The orchestra won but practice stayed in the school stairwell.

## The Winter of '62

*Savoir faire* may sometimes flow from a certain sensitivity, but such sensitivity can be dulled in a 14-year-old boy by an awkwardness of age. If the boy is 2 years younger than his peers, that awkwardness can be made worse, and how he relates to peers or gleans social adroitness will be done from a lower vantage point—social evolution will be governed like good port by time and by the inadequacy of inter-relational experiences. By default, parental prominence will loom large.

I did not invite a girl to the high school Football Dance; Nancy Brown invited me, 6 days before the ball. I had overheard a number of classmates remarking on their going and had heard them speak of appropriate dress. "Semi-formal" was a concept I did not understand and I looked to my parents for guidance. They were quick to instruct me on proper taste.

One thing my parents dismissed was the thought of a corsage. My mother directed that I was not to buy one, since it was I who had been invited. As for clothes, I mentioned "semi-formal" and my parents presumed to know the decorum. I possessed no suit of clothes and had only a dress jacket, black with burgundy stripes but was told it was "quite snazzy." I had one pair of trousers, gray and was told "appropriate" and my shoes were school ones—black and suede. My tie was black and told to be quite right, socks were dark but short like my father's, and I had never heard the expression "Leg shows are for ladies."

Away I went to pick up my first big date. When her front door opened, Nancy's smile strained as she eyed me. Her mother quickly composed a corsage from her home's front room flowers and off we walked the mile-and-a-half to the high school's Football Dance. Before entering the school, I caught sight of classmate Sean McCartney and beneath his open coat was a black tuxedo. Once in the school, I noted only one other male not dressed black tie. He was "Dickie" or at least that is what cruel people called the poor fellow, cast by many as the school boor. He had on a blue suit that looked black at the dance.

Nancy rushed to gab with the girls, but one came to within 3 feet of me and said aloud, "You didn't read the invitation, dear?"

By 10:00 p.m., 2 hours had passed and friends were talking of places to go after. Go after? Except for bus fare, I did not have enough money and said so to Nancy. To her credit, she stayed with me, and back we hoofed it to her Lawrence Park home. Her mother was still up and looked askance at our early arrival. Then she looked again at my clothing.

## The Years 1958 to 1962

Being close to the front helped, but by the end of Grade 9, I could not see the blackboard. I was borrowing glasses to see the teachers' notes, had not seen clearly for 3 years and my vision had worsened across each school term.

The first time I had noticed had been during a 7th grade eye test. I had lifted my hand from my left eye to see what I should have been able to see with the right, and no one else would later take seriously, bespectacled Billy Clifton's catching my cheat. In the years thereafter, I dreaded the thought of wearing glasses but it never escaped me. By the time I reached North Toronto Collegiate in Grade 9, some senior students wore glasses and needing them was more acceptable than it had been at Hodgson. Already I was rationalizing.

By the middle of Grade 10, I asked in hurt for my eyes to be checked, but my mother balked at what she said was my desire to be sophisticated and superior to the rest.

I could still see words in a book but not beyond. I dropped balls in sports, missed girls' smiles and relied on my ear in music. My school marks slipped. Neighbor Mrs. Brethren told my mother of her own son's marks dropping in school because he had needed glasses.

After another 18 months and year 4 of my needing glasses, the eye doctor was astonished I had been so long in coming. I then wanted to buy unobtrusive caramel frames but was stopped by my mother. "The only reason you want expensive frames is because you want to be sophisticated."

With each new day, I plastered on big black plastic frames and the marks kept going down.

## The Spring of '63

The hardest part was carrying it out in secret—I performed it in the bedroom but occasionally would get caught, when a parent tore away from the television long enough to go to the bathroom. The parent would thrust open my door to probe the sound, and I would scramble and try to change my position. But each time, I was made to feel shame. By the time I reached 15 in 1963, my night-time practice had been going on for 10 years and had escalated from 15 minutes to over an hour.

I don't know how it had started. It had begun one Sunday morning when I was very young. That day as always, the television had been loud enough to snuff out most other sounds and I would have pulled off my act unnoticed. But on that wet March morning, I had not wanted to do it at home. I had been only 5 at the time but the drive would not go away. It had been a need that I felt only one other place could have afforded me the solitude to satisfy—my church. The need had been spiritual.

That morning, while family members had been worshipping TV, I had trudged the half-mile hill through March rains, to my church. I had known my need not to be Uncle Jerry's Club or old Shirley Temple movies.

The practice had started almost immediately after that. At first, not in secret—it seemed that anything up to 15 minutes of text-book prayer before bed was "fine" but when I had begun creating my own prayers and picking out my own passages of the Bible to read, it had soon been made known to me that I had carried my rituals too far and was becoming a fanatic. As the mockeries of my "rituals" had increased, so too had their degree of concealment and each mockery drove further, the push in me for spiritual strength.

I cannot begin to explain where the need or even curiosity had come from. My father had barely seen the inside of a church and my mother went from time to time, I suppose to flaunt her purity. My elder brother laughed at the idea, my younger brother was officially sick and none at church had urged me nor had any friends. No one had put upon me the daily praying and study of religion and I would have been ashamed to tell anyone.

I prayed at short silent intervals during the day, prayers of thanks and help for others, prayers of forgiveness when I heard another boy lie or steal or swear, and prayers for strength to continue my prayers in freedom and without the embarrassment I was made to feel. There were 10 years of it, an hour a night, at intervals during the day and at 2 Sunday services, done despite ridicule and in secret, to minimize mockery and shame.

I knew not the source of my motivation. I knew not why. But late that spring of 1963, my mother decreed in front of extended family that it had all been done "just for show."

## The Pre-Christmas of '63

Of all the turns I made in life pre-crash, 2 stay stuck in my mind. In each case, outside influences were at play but I still fault myself. One was not taking a year-long course for the world's civil service élite and another happened after I turned 16 in December of 1963.

The world was going dark at the time. The Protestant-respected Pope John XXIII had died and with his death came fears that his visionary steps of Vatican 2 would be stopped. In late autumn, Toronto's young Mayor Donald Summerville had collapsed after a charity hockey game and at the same time as his funeral, U.S. President Kennedy had been shot. The Beatles had not quite debuted on *The Ed Sullivan Show* and life felt tentative.

I was halfway through Grade 12 that December and was

planning to leave Toronto in 6 months and head for Windsor across from Detroit, to start a one-year enrolment at Windsor Teacher's College. I would never see home again.

During the autumn, I had been dating a girl 2 1/2 years my senior, and my parents had hurt me with false accusations and blistering sarcasm. On weekends, they'd used sleep deprivation.

I remember my parents' giving me my first watch on my 16th birthday. They made some comment about the watch marking a first step in my long road toward maturity. I winced but stayed calm, my dreaming of the day when I would never have to hear from them. I would be 16 years old, possess an Ontario driver's license, have my Grade 12 Junior Matriculation and be in Windsor Teacher's College, beginning life anew.

I did not go west the 250 miles to Windsor. Instead I was barred inside.

## The Years 1963–1964

Mid-way through the 11th grade at the beginning of 1963, I had turned 15 and found myself locked up behind bars, day and night.

Braces. At a time when confidence had already been hurt by my being younger than others, by the start of eyeglasses and the building of pimples, I suddenly had a mouth full of metal and interconnecting elastic bands. The metal and rubber harbored old food, odd sights and foul breath. People previously jealous, made jabs.

Solo desk had gone, recitals had stopped and the French horn was soon to go.

I could not get the bars off. Orthodontist Dr. Penguin had said 12–18 months but a year had gone by and I was told "…2 more."

I took to the house cellar and with chisel and stone, tried to grind off the braces. The pain was like none I had known and the damage meant more orthodontics.

— • —

I entered Ontario's Grade 13, at 16 years old. I begged Dr. Penguin to take them off, and he said he would not remove a brace until my father paid his bills. He began to preach about my "…poor-mouthing father's Cadillac" but then without warning, seized my mouth and ripped off the braces, one by one. When finished, he swiveled around in his chair and spat, "Out!"

After 2 years through all of ages 15 and 16, the metal bars were off.

## The Autumn of '64

"Alan has a good mind."

The comment was made to my mother on high school Parents' Night by the legendary Betty Bealey. Miss Bealey was an English guru and my home room teacher, and was known for her knowledge of language and care for her students.

My mother relayed the comment but suffixed, "If only she knew the sorts of things you and Cousin Buddy talked about late at night."

My mother did not know that she was revealing her denied snooping on Buddy and me. One August night in 1964, my Chicago cousin and I had been listening to the radio's WLS in a one-room shack, some 100 feet from Papa's northern Ontario cottage. I had been talking about a spring '64 incident in which classmate George Summers had smelled something, turned to me and resignedly said, "Oh, no. Some girl forgot to change her pad."

Buddy had guffawed and had moved to urinate out the shack's door. Before he found the knob in the darkness, Buddy and I had heard a rustling outside the cabin, "An animal" we had thought.

When Buddy had found the knob and creaked open the shack door, he and I had heard the rear door to the cottage shut.

---

## The Spring of '65

Four years earlier at the start of high school, I had wanted to take acting but drama was not to be thought. The study of vocal music had also been out of the question, with singing seen as sing-song and relegated to 9F. The 9A brain class was designated for brass and woodwinds, and I had been slotted into 9A with the future leaders-to-be.

By the end of Grade 9, I had become fluent in French and fast in Latin, and as late as Grade 12 with marks in steady decline, I could still stand up, hear a long English sentence and to gasps of the future leaders, translate it into perfect Latin. I could mimic, and students labeled me Canada's second Rich Little. Interior design was so much a love that within my childhood home, I spent hours rearranging and juxtaposing, for optimal use and appeal.

Every area where I exhibited talent was held in contempt at home.

"What can you do with music or language? You're not creative enough for architecture."

My elder brother had been scraping through each year ahead of me but showed some skill in real-man math and science. After he repeated Grade 13, he went into Engineering. I was blackmailed into chemistry, physics and the natural sciences, and pressured to drop subjects deemed effeminate or impractical.

I turned 17, was nearing the end of Grade 13 and my hopes for drama, music, languages and design were all gone. In an attempt to earn acceptance and follow filial example, I accelerated my 4-year downward spiral and failed grade 13.

## The Summer of '65

I had not seen Jo-Anne Gardner for 12 months. The anticipation of seeing again my first love gripped me on the days leading up to our rendezvous.

Jo-Anne was the most beautiful girl I had ever seen, with radiant health, rose complexion and an oval face. Her eyes were soft, her eyebrows unplucked and she had a cute upward nose. Her teeth were flawless, she wore no lipstick or makeup and her face was wrapped in hair of untouched brown. Jo-Anne's figure was smooth and her skin immaculate and tight.

Jo-Anne had an innocent beauty that had touched my sensitivity whenever she and I had appeared anywhere. Heads would turn, smirks would be seen and quirks not quite heard.

I was gripped with fear over our forthcoming re-encounter. How would Jo-Anne receive me? After all, I had been the one to break it off. The pressures against us had been just too great. I had been only 15 years of age in the summer of 1963 when we had met in cottage country and Jo-Anne had been one month short of 18. My parents, in particular my mother, had not approved of the age difference or of Jo-Anne's good looks and broken-homed background. My mother was an ex-schoolmarm from that same Northern Ontarian country, and from the moment I had met Jo-Anne, my mother had embarked on researching the poor girl. Despite hours of seeking gossip within the small community, my mother had found Jo-Anne guilty of no sin other than that of being gorgeous. For a while, my mother's dredging had rekindled local speculation about Jo-Anne's virginity and willingness to put out, but the locals had concluded she was still a Big V and thus a hopeless chance.

During the school year following that 1963 summer, Jo-Anne and I had attempted to overcome our new separation of 40 miles and keep open a fragile line of communication. Dedicated writing and long distance phone calls once per week had been the regimen, and then she would come into Toronto each Saturday, to overnight at her Grandma's.

I had been filled with disillusionment by my mother's snooping in on our date confirmations and her sneaking into my dresser drawer to read Jo-Anne's heartfelt letters. Perhaps my mother's acts had been done in part to satisfy her own sexual needs—late each night, while her husband had lain awake in bed, puffing away on cigarettes and circling key points in his *Racing Forum*, my mother had ostensibly done ironing downstairs, while pouring over any smut she could have bought at the grocery counter. The scandals she had read about, whether they involved Elizabeth Taylor or the Kennedy family, were ones on which she had later pronounced judgment, without revealing her source.

One night in 1963, my mother had shattered a covenant held precious to me. She had accused me of acts that I could not even fantasize and had proven herself underhanded beyond anything I could accept from a woman in whom I had lived for the first 9 months.

Both parents had begun to gouge me with their insinuations. With no supporting evidence or attempt at understanding, "You're making a fool of yourself with that glamour puss" would come from my mother; "You're up to no good with those godawful hours that you are keeping" would come from her husband, as he kick-forced me into a premature awakening from my late Friday night. And again from my mother, "Girls from broken homes wind up in broken homes. "Things can happen. I know they can. I've seen it!"

What things could happen? The relationship had been born and had grown in the sincerity of a love genuine yet brimming with the innocence of youth. I had not kissed Jo-Anne until the third date and it had been 6 months before we had approached anything so daring as a French kiss. Often our date to a movie would have ended early and we would have sat on her grandmother's sofa, holding hands and smiling at each other. Then I would have begun the many hours walk and streetcar ride back from her west end home.

Jo-Anne and I had struggled for a year that way, into the summer of 1964. Thereafter, her father had grounded her at the 40-mile distance from Toronto and me. Beginning in September, he had begun using her as housemaid until his fiancée moved in. At that point, Jo-Anne was to be encouraged to terminate her studies, "…find a man more mature in years and marry him." To the delight of my parents and her father, and to the utter despair of Jo-Anne and me, I had terminated our togetherness.

Throughout the following Grade 13 school year, my thoughts had wandered back to Jo-Anne. I had stood at the high point of land near my parents' North Toronto home, gazing westward, hoping to absorb some vibrations or high frequency message from Jo-Anne's eastbound thoughts. I had been 16 in grade 13, years ahead of myself in formal learning but still very much a young boy, longing for the tender affection of his lost first love.

On New Year's Eve of 1964–65, I had been totally alone, listening in bed for 3 hours to the ringing in of the new year across to the Pacific. During those hours, I had felt the urge to call Jo-Anne but had not; nevertheless, I had come to feel that something was going on with her that night.

The following 1965 spring, I charged westward on a Saturday morning, leaving my father without his car for the horse races. If I were to work up the nerve to see Jo-Anne, it would have been our first contact of any kind since September 1964 and I wondered what she would be like. Would the hurt of our split-up have made her vulnerable to a new boyfriend? Would her beauty have helped her or have harmed her? Would she still have retained her sweet innocence or would someone now have touched her?

I was to get as far as Port Credit 15 miles east of her home, before stopping to coat my gastric acid with a milkshake. There in a car at the Dairy Queen was a young football jock wearing a jacket from her high school. I shot to him that he was a long way from home. When he asked how I knew, I mentioned Jo-Anne Gardner. He swiveled his head to meet the sly grin from his buddy on the passenger side, and then he turned his head back.

"How do you know her?"

I replied that I had met her at a party and the jock snapped that it must have been some party. When I then queried "Why?" he loudly retorted, "She fucks!" I did not continue.

The Dairy Queen encounter cut deeply. I wrote Jo-Anne a letter and to my shock, received in short days a phone call. Shaking in heart, I listened to her assurance that the jock had merely been slandering for her refusing to date him. Jo-Anne's voice sounded reckless, harsher, but no matter. She seemed safe.

We agreed to keep in touch by letters over the next 2 months until the end of high school, when Jo-Anne landed a summer job as chambermaid at the grand resort, Bigwin Inn. I secured a job as a glue-sealer in a cardboard carton factory.

The factory work was hot and grueling, and my correspondence with Jo-Anne was the only break in days of monotony. I would arrive home at midnight after an 8-hour shift, see a letter from Bigwin Inn, rip it open and absorb every word. Jo-Anne would talk of the never-ending excitement of Bigwin, the exotic summer weather at postcard Lake of Bays, the Bigwin staff of 300 between the ages of 18 and 25 and the wild parties—"They go on until 4:00 or 5:00 in the morning, so you can imagine how wild they are!" The picture contrasted sharply with the life of a shift worker, grinding out 8 hours each day in a sticky factory, where the only glimpse of trees or river was that of the Don Valley, beyond a dusty parking lot.

I would reply to Jo-Anne's letters at once, often writing for 3 hours until early morning but her responses were less prompt and never addressed any of the issues of my letters—never an acknowledgement of the dangers of Bigwin Inn, never a soothing sentence to lessen my worries about the "late night parties."

With the August holiday weekend approaching, I suggested I pay her a visit. It would be the first time I had seen Jo-Anne in almost 12 months. She assured me that my lodging arrangements for the Saturday would be taken care of and I should meet her at the Bigwin ferry dock at 5:00 p.m. on the agreed day.

The week's leading up to our renewed togetherness was frenetic, and I bought clothes I could not afford—lush cardigans, French shirts and Swiss shoes.

I tried sleeping after my Friday shift ended at midnight but could not. Finally at 3 o'clock Saturday morning, I departed in my $200 Morris Minor with my $300 of new clothes.

I arrived at the Bigwin ferry dock at 6:00 a.m., 11 hours ahead of schedule but precisely on time to catch the first crossover to the island resort. As I was ushered across Lake of Bays, the affluence arose before me and Bigwin sprouted like a castle out of the tall green forest.

The early-rising patrons in the vast round breakfast room were already being served by waiters in red tunics, and I sat down and ordered my morning meal in as adult-like a manner as I could. I asked my waitress where I might find Jo-Anne Gardner, and she gave me a start that made me feel young and unimportant. The waitress then pointed to a long dreary building far off in the distance at the resort's rear and said that I should try the female staff quarters. My subsequent query as to the rules for allowing males into the ladies' quarters was met with the waitress' crooked smile.

"Up here, the rules are enforced by an old drunk and he's out between midnight and noon."

I entreated the waitress nevertheless to go to the women's quarters on my behalf, my presuming that by 7:00 a.m., Jo-Anne would be getting up.

After a period of tense waiting, I saw Jo-Anne walking down the path from the maid's quarters to the breakfast room. Without a halting thought, I bolted out the door to greet her and grab her hands. I then went forward to embrace her but stopped short, fearing I had been presumptuous in such aggression after a year's hiatus.

Jo-Anne was no longer free of makeup and the pureness of her face and eyes was now complicated by mascara, eye shadow and glossy lipstick. There were adornments where none was needed and cosmetic beauty where nature sufficed. Her slacks and turtleneck were now ultra tight and revealing in detail all of the moldings of her flawless figure.

After a moment of her poster-white smile, Jo-Anne grabbed my hand, brought it against her left hip, held it there and exclaimed, "Shit, you're early!"

"Shit?" Jo-Anne had never mouthed a 4-letter word in all the time I had known her. She picked up my wince and apologized, then broke into excited schoolgirl chatter on everything, from how glad she was to see me to what a swinging place Bigwin was, to what a great time we were going to have.

Jo-Anne was anxious to leave the island on which Bigwin was situated and noticeably steered me away from several male staff along the paved footpath to the ferry dock. Once there, we departed for a day of lunch, sightseeing, a movie in the town of Huntsville and a dance at famous Hidden Valley.

While crossing Huntsville's main street toward the cinema, we were greeted with a round of catcalls from locals. In indignation, I turned toward them but Jo-Anne pulled me back and urged me into the movie house. Once seated, I reached out for Jo-Anne's hand and she clasped mine and took it to rest on her right thigh. Where once shy, she was now forward and in charge.

I don't remember the movie, only thoughts racing through my mind. I finally asked, "Jo-Anne, your letters, you talked of wild parties."

"Oh yeah, Alan, you should see them, 4:00 in the morning."

"Your letter of July 16th said 4:00 or 5:00 in the morning."

"Yeah, something like that. Some have to start work at 6:00. I have 'til 9:00."

"Do you have a boyfriend now? A guy you have been trying to avoid my seeing?"

"Oh, no. I go out with a different guy every night."

My heart vented. No boyfriend meant no involvement and thus no intimacy.

"I had a boyfriend this past year and, no more!"

No more? What had happened? I felt a need to be reassured that she had not gone beyond French kissing with anyone.

"Have you been intimate with anyone?"

"Oh sure, a few."

I could feel myself tightening. In an attempt to put me at ease, Jo-Anne rested her hand on mine and raised it up her left thigh. I went tenser still. "What have you done?"

"Well, I've done it with a few."

"It?" What was...It?" My pulse raced. Had she gone beyond French kissing with a few? "What have you done, exactly?"

Her face turned from the movie screen to meet me and she pressed her hand on mine. There, my hand rested uneasily on her inner thigh and she pressed again.

"Why d'ya wanna know?"

The tension was unbearable but I tried to assure her with a forced smile of worldliness. "You can tell me. I've been around."

"Well, this guy in my high school...he...got me."
My face flushed.

"Got you?"

"Right. He was the first. On New Year's Eve. We had sex."

"Sex? Do you mean he felt..."

"Sex. Sexual intercourse."

My palm on her thigh went clammy. "(That New Year's when I'd...)". She tried to console.

"But it was no more than 10 times or so after that."

I thought "(Ten times!) Or so?"

"Don't worry, Alan. He was a creep and we've broken up. I couldn't even come the few..."

"But your phone call in April said nothing...had happened."

"Almost nothing...well, until Bigwin."

"Bigwin?"

Jo-Anne's hand again pressed firmly on mine and she began to rub my hand up and down her left thigh. My peripheral vision caught her coy smile but my pupils held fixed on an area of air somewhere in front of me.

"Well." Her face turned toward the area of my focus. "I'm not sure how many felt me up." She gestured. "That's nothing. I didn't take off my clothes with everybody. Almost nothing happened then, except for a few guys at school parties. You should see these big houses!"

"Happened?"

"Right. Sex."

"Sexual intercourse."

"Well at one party, the guy I was with had closed the bathroom door but it was pushed..."

"Bathroom?"

"The bathtub, away from the party, with this guy I like. But creepo Mitzi barged in."

"...And?"

"Well, the nice guy had been using a Fourex, the kind where you can feel everything—they're really great—but Mitzi came along."

"What happened to the nice guy whom you liked a bit?"

"He was smaller than Mitzi. We never dated again."

"Who were the others?"

"There was only one good enough to look at, so don't worry, Alan."

"Weren't you…afraid of your high school reputation?"

"Well, the ugly, skinny guy who'd done it to me 20 or so times over the winter…"

"You said 10!"

"Oh right, 10. He spread it all over school, so even the girls heard he'd f'kd, sorry done it to me and I kind of figured all was lost."

"And of…the rest in your school?"

"Oh, they weren't all from school. Most of the guys from school were too…"

"So, if not from school, from where?"

"Well, our next door neighbor was a married guy I'd babysat for. Let's see…oh yes, there was the guy at our drugstore. He used safes but not the nice ones and there was a school…"

"…Party?"

"Some of us had been drinking rosé. Or was it sparkling rosé?"

The difference had not been of issue to me.

"Someone turned off the lights but I could see 2 girls with guys' hands under their sweaters."

"And?"

"And I felt, well, lubricated and a little drunk."

"And?"

"I stripped down, and then someone threw the lights back on."

"And did you get dressed?"

"Of course! People saw us but that wasn't fair, because the lights had gone back on."

"But you got dressed!"

"Not at…Everyone had a chance to see us. I was told I had a gorgeous body."

"Lying there?"

"Well, we didn't get a chance to finish."

"Fin… then school was over?"

"Yes, oh, but for the final day when 2 younger guys both 16, told me that I was very pretty and had a nice personality and didn't need to give my body away to everybody. Oh wait, that was up here."

"So?"

"So, I really couldn't be seen dating them, because they were much younger."

"…And at Bigwin. Everyone?"

"Of course not! One guy tried when I first got here, but I told him I was not that type of girl. I like to keep people guessing."

Jo-Anne put both my hands between her legs and closed them on my hands.

"How many…have there been here?"

"Oh, up here? Well let's see, do you mean that I've gone all the way with or part way?"

The distinction was one I'd never had to make.

"Both."

"Well, one guy up here, Hosé, I consider my boyfriend. He has done it to me on my period when we didn't need safes and when I'm at my hottest. Another is a guest who later tipped me $20 for cleaning his room…"

I was choking but had to hear it all.

"And oh yes, a guy came up from Toronto last night and he was set up with me on a blind date. We met at this cabin he had rented but never did go out. He got me drunk on 3 screw drivers and then he did it so 2 other couples could see. That creepo didn't use safes either, so I made him come on my stomach. The oth…"

I breathed in, loud enough to interrupt.

"How long did you know him first?"

"I guess about an hour."

An hour! A year! 12 months! An hour!

"What was his name?"

"I don't remember. He was nothing to look at."

My gaze moved to the movie screen and something was playing but I had to urinate. I excused myself to the washroom where I tried to self-collect and then I returned to my seat, wobbling under the weight of my body.

"Alan, you're upset, aren't you?"

Jo-Anne tried to make me feel better and eased both of my hands to her upper thighs while squeezing her legs closed. I was physically forced to face her.

"Alan, you can do it to me tonight. I have arranged for you to sneak into my room."

I stammered, "I don't have any protection."

"We don't need safes. I just finished my period, so I'll sit on you. I can lean back and put my hands on your ankles so you can get a really good view. I used to be concerned about my big pubic bone and smaller breasts than my younger sister but I've got over that. Just think, my little sister almost 2 years younger than me and she lost it a whole year before I did."

We left the cinema to go to the dance but I avoided slow dances where I would betray my trembling. All eyes could be seen focusing on Jo-Anne's middle, while she thrust out and around her prominent pubic bone and button bum.

We arrived back at the maids' quarters at 2:00 a.m. Jo-Anne smiled teasingly and removed her clothes, revealing what I had never seen but many had.

"Have a good look, Alan."

Terrifying beauty. I felt young and alone.

Nude, she adjourned to the hallway washroom and when she

returned, she had to push a male back out of her room's partially opened door.

I was tired and Jo-Anne expressed empathy, saying she preferred to do it in the mornings.

Before bedding down nude for the night, she reached to the window sill and pulled in a bottle of vodka. Then, with tap water from her old bedroom's sink, she mixed a tall glass and downed it without stopping. I accepted her offer of a sip, in the hope that my first non-church-communion contact with alcohol might calm me down. It did not.

I lay down on my back in the bed and Jo-Anne fell asleep. My long stares began alternating between the aged ceiling and Jo-Anne's face, lit by moonlight peering in through a rip in the blind. Asleep, she seemed to return to her innocent self and her raw beauty shone through.

About 3:00 a.m., the night's silence was interrupted by a pound on the door. Too dazed to worry about the security guard, I arose to answer, and when I opened the door, a stud stood semi-drunk in front and looked at me with surprise.

Stud : "Haven't seen you around here, before."

A. : "I'm Jo-Anne's boyfriend, from Toronto."

S. : "Oh, well I was just paying a social visit. Bye."

J. : "Who was that?"

A. : "I don't know."

J. : "Oh, I forgot about Sharpy. The girls up here really like him. Alan, please get something to drink next time."

Jo-Anne fell back asleep.

When she awoke the next morning, there were only 10 minutes for her to get dressed and report for chambermaid duty. She slapped on renewed lipstick, shadow, mascara and assorted coloring. I had one final question to ask her before we parted.

"Jo-Anne, aren't you afraid of getting pregnant?"

"My father wants me to get pregnant, so I can trap a man... Wanna have a quicky?"

A quicky? "Jo-Anne, my long letters. Didn't you take to heart any of my warnings?"

Jo-Anne's smile waned and her eyes dropped to the bedroom floor. "Alan, I have a confession to make."

"A confession? "Yes?"

"I can't read your handwriting. I never could. The slant is too strong. I was afraid to ask someone else to help, for fear they disclosed something too personal."

"Too pers..."

"I know they were long and beautiful, but I had to burn them all."

— • —

In subsequent weeks, I was unaffected by the factory noise and heat.

## The End of The '60s

In an act of protection and attempt at acceptance, I tried to save Jo-Anne. I took her to non-sexual socials and in her new school, she became queen of the prom. I was back in Grade 13 and it did not matter that I was still a virgin—I was being seen with drop dead Jo-Anne and her reputation had shot across Toronto. Jocks were now my admirers, girls respectable steered clear of me but naughty ones tried to ask me out. When I declined, my mystique shot up. I was accepted and endured the male barbs, and people could not see the sensitive, young boy or his virginity—only the stick man of North Toronto.

A year later in 1966, I slid into a General BA on the low rung of the University of Toronto. Subjects exploring human behavior were made suspect by a fearing family and I was shamed into calculus and the masculine business of economics. I snuck into philosophy and political science, but soon fell into family feuds on everything from Vietnam to Nixon.

My mother began to shift her snipes toward my younger brother. Until Jo-Anne got pregnant. I took the blame and Jo-Anne let her family think I had taken advantage of her innocence. A son was born December 26, 1967 and was at once adopted.

I took to studying religion that autumn of 1967 and my mother misread my being born again. I liked my Professor Waters, and at a time when Jo-Anne's pregnancy confirmed to my mother that I was a dirty rotter, I came first in religious studies. In my final school year of 1968–69, my marks were coming back and I began to think of law school. I was also invited to go on scholarship to Harvard, to study theology but came down with mononucleosis. I was given the year but denied further entrance. With my parents' stamp of approval, I went into something done by my father a generation earlier—apprentice accountancy.

## The Spring of '68

"Where are 'ya, yo'l goat?"

When I could not see her as I entered her house, one of the ways I could gauge how well my grandmother was, lay in her response. If it were a giggle, my mind would ease. Gramma had a sense of humor and despite her rural roots, an awareness born from common sense.

In my last spring-summer before graduating from university, I was a park ranger and lived with Gramma. Her tiny house sat in the village of South River, 200 miles north of Toronto and 8 miles east of the Ontario Park where I worked. When I came home each day, we would talk about whatever, until it was time for her to go to bed and me to roll out the chesterfield.

One evening, I remember her saying that she had to straighten out the sheets on her bed. She said that she "...simply could not sleep, if (her sheets) were at all undone." Sometime between 9:30 and 10:00 p.m., while I folded down the couch and made my bed in preparation for the 10 o'clock news, "Gobby" waddled the 12 short steps to her little bedroom. As she entered it, Gramma let out a sigh when she looked down at her sheets.

"Well, at least I won't have to press them again."

She reassembled the bed with care and tucked in the lower corners of each sheet, then after realigning the blanket, she issued a "There!" which she thought only she could hear.

I decided to do a bit of mischief. I moseyed into her off-limits boudoir and shifted past her. I grabbed each sheet at its bottom and rooted it out of its groundings, then proceeded to ruffle up her blanket and pillowcase.

Gramma giggled and headed straight for my living room bed. I could not get around her sturdy frame, because the snickering little lady started flailing her elbows in every direction. When she reached my bed, she tore off my blanket and sheets, and flung them over the head of my bed. Then she broke into a "Tee hee" laughter. With smiles, I went to retrieve my bedclothes.

Gramma made her way to the television set and shut off the TV. She flicked askew the news channel and rearranged the rabbit ears, then turned around to face a grinning me. She made a "Ha, ha!", worked her way back to the bedroom, closed the bedroom door behind her and made another "Ha, ha!" Then she turned off her light and went to bed.

A sweetheart. I loved her. My mother's mother could cut through nonsense and discern what in life she was enabled to be.

## The Seasons Thereafter

A 21st birthday marked in those days, a sort of coming out for Canadians—a person could vote, legally drink and be officially responsible for one's person. Friends got abstainer me drunk. Until then, I had not broken the legal drinking age, except for a non-church-communion sip at Jo-Anne's Bigwin Inn, and while university classmates had made visiting the pub a regular thing, I had not and had been dismissed as a goody-goody.

Post graduation in 1969, I survived 2 1/2 years of apprentice accountancy. My bones were broken by a bad driver and they kind of mended but the mononucleosis of 1969 meant my being run down for 10 years.

If you dear reader are still with me, I hope you have gleaned something of the skew that one's mind takes with an impossible-to-articulate personality change. Certainly the ego becomes more fragile. Recently, a long incommunicado cousin phoned from New York and tried to remind me of happier times playing cottage shuffleboard, speed boating and going to the Toronto Exhibition. I had forgotten. Classic left frontal lobe symptoms.

You may have noticed how the stories and scribbles that were started after the car accident were sometimes pre-occupied with my pre-accident abilities. Such self-adulation is also known to neurosurgeons and neuropsychologists but the ability to critique it, I leave to you.

# BACK TO THE PRESENT IN 1985

Recruiter Sandra Font of the prestigious Canton Group phoned. She asked how my recuperation from the accident was going. She also talked of my black book. I tried to speak reassuringly and won the chance to interview for a VP Marketing job with a Canadian Government Crown Corporation. That same March 1985 week, another recruiter suggested I meet with the head of advertising agency Benson & Bailey. The second recruiter first confronted me with my car accident, memory impairment and Blimiss Hope firing but spoke too of the superb marketing record I'd had in the past.

Before my 2 interviews, I received a call from my old friend Peter Shaunessy, Director of Research for Warner-Lambert. Peter told me he had heard from Warner employee Lawrence Masteson who had in turn heard from Mary Falwell who had heard from General Foods that Alan Cooper had been fired from Blimiss Hope after his nervous breakdown, caused by his bad memory from the car accident. A second call came from my mother who phoned to say "Dad had a stroke." I failed both interviews.

My relocation counselor John Bridge had found out through reference checks about my neurological problems, and I knew Bridge was reporting back to Blimiss Hope. I feared the neurological news would cut off severance and I had to get a new counselor.

For the next 3 months at the new outplacement firm, I worked hard to get a marketing job of the kind neuropsychologist Dr. Winter would later confirm I could not do. I think I already knew and began trying to land more junior jobs, including one at my old Ministry of Food. Cork had been ushered out, but not before circulating another false rumor that I had been forced out of the Ministry because of political involvement. It was a lie, nevertheless used later against me at the highest level in court. My attempts at jobs in the Ministry did not go anywhere nor did any of the other lower rung tries. People knew about the car accident, and my applying for junior jobs had them further doubting my very ability.

I sent out hundreds of applications and attended dozens of interviews but received no job offer. July was coming and with it the summer closedown of marketing openings. My lawyer Dour said he would not do a minute's more work until I paid my huge legal bills; again he added the salt that he thought the other legal side might "come back at malingerer me." Dour did not believe I was applying for jobs at all and Dr. Fisher had to show copies of all my applications to him. Dour then said my letters were too coherent and positive for a person truly brain injured. My severance was to run out in September and there was no job in sight.

I left the theatre of marketing and crawled down to burlesque, my seeing no choice but to take a job at Lord Advertising, working for Lord himself. He was an American, slushing both sides of the border, writing his own copy and meshing his Wharton financial skills to produce creative accounting. My associates pleaded with me not to take the job.

My title was to be Executive Vice President, but when I arrived I was shown to an office tinier than that used by Lord's most junior person. No mandate had been announced and soon I was told to go solely after new business. Lord had checked my references only after his offer and had then tried to wriggle out of the contract. He cited my brain injury and argued that he had bought a car without an engine. Lord would renege on severance.

It was to become January 1, 1986. I was now fired from the bottom and was the same brain-damaged self. No further recovery had taken place and 4 years earlier, Dr. Steve Jensen had made long term disability payments through the Ministry's insurance, impossible.

## Robert

On September 11th, 1985 and day 2 of my being with ad man Lord, my son Robert had been born. Robert had a birth weight of 9 pounds, 12 ounces and an apgar rating of 99.

Robert would prove the kindest person I had ever met. Multi-talented, yet humble, he seemed to occupy some vantage point from where he could help others down below.

When Robert turned 2, he was sitting on my lap and listening to nursery rhymes, when he caught sight of what he considered my oversized stomach. My 2 year-old son Robert then looked at me and whispered, "Oh, Daddy."

I looked down into his gentle eyes and he entreated. "Share, Daddy."

Whenever I had doubts about myself pre-injury, Robert would remind me of the kind and gifted person people told me I had been.


## Emmanuel

For as long as I can remember, I had been pulled by the spiritual. Good acts embraced for me a sense of logic, and as early as toddlerhood, I had felt the high of helping others. Kindness held a symmetry to soothe both giver and receiver and perhaps from early childhood, kindness had revealed to me the selfish joy of giving. Not self-centeredness but self-fulfillment compatible with others. And far reaching. Sometimes it was difficult to see the growth from helping others, but this act of giving did build and move to new plateaus upon which to build further.

Armed with this idea, in January of 1986, I chose to harness my remaining talent and energy towards a thrust whose focus was the betterment of others. The ultimate contribution? I fear I felt so, because the words "the" and "ultimate" connoted for me exclusivity and a defining of realms beyond people's grasp. Exclusivity suggested to me something territorial, and attempts to define the infinite betrayed to me a human need to harness all that is limitless, using the human mind as harness. I chose instead a vehicle I thought rooted and structured on principles—The United Church of Canada. I entered the start of United Church ministry and its Emmanuel College.

During that first term of 1986, I fought a lot in my study to be a minister but never in any personal way. I could not imagine anyone unable to separate intellectual wrangling from spite. Was faith's enemy not doubt but fear? Why then fear questions? Principles strengthen questioning. I was rooted in the 1960s, so I questioned.

I sensed fear first from one professor, not my fear but his. The professor's roots were not in the '60s, at least not in those late '60s. He was a little older, but not much. I had not known that while he had been degree-building in the late 1960s, he had then completed only the last of his degrees, his doctoral work. That work had been done in the rigidity of central Europe where professors had been revered by calling.

In the first months of 1986, each time I questioned, this professor looked not at me but at the class and he preached over my question to the audience beyond. His pattern did not break but I remained insensitive to his defensiveness and unaware of the possibility that he might feel threatened.

Threats? Not possible! This professor at the University of Toronto, this teacher of mature students, this dispenser and grader of information from the professedly principled United Church of Canada, threatened by my questions? I could not see that an institution of the highest form of learning and a church founded on principles could produce anything less than the highest form of thinking, always free to absorb and assess new ways.

Professor David Frisch was bent on liturgy and I had left much of it behind. In the first lecture, I asked Doctor Frisch if liturgy could not confine or cloud spirituality. The Professor snapped back not to me but to the class, "It can enrich," he said.

I heard his words and volume, and watched him turn to the class but I did not link together his words, loudness and face, and I continued. To my expressed concern for the risk of prejudices being shaped by liturgy, the Professor again faced the class and said, "Prejudices shape such questions."

I responded, "Possibly," and was set to continue when Frisch cut off my words without so much as a turn to me. "Definitely," he said. I then sat in silence with all the others, and did not know what the professor meant.

During my second class of 1986 with David Frisch, I again questioned.

"David." He winced at my use of his first name. "Is not talk of correctness for a minister, of scents, candles, mystery-shaping lighting and the need for a richer liturgy like that of more orthodox denominations and a wrongful prioritization within our United Church? I just left Anglicanism and more orthodoxy, richer in liturgy only if richer means buildings wallowing in bigness, spattered with ornaments and one governed in great part by such a superficial show."

Gasps preceded a hush over the room, while David turned away. I questioned no more that day.

In class 3, I made a joke suggesting Astroturf for weatherproofing the floors of the sanctuary but my quip was not received in the spirit in which it was given. Some students snickered but David did not, and again he turned his face to lecture the group, this time on taste. My God had a sense of humor. Did David's?

For classes 4, 5 and 6, I was going to say nothing. Prior to these classes, I had talked to my old professor friend Regis Waters, who had counseled me to say nothing in public against Doctor Frisch but instead go to him in private and ask for his help.

Within David's chambers, my eyes ran over his rows of books on liturgy and I felt in the presence of cemented learning.

"David, thank you for seeing me. I wanted to ask you why you had written your feelings of disappointment on my first paper."

"Yes, your liturgical diary is not written in the format that I have prescribed for the class." His voice was barely audible. "It deals with your being fired from your business-world job and your subsequent enrolment in our school but does not deal with liturgy as I have taught it to the class. It does not give sufficient indication of your having done the prescribed readings."

"But David, I included my firing to point to the acts of conscience contained therein, and I drew focus to my feelings in highlighting my spiritual searching within the school chapel, my reaffirmation of faith in Clair Park Church, my private prayers in Clair Park's chapel, even my relationship to this Emmanuel College. My discussions on liturgy, perhaps too much my own, given your prescription, touch each point of that period. And yes, I have done the readings. I could not have done the diary had I not done them."

Frisch's eyes did not meet mine and I left him within the half-hour, with his directions for the course on church liturgy. I then pondered his voice when he had whispered about my being fired. I wondered what picture this image-conscious man had of the person fired or what image I was to take from his "business world?"

Humor sunk me again in lecture 7. I was appalled with Professor David Frisch's monologue on the Eucharist and with his final question of whether or not one was literally eating the body of Christ during communion, I could not resist my caustic question, "Why does not the minister simply cop out and say he can't talk with his mouth full?"

In lecture 8, Frisch was talking about the sacred rite of baptism and the issue swung to not always knowing whether one were baptized as a baby. Against a backdrop of not knowing the specific church teaching, my question was met again with a class gasp.

"David, if one is not sure, why not simply get baptized again?"

"No! That would be a direct affront to God. It can be done only once. To do otherwise is to make a mockery of entry into His church, to insult God."

"Well, David. I have difficulty seeing your…"

"It's a sacred rite of the church!"

"Whose church?"

Frisch looked over the class. "Ours."

"Well David, please let me finish. If I carry out such an act reaffirming my faith and make a technical error in so doing, my God will not get His territorial tail feathers ruffled but will take the high road and see my act in the spirit which I intended. For one to think God would be insulted is, I submit, to have a very low opinion of God. I suggest that to project human frailties onto God is to fall prey to our slotting God into our own compartments. David, I respectfully suggest that to think God would be insulted by an act rooted in good faith is a far greater insult."

— • —

As part of the course's curriculum, I was involved in a worship workshop with 4 other classmates, and classmate Bob took charge from the start—Bob from the stage. He had been in the theatre in New York as a shaper of impressions and now he wanted to shape everything.

The first and second group meetings produced little. In the first, Bob inventoried the participants' backgrounds, but I stayed in reserve, quietly reciting my past and closing my eyes to people's disdain for my dressing out of uniform. The second meeting sparked reaction in peers when I proposed steps, minor steps I thought, but in fact major, as nothing had been done in the 2 hours of previous meetings. Major too, because I not Bob, had voiced them. Bob steered their quashing.

By meeting 3, Bob took command. I felt a sense of relief, because the group started making decisions. But I also felt a kind of hurt, not from my subordination as I did not wish to assume leadership, but from a clear sense of a growing group hostility towards me, now funneled through its risen leader.

Though I arrived on time for meeting 3, stage director Bob had begun the meeting early and I entered late. As I approached, Bob's head lowered and his eyes missed mine. Two others turned to view group member me dressed in gray suit, white shirt and tie.

"Sorry, I'm being presumptuous. You were obviously in a discussion. Please contin...."

Group member Lucy Vlangwedge responded before I finished, "No, not at all...," she said.

I sat down and placed the book *Resistance to Church Union* on a side table. Leader Bob eyed the book's cover.

Lucy continued. "We were just discussing inclusive language and South Africa."

Leader Bob then spoke.

"When in fact did you start here, Alan?"

"January of this year, 1986."

William Patrick then felt the need to speak.

"Oh, January. How many courses are you taking, again?"

"None again."

"Are you in the program?" William Patrick asked.

"Sorry. 5. Yes."

Leader Bob asked, as he stared over at *Resistance to Church Union*, "Is this book for Professors Huntington and Cushet's course?"

This question sparked a class dialogue.

| | |
|---|---|
| William: | "Yes, have you read that book?" |
| Alan: | "Just. I finished it this morning, along with another, Hoekstra's *Demise of Evangelism in the World Council of Churches.*" |
| Lucy: | "What are your opinions on the subjects?" |
| Alan: | "I'm having some difficulty with my opinions on the United Church, particularly since having read *The Resistance* book." |
| Lucy: | "No, I meant on inclusive language and South Africa." |
| Alan: | "Sorry, I misunderstood. I'm not sure I understand the relationship." |
| Lucy: | "Well, there isn't one, really. Unless one considers women to be oppressed in our society, like South Africa's Blacks." |
| William: | "Oh, but Lucy, you can't be suggesting that women in North America are the same as South Africa's Blacks." |
| Lucy: | "Maybe not to the same degree, but women have no more control over the reins here than do Blacks in South Africa." |
| Alan: | "Women have made substantial strides in say, the last 12 years, in Canada, particularly Toronto." |

Hearing our group's noise drift into the library, non-group member Elizabeth Sen abandoned her studies to join us.

| | |
|---|---|
| Elizabeth: | *Liz Sen Smiling:* "Are you a candidate for the ministry, Alan?" |
| Alan: | "I hope to be." |
| | *I too smiled.* |
| Lucy: | "So, how do you feel, then about inclusive language?" |

| | |
|---|---|
| Alan: | "I'm not sure I understand what is meant by the term." |
| | *Silence.* |
| Liz: | "What effectively is meant, Alan is the de-sexification of verbiage in our liturgical books. 'Humankind' instead of 'mankind,' for example." |
| Alan: | *Pausing:* "I'm not sure that the subject warrants the energies being expended against it." |
| | *All heads turned directly toward me.* |
| Alan: | "It's my view based on what I have observed at Emmanuel, that its women have a perception of their human condition in Canada out of sync with their times. Were for example, many a young female lawyer, architect or doctor to be confronted with not only the issue of inclusive language, but also the zeal with which Emmanuel embraces it, she would chuckle to herself." |
| Lucy: | "So you don't believe in inclusive language?" |
| Alan: | "I believe that non-inclusive language, as you've defined it to me, is perhaps symbolic of historical male chauvinism but as sexual discrimination becomes less of a fact in Canada, so too will the need to do away with its former symbols. They will simply erode in meaning to the point where women, confident of their new positions, feel no threat from them." |
| | *Again silence.* |
| Liz: | "You feel, therefore, we're out of touch with the current reality, Alan, and should focus our energies elsewhere?" |

| | |
|---|---|
| Alan: | "That's my opinion, yes." |
| | *Lucy Vlangwedge looked with curled lip at my gray suit.* |
| Lucy: | "Then on what, pray tell, would you, the newcomer, have us focus?" |
| Alan: | "From all I have learned to date, the United Church has a resolve to live Christianity through the principles of love and justice. Both principles call the Church to social action. Given that the United Church's mandate is to try to focus its energies always on means to manifest Christian love and justice, any activity which compromises that manifestation is compromising the Church's priorities. Going from the general to the specific, one can conclude that any concentration for a sizeable time on inclusive language, though the subject may be a worthwhile one, is penalizing an area of higher priority in executing optimally the Christian principles of love and justice." |
| William: | "I must protest on behalf of my women friends." *His voice grew louder and his head panned the group.* "What can be of a higher priority to Christian love and justice than our saving the one-half of Canada's population to which gross injustices are being done?" |
| Alan: | "I am sorry but I can't answer that question." |
| William: | *William smelled victory and shot back,* "And why not?" |
| Alan: | "Nothing constructive can come of either rhetoric or a response to it and I would respectfully suggest that you, William, have a |

moral responsibility not to use rhetoric when addressing such serious issues."

*Lucy Vlangwedge resumed her looks of disdain at my gray suit.*

Lucy: "Still haven't answered the question. On what would you have us focus?"

Alan: "On those issues which afford us as United Churchmen ..."

Lucy: "United Church people!"

Alan: "United Church people, the opportunity to achieve excellence in our manifestations of love and justice."

William: "You're speaking tautologically."

Lucy: "Yes! What are these higher priorities on which you would have us focus?"

Willam, Bob: "Yes, what?"

Alan: "You do not know?"

Lucy William, Bob: "No!"

Lucy: "Women's rights!"

Bob: "Women's and Gays' rights! What could be closer to the here and now, with which we pastors must deal?"

Alan: "Alcoholism."

*All groaned, except Elizabeth.*

William: "We've dealt with that problem. Dead. Conquered."

Bob: "That's passé."

Lucy: "Alcohol was one of the earliest subjects, the United Church dealt with!"

Liz: "What is contemporary about alcohol, Alan?"

Alan: "Raw, up-to-date data. Statistically staggering. We have an epidemic on our hands."

William: "We had an epidemic with the Indians more

|  |  |
|---|---|
| | than 100 years ago, before the United Church of Canada was formed. What is new? Drunk driving? Something is being done about that." |
| Alan: | "No." |
| William: | "Yes." |
| Alan: | "No." |
| Lucy: | "Yes, something is being done about that." |
| Liz: | "Are you saying 'No' Alan, to William's question about impaired driving being a new issue?" |
| Alan | *Sighing*: "Yes." |
| William: | "Then, why didn't you say so?" |
| Alan: | "I did." |
| William: | "We didn't hear you." |
| | *I looked to Liz Sen with gratitude.* |
| Lucy: | "So what is new with alcohol?" |
| Bob: | "Does it cause AIDS?" |
| Alan: | "I don't know." |
| Lucy: | "So what's the rage on alcohol?" |
| Alan: | "But you have been here for so long compared to me. What can I possibly bring to you in terms of priorities of the United Church? Have you not exhausted the key issues of the day, issues in which we United Church people have a significant role?" |
| Lucy: | "United Church people!" |
| Alan: | "Church people." |
| William: | "Yes! We've torn to pieces all the major issues—Star Wars! Homosexuality in the ministry! Gay rights! AIDS! We're as contemporary as possible!" |
| Alan: | "Are you?" |
| Bob: | "You would deny full rights to Gays?" |

| | |
|---|---|
| Alan: | "Again, rhetoric, but I will answer, nevertheless. No." |
| William: | "Is Star Wars not an important issue?" |
| Alan: | "Again, rhetoric, but I will answer. Yes." |
| Bob: | "AIDS is fatal! AIDS kills!" |
| Alan: | "Many diseases, incidents, kill." |
| Bob: | "Alan...or is it Al? Do you know?" |
| Alan: | "Yes." |
| Bob: | "I think you should understand, there are homosexuals in your Church." |
| Alan: | "Thank you, I do." |
| Bob: | "Homosexuality is active in your Church." |
| Alan: | "Thank you." |
| Bob: | "Alan! I think you should know that *I* am a homosexual." |
| Alan: | "Bob, I think you should know that *I* wear glasses." |
| William: | "Well, I'm not! And you have shown me only ignorance and monetary superciliousness." |
| Bob: | "Name one issue more pressing than AIDS, homosexuality, Star Wars." |
| Alan: | "Alcoholism is not a current rage, in terms of either anger or (*looking at Lucy*) rage as high fashion." |
| Liz: | "Should there be rage, Alan now in terms of anger?" |
| Alan: | *Smiling:* "Yes." |
| Liz: | "Is there new information that we don't have?" |
| Alan: | "There is a wealth of information, much not new and I can't say, Liz what information you don't have." |
| Liz: | "Please try us." |

| | |
|---|---|
| Alan: | *Turning to Lucy:* "What is the current conservative estimate as to what portion of Canadian families is damaged by alcohol abuse?" |
| Lucy: | "That's easy—somewhere near the portion of the population, 1/25th who are alcoholics. Given the average Canadian family size of 3.2 (*her reciting with open pride, her knowledge of the sociologically based number*) approximately 1/25th of all Canadian families would appear to be directly damaged by alcohol abuse." |
| Alan: | "No, I'm sorry. The number is much higher." |
| Lucy: | "1/6th? 1/5th?" |
| Alan: | "Conservatively, between 1/4th and 1/3rd of all Canadian families is damaged by alcohol abuse." |
| William: | "I can't believe that one quarter of all Canadian families is directly damaged by alcohol abuse." |
| Alan: | "*Between* 1/4th and one 1/3rd. And that guesstimate is conservative." |
| Liz: | "We failed the first question, Alan. That number is shocking. Are there others on which our thinking is distorted?" |
| Alan: | "I would guess, Liz, many. Hospitals and prisons, for example." |
| Bob: | Rising to a stance: "Careful here! I have just completed 7 months of field education where I was working with prisoners." |
| Alan: | "Then, you know." |
| Bob: | "Alcohol has been a problem, granted with some prisoners but given our prison conditions, that is readily understandable." |

| | |
|---|---|
| Alan: | "Before Canadian prisoners enter prisons, before they commit the crimes that send them to prisons..." |
| Bob: | "Who says they deserved to be sent to prison?" |
| Liz: | *Turning loud*: "No one here, Bob. What proportion of prisoners, Alan?" |
| Alan: | "Of male prisoners who constitute the overwhelming majority, between 1/4th and 1/3rd report serious drinking problems." |
| Liz: | "And hospitals?" |
| Alan: | "Of adult males in Canadian hospitals, 1/4th is there because of alcohol." |
| Bob: | "But alcohol erodes the body slowly, sometimes taking decades to even show. AIDS, on the other hand, kills. We are confronted with an epidemic." |
| Alan: | "*Alcoholism* is an epidemic. To date in Toronto, fewer than 150 have lost their lives from AIDS. Last year 1985, we lost that number from alcohol-related deaths in home fires, more than that number from alcohol-related drowning and roughly 50 times that number from alcohol-related traffic deaths." |
| William: | "That's why we're now clamping down on impaired drivers. We're already doing something about that problem." |
| Liz: | "The problem is not impaired driving. That is not what Alan said." |
| Bob: | "Alan sounds rather puritanical in his condemnation of alcohol." |
| William: | "Yes! After all, non-Anglo Saxons who have grown up with alcohol, have a respect for |

|         |                                                                              |
|---------|------------------------------------------------------------------------------|
|         | alcoholic drinks and a maturity in say, their consumption of wine."          |
| Alan:   | "Non-Anglo Saxons? Outside of the Canadian Native, it is believed by the World Health Organization that Poles and Russians have the highest rates of alcoholism in the world." |
| Bob:    | "Not surprising, given what we have done to them."                           |
| Liz:    | "What have we done to contribute materially to their alcohol problem?"       |
| Bob:    | "Whites have taken their land, their livelihood and their culture. Why wouldn't they drink?" |
| Alan:   | *Looking at fine person Elizabeth*: "Thank you for trying, but if the receiver is malfunctioning, the transmitter cannot deliver the message." |
| Bob:    | "So, perhaps we should be stepping up our focus on the plight of our Canadian Indians and how we can help them?" |
| Liz:    | "Alan was talking about the alcohol-related problems among the 'non-Anglo Saxon' Poles and Russians." |
| William:| "Well, I'm not sure we can do much to help them."                            |
| Liz:    | "I believe that Alan was attempting to address your comment, William, about non-Anglo Saxons who grew up with alcohol in their families. Were you not, Alan?" |
| Alan:   | "I was, thank you."                                                          |
| Bob:    | "But others in our midst, Italians for                                       |

| | example, grow up from infancy with wine and have few alcohol problems." |
|---|---|
| Alan: | "French grow up from infancy with wine and have the highest documented rate of cirrhosis of the liver in the world, 10 times the rate of Germany or the U.K." |
| William: | "So now we're condemning the French?" |
| Lucy: | "Are you suggesting that we ignore the problems of women's rights, gays' rights, the atrocities of prisons, the atrocities of South Africa?" |
| Bob: | "AIDS?" |
| Alan: | *Becoming tired:* "No." |
| Liz: | "Are you attempting to build to a suggestion, Alan, that the United Church's priorities need re-examination in light of the devastating statistics you are providing on alcohol problems in Canada?" |
| Alan: | "Yes." |
| William: | "I don't think anyone is denying that alcohol is a problem, but The United Church in its socially active policy of practicing Christianity in our times, must be prepared to address the key issues of the day." |
| Lucy: | "Yes! You must agree, Alan." |
| Alan: | "Yes." |
| Lucy: | "Then what of inclusive language?" |
| Alan: | "It is late in the winter of 1986. As we have spoken, as we now speak on inclusive language, more Canadians have died and more Canadians have entered hospitals from alcohol than from all the recorded Canadian cases of AIDS to this moment. For each hour |

|            |                                                                                                |
|------------|------------------------------------------------------------------------------------------------|
|            | we spend discussing inclusive language, we lose an hour of attempting to deal with problems related to alcohol abuse." |
| Lucy:      | "Are you saying that inclusive language is not an issue?"                                       |
| Alan:      | *Becoming more tired*: "No."                                                                    |
| William:   | "We have discussed alcohol abuse. In fact, the United Church's stand on alcohol abuse is well known and documented." |
| Liz:       | "We at this table are future leaders within the United Church and did not know any of the alcohol-related information that Alan highlighted to us." |
| Alan:      | *Smiling at Liz*: "And documentation? The Emmanuel library is virtually void of books on alcohol-related problems written since 1970 and that is 16 years ago. During those 16 years, the information base on alcohol-related problems has increased exponentially." |
| Bob:       | "As have other problems. AIDS was unheard of in 1970."                                          |
| Alan:      | "*Alcohol* problems seem unheard of in *1986*."                                                 |
| Bob:       | "Well Alan, we appreciate you comments on alcohol. Obviously you feel very strongly about it as do we on AIDS or inclusive language. Not dealing with AIDS or women's rights shuts down the Church to the input of many in our contemporary society." |
| Several:   | *Heads nodding*: "Yes!"                                                                         |
| William:   | "And the Church must stay contemporary."                                                        |

— • —

The Group's meeting #3 on liturgy ended and liturgy had not been mentioned. I rose to go to Emmanuel's library and sat down to continue a paper on N. Keith Clifford's book *Resistance to Church Union*, the 1925 union to create the United Church of Canada. I opened the book to read what I had earlier highlighted. The first was on page 43:

> *"Throughout the debate the unionists had implied that only the old reactionaries were opposed to union and that anyone with a degree of common sense could see that organic union was the obvious solution." (University of British Columbia Press, Vancouver. 1985)*

I turned to the next yellow stickered highlight on page 47:

> *"(The unionists) left little doubt that (they) believed they were on the Lord's side and that for them there was only one side of the question worth considering."*

From page 48, I had earlier noted on scrap paper:

> *"No one apparently foresaw that the immediate effect of (unionists' methods) would be to deny the dissidents any reasonable hope of having their complaints heard within the...Church."*

I recalled from my readings, the 1930 request from a New York City student to study The United Church of Canada's 1925 union. Reaction to his criticism of the United Church's actions, which had already been self-evaluated as tolerant and thorough, had been almost immediate. A Church committee had noted the student's limited comprehension and had stressed deeper forces within the union. The committee had said the American was an outsider of inadequate awareness and had failed to appreciate the spiritual intellect, passion and glow that were animating many of the participants in the union.

I peered through Emmanuel library's windows of Scottish stonemasonry and thought Scottish thoughts. I thought of Hoekstra—though I strenuously disagreed with the evangelical fundamentalism preached in Hoekstra's *Demise of Evangelism*, I empathized with the étranger feeling which Hoekstra had experienced. I thought also of the double-mindedness in the Church he had joined, and thought of Voltaire's 'I disagree with you but will defend to the death, your right to say it.'

With the end of winter in 1986, my first term courses in the United Church of Canada were coming to a finish. Knowing from the start that I would have extreme difficulty in absorbing and recalling because of my brain injury, I had gone into courses demanding heavily on essays and nil of recall. My term marks in April were good but for one, that one being liturgy with Professor David Frisch. He gave me a C and talked of my disrespect when I wrote of Jesus in part as follows:

## JESUS: A LOVING JEW

It is not important, I believe to understand Jesus' resurrection as a concoction. What is important, I posit is understanding that a religious institution should never be allowed to cross-pollinate into statehood. Such temptation is, I submit the work of our human minds' conceptual devil. Jesus received death, I think because people misunderstood his principles, their intent and the power construed thereto. He threatened an establishment in which religious fundamentalism was the government's strong arm.

Jesus was by no means alone in his questioning, doubting and acting with conviction. Imitation does not have the guarantee that religious fundamentalists would have us believe. What is imitated is a humanly imperfect, linguistically limiting set of rules put in place to expedite some things, many of those things questionable as to their worth in world help.

Another paper entitled "The Net Effect of Christian Missions in Upper Canada During the First Half of the Nineteenth Century: Positive or Negative?" sunk me deeper. At one point, I praised Canadian Natives for their steadfastness in resisting missionaries' push of the profit motive, and the marker flung back that he was shocked by my attitude, given my profit-motive business background.

— • —

Whether I were a healer by birth or a newly wounded one, whether a challenger by learning or just a person spent of reverence for authority, I don't know. As a youth, I had helped bring out the girl wallflowers and shy guys at school, and had wanted to help those less fortunate. I had felt some need to stand up for them, though I think my brain damage now gave me an empathy that would soon govern much of my life.

# 1986

By May 1986, Emmanuel's winter session was over. Maria was in conflict with yet the 5th of our nannies and a chance came for me to be a stay-at-home father with James and Robert. It was a chance that I had not dared allow myself to appreciate, and for the first time since my brain damage of 4 years earlier, I began to feel a sense of worth. If my formal learning had not already taught me, I came to know that the more love and listening we give to a child, the more we receive back in return. It thus became impossible for me to conceive of any circumstance in which a child should be struck. Children love us from the beginning and they do so unconditionally. They trust us and if we trust them, they grow to know a world of mutual respect that is forever.

What little peace I had in staying home with James and Robert was attacked by bourgeois bitching under the camouflage of professional pretence. North Toronto mothers were the worst. They just could not handle my invading their territory or that of their nanny help. With the exception of kind neighbors, the Goldrings and the Grosmans, not one other person had a non-condescending comment. I was ahead of the social game but my neighbors echoed my family, that I was at home because I could do nothing else.

A job was advertised in Toronto newspaper *The Globe & Mail* and I applied. It was for Vice President Marketing for Central Trust, a giant financial institution headquartered west of Toronto in London. A call also came from Ottawa and I soon found myself being interviewed for the role of an all-encompassing communications strategist for the Canadian Government.

The Canadian Government job fell through but the Central

Trust one marched on. When it came time for reference checks, feedback caught up with the facts and Central Trust wanted to see the neuro-psychological tests that had been done on me. My lawyer Dour would not release them and Central Trust was forced to contract for its own.

I drove to London, saw a psychologist, Dr. Pin, and told him about my difficulties with word selection and absorbing new information. Pin asked where I still felt strong and I said numbers. Then Pin said Central Trust was impressed with me and he did not want to stand in the way of my getting the job. Pin tested me on numbers and deliberately avoided areas where I said I had deficits. He administered a Minnesota personality test and late in the evening when he wanted to go home, took the answer sheet and asked me to voice my choices. At one point, he lost his place and said he wasn't sure where he had begun misplacing answers on the marker card. I never saw the results.

At the end of the summer, Central Trust offered me the job. Then the vacillating started. Maria started talking of loving her own new position in Toronto. I knew the tests that Central Trust had paid for on me were bogus. House moves were in the works and the logistics were being handled by brain-injured me, while I cared full-time for James and Robert.

Inside a prospective home in London, Maria said she did not want to move. I knew my new job chances were 50–50 if I worked 60 or more hours per week, but without spousal support, the chances Dr. Fisher said were nil. I saw the images I'd had after being crushed by Blimiss Hope and of soon being the sole bread winner in a strange city, fired, with 2 toddlers and no hope of getting back to Toronto.

I did not know then that the left frontal lobe has a monitor to aid decisiveness and mine was broken. That injury had also been at work in my on-and-off jobs from 4 years earlier.

I said "no" to Central Trust.

I began to feel a future where I could not provide. The Goldrings and the Grosmans up the street tried to tell me of my excellent fatherhood and how confident my sons James and Robert were with me, but little else allowed me to see the gift I was giving my children.

The better I became as prime caregiver, the more jealous Maria became. With her now controlling the purse strings, she flung vicious notes if I had one $3 call on the phone bill. Gone was her remembering how generous I had been, or how forgiving of her fender benders and many monetary misplacements. Weekends, she would accost the children, saying I'd had my chance to enjoy them during the week and now it was her turn.

I did not agree with how Maria kept the children up late every night, her talking first at 9:00 p.m. on the phone with her sister, then showering while she yelled to J and R that she was not far away and would be right back to tuck them in. She would eventually return in 30 minutes and our tiny tots would have been kept awake until 10:00. Then she would leave their lights on low, despite the pediatrician's saying they needed blackness, and also a light on outside their rooms to keep them as she said, safe. No pediatrician or doctor could convince her otherwise. On toddlers' going to bed or any other child issue, Master of Social Work Maria over-ruled every expert and went with the dictates of her mother.

At children's bedtime, I resigned myself to the basement and kept current my black book. But by late October, after Central Trust was dead, I started after 10:00 p.m. to drink. On Halloween, I took J and R out trick-or-treating, and then at 8:30 went out to buy liquor. Along the way, I caught sight of a Halloween party going on in a pub and I poked inside. I left at 8:50 to go to the closing liquor store, before returning home to kiss James and Robert good night. I phoned Maria to let her know I was going to be 15 minutes late, but when I arrived home to enter via the back door, I heard her car pull out of the driveway in front.

## November 1986

I began to wake up as daylight hit the basement window. My eyes were waxed stuck and my kidneys felt cold on the stone floor. A rush of fear gripped me and I reached with closed eyes for a half-full bottle of vodka. As each second crept forward, I started sensing the worst and within a minute knew again what had happened. The thought of losing James and Robert made me want to be unconscious and down went the vodka.

An hour later at 8:30 a.m., I awoke but this time found the bottle empty. There was another vodka but I would have to crawl in the dark past the oil furnace to fetch it. My mind held back an insidious dread and my mouth craved for water. Once the new vodka was in me, I made my way back on all fours through the furnace room, lugging the new bottle. When I got to partial daylight in the basement hall, I eyed the unlit laundry room. I reached its sink, put my lips around the leaden tap, and an industrial flush of water hit the insides of my mouth. I managed 4 gulps but then the dread came back. I quaffed more vodka, then with bottle in hand, made it to the bottom of the basement stairs.

It was brighter now and the clear November sky was beaming through the back door window, half-way up the stairs. The door at the top of the basement stairs was open.

The kitchen looked spanky and seemed to glare at my shabbiness. I dared not go beyond, for I feared the emptiness I would find. I went to the fridge and downed 2 raw eggs, and then pried out a piece of pita bread and started chewing it. Again I felt thirsty and poured a carton of orange juice into a salad bowl, then emptied some vodka into the orange juice, finger stirred the bowl and tipped it to my mouth. The mix trickled down my chest but most of the mix got in. I tipped and tipped again until I felt a sense of soothing and then I phoned the police to ask about James and Robert. But nothing.

The dining and living rooms looked like a turned-out funeral parlor. The stairs grumbled as I one-stepped it to the second floor. There, cluttered clothes were laid waste, like the battlefield of a losing side. I went to Robert's room but he was not there. I went to James' room but he was not there. I went to Maria's-and-my room, and its contents were sprawled all over. Maria had kidnapped J and R and taken them to her mother. I never knew that a human being could love another human being as much as I loved my sons James and Robert.

I was still in safari pants and hiking boots, and I worked my way back downstairs. I went to the closet and tried to pry my parka from its hook. It fell to the floor and when I tried to pick it up, I fell on top of it. An hour later I awoke to grimness, took to the kitchen, had 3 more gulps of vodka and 3 mouths of water from the tap. I put vodka and orange juice into the juice carton, and off I went with the carton for the tromp to the liquor store.

Before the store door, I downed the carton and trashed it, then bought another vodka, trod halfway home to a bench in Eglinton Park and opened up the bottle. It was 45° Fahrenheit and I soon felt the belying warmth that ethanol gives while heightening exposure. Leafless trees swayed around me and I began again losing consciousness.

I lifted my body off the bench and pressed south the 150 yards to the house, then negotiated my way through the main hall to the basement entrance. I began the climb down to the warm furnace but when I started to slip, I had to crawl. I got to the furnace room and there lay down on an outdoor lounger, stored next to the oil burner. I drank 4 gulps, eased the vodka onto the stone floor, curled over in the darkness and passed out.

I awoke that same November 1st 1986, this time in the afternoon, to realize the 4 o'clock sun was streaking a shaft through the furnace room's one window. To spare the effects of sunlight, I reached for the vodka and got myself out cold again in a matter of gulps. I awoke again at suppertime and rallied to repeat the liquor store process.

To face the daylight of November 2nd, I had enough vodka to steady me once again for the trip to buy more. This time I skipped the park and went straight home to phone the police. But nothing. I telephoned Maria's mother but received no answer. From November 3rd-14th, I phoned. James and Robert had been taken.

On November 15th 1986, I managed to get out of my clothes and tried to lie down in the upstairs marital bedroom. I physically could drink no more. Alcohol had reached so far up my spinal fluid that with each new sip, the alcohol would begin touching the back of my brain. To protect itself, the brain would instantly command my stomach to vomit. Any water going into my mouth would produce the same effect, with the combination of water and alcohol in the spinal fluid triggering the brain command to vomit. My body was severely dehydrated but could not take in water.

Shaking out of control, I let my bathrobe fall to the floor and tried to lie down naked. Under the duvet, my pelvis bounced up and down and then came the sweats. I hurled off the soaked duvet but then felt chilled. I pulled it back on, and there lay bouncing under the sweat-drenched down. My eardrums boomed as if there were a bass drum coming from within and my arms fired off baby firecrackers, with each firecracker kicking out the skin. Then the baby crackers began firing off inside my thighs.

I flung off the duvet and began crawling the 16 feet to the bathroom. Now, I thought I heard low voiced laughter from the furnace, 2 floors below. I pulled myself up to the sink, looked into the mirror and wretched. I fell down to my knees, turned to the toilet and ripped out my insides. I collapsed on the floor, trembling next to the toilet. I kept "hearing" the furnace but now also thought I heard men on the main floor, murmuring in baritone.

I crawled to the sink, climbed up its front and tried mouthing from the tap, a drink of water. I took one gulp and spewed. I tried to straighten up but fell back into the bathtub, hitting my back on the tub's far side. I reached for the tub's taps but scalded my hand. Slowly, I rotated my torso around, reached with my other hand for the cold tap and from a crouched position, took a cold shower and washed away what I could.

I was in a withdrawal out of which some never come. I spent the next 2 days trying to get water into me and late on day 2, took a bit in without vomiting. Day 3 was a nerve end better and I began to realize I was not going to die. By day 4, I got to the phone and tried to get myself into detoxification. It was mid-week and the detoxes were full but I did manage a talk with one detox director, an old alcoholic lady who gave me acceptance.

I tried to shave and then with shredded face, showered. Then I spent 20 minutes trying to coax on fresh socks and underwear. I walked to one of Toronto's 400 weekly AA meetings and there was received by kind faces, pouring forth their empathy.

Vegetable juice first, then grapefruit juice. Days passed. Then a banana, then watercress, then spinach. I walked Toronto, sometimes 15 miles. Then the university Hart House pool and a shower, then off I would walk to an AA meeting. For 3 weeks, until my December 8th, 1986 birthday and age 39, life was little else. Swimming built to one mile per day and during the hour of swimming, my mind was allowed to drift. I thought of James and Robert and how, broken brain and all, I might still contribute.

## The Pre-Christmas of 1986

I went late that fall of 1986 to my old friend Regis Waters, the one
who had counseled me to say nothing against Emmanuel College's
Dr. David Frisch in public, but to go to him in private and there
ask for help. Regis had taught Frisch and had taught me. Regis was
a Protestant but had assisted in marrying Maria and me in a Roman
Catholic Church and had baptized James and Robert. Reg had
challenged my 25 years of doubt and had, in early 1986, catalyzed
my public reaffirmation of faith and entrance into Toronto's Clair
Park United Church. Reg was a selfless healer and a man built on
roots deep and happy.

I had finished that 4-month first term at U. of T.'s Emmanuel
College in the spring of 1986 and you will recall my marks had
been excellent but for one—a flat C from Professor David Frisch.
I had made friends: a Mexican priest-to-be who had wanted his
Roman Catholic traditions tempered with both an understanding
of Luther and a greater sense of freedom as embodied in
Emmanuel's liberal learning; a veterinarian who had wanted to give
new dimension to his help to living creatures; a lawyer who had
longed for greater scope around her talents and compassion; a
male gay who had shared my view on the United Church's sometimes confused priorities in latching onto the trendy.

At the end of April 1986 and before Central Trust, I had been
slotted into Emmanuel for September to resume full-time studies,
but pressure on finances, a prepubescent-acting wife and an inde-
cisive broken brain had made me say, "Thank you, not now."

Beginning in May, I had lived the fatherhood I described.
James and Robert had taught me an unconditional love I had not
dreamt possible: James' plea to be taught new words; Robert's glow
as his face locked onto mine and my 2 sons' deep hugs.

Two weeks before Christmas of 1986, I returned to the Registrar of Emmanuel.

"Bobby, let me thank you for your kindnesses in September. Others too have been kind to me since then. Bobby, I can come back."

Registrar Bobby gave me a blank face.

"We have heard of your pain, Alan."

I smiled in gratitude.

"Courses begin again in January as you know, for the 4-month winter period. Have you looked at which ones you would take?"

"I have. And have found 5. 'Sexy' ones, I think."

Bobby's smile tightened as did her tone.

"We do not have sexy courses here."

I have never understood confusion by educated people in receiving some metaphors I used. I did not reply but assumed she had grasped the extended meaning of my "sexy" and was merely responding to my dryness in kind.

"Alan, how are your finances?"

"Bad, Bobby. I would love help."

"Again?"

"Bobby, I know I joked a lot with you last year and I appreciated your help then, but finances are still no joke. You know I had to cancel with monetary penalty, all summer courses I had chosen and it was I who was our children's nanny."

"I can't promise, Alan."

I issued an "I understand" out of gratitude, my not being conscious of her hidden meaning, and then Bobby and I worked through my choices and I registered.

— • —

Two days later, a phone call came from Bobby and I was in her office within the hour. She had an absence of smile.

"Alan, I am afraid we have had to turn down your application."

No previous pains had tempered me enough for this new hurt. There was little neurologically wrong with my ability to fantasize but I had never conceived of such an outcome. For 6 seconds, I stared not at Bobby but at the gap between Bobby and me.

Bobby's tight voice continued across the big desk between us.

"We are too heavily enrolled and professors are complaining of their burdens. We cannot accept new students now."

"*New* stu...? Bobby, I want to come *back*! I pray, is there something, anything I can do?"

"Well, the school has had to consider your finances where we are also overburdened."

I perked up. An antique furniture restorer had been trying for years to buy back the dining room suite and had recently heard of Maria's leaving.

"Bobby, I may know of one source of money—the selling of our dining room suite. It comes from a time when..."

I failed to read her look.

"I can have the money by January, Bobby."

Her tightness held.

"Bobby, is there something I can do to persuade the school that I will help, not burden?"

"Well, our statutes allow for an appeal of a decision on admissions, if new evidence surfaces to affect eligibility. And you're now telling me that you have suddenly come into money, after having just been turned down."

I had not realized how my words on the dining room suite had been distilled.

"You could appeal to the Admissions Committee, given your changed circumstances."

"Admissions Committee?"

"Yes, but we would have to receive the appeal almost at once, since we cannot act beyond next week."

"Bobby, I will write my appeal here in Emmanuel's library and will give it to you in 30 minutes."

"I will advise the Committee that it is coming. Make sure you draw attention to your newly found ability to finance yourself."

"Thank you, I will do so. To whom should I address my appeal?"

"To the head of the Admissions Committee."

"Who is ... ?"

"Professor David Frisch."

"David Fris...", I murmured.

The next 4 days were not my friend. As best I could, I prepared for an appeal.

Regis Waters was once more balm. He wanted to talk again to his old student, Frisch. He had known of Frisch and me but I worried over Regis' offer. I felt Frisch to be a man wracked by his own low opinion of God and people, and I stewed that David Frisch could view the Dr. Regis Waters call as a political maneuver such as Frisch himself might pull. Regis assured me this was not so and I let him call.

With Regis' assurance, I telephoned another old friend Brian Alexandra. Brian had been with me in Regis Waters' class in the undergraduate 1960s years and had agreed with me on many important ideas. Brian had also shared that 3-week voyage in 1972 down U.S. Highway #1. Later he had settled 160 miles east of Toronto in Kingston where he had been a chaplain in the maximum security penitentiary. Brian had come to my wedding.

Recently, Brian had become Queens University's Chaplain in Kingston. He knew an emigrant from Queens, a Professor Classtick who by September 1986 had become a professor at Emmanuel. Dr. Classtick had replaced retiring Professor Puer, whom I had enjoyed as teacher of pastoral healing, and I had to believe that Emmanuel's criteria for such a replacement would include trying to approach those heights attained by Dr. Puer. Brian assured me, too, that Classtick would not view his call badly.

Two days later, my phone rang and it was Regis.

"Alan, I remain reassured. In fact David Frisch voiced surprise at your expressing any chemistry problems with him and went on to talk of his personal concern for you, having heard of your recent marital and vocational difficulties. But David did wonder about your sincerity, Alan, having just been turned down for a high-paying job."

"Regis, I was *offered* the job as you know! And high pay is not my priority."

"Well, David's assumptions in this instance are wrong. But he also spoke of your workshop group's seeing him to ask you out of the group."

Seconds passed amidst this new negative revelation.

"Reg, I'm not sure I can offer anything on that issue. You see, the group's leader...no."

"Well, David relaxed me on my concerns. He will not let that feedback on you influence his professional judgment, but David did address your poor academics."

"Reg, my academic record was excellent but for David Frisch's C."

"He spoke of some course you did not complete."

"Not complete?"

"Yes, Professor Doris Cushet's course which included a major paper."

"Regis, I *did* complete that course! I was given a 3-day extension, because I'd had the flu but I met the extended date and was given the final paper's mark, only days thereafter. A good mark."

"Well, that's certainly something you should straighten away with Emmanuel's Bobby, since that unfinished course is raising questions. Incidentally, you told me that you'd had a glowing relationship with Professor Cushet. She too had some comments about you."

"Doris did?"

My question came before this new hurt hit. I could not believe that Doris could have said anything against me. I thought we'd had an almost ideal student-teacher bond.

"Doris complained to David of your infringing on her home time, with phone calls."

Three, 4 seconds passed.

"Regis, you yourself told me of your enlightenment in discovering that your own professors had really cared. I was following suit. And my phone calls were only 3, were short and one related to my flu and 3-day extension. And of my 5 courses, a full 3 were with Professor Doris Cushet."

"Well, that's completely different and I'm not sure David understands those circumstances, either."

"Regis, David Frisch and the Admissions Committee are about to pass judgment on me and have wrong, key facts."

"Let's be calm, Alan. David Frisch has assured me that he will talk with you—I talked with him for over an hour—to give you a chance to discuss your areas of misunderstanding. I was able to set him straight on one important fact—David had been under the impression that you and I had just met in January when you joined Clair Park. He had not looked at the reference letter I had given Emmanuel at the time. David is now clear on that point. He did say, however, he could not guarantee anything until he conferred with the rest of the Committee. He seems a good sort, knows of your difficulties and again stressed his strong, personal concern for you."

By day 4, Emmanuel's Bobby phoned and asked if I could see the Admissions Committee in 2 hours for a meeting. It was only 4 days until Christmas. At 3:00 p.m. on Friday December 21st, 1986, I arrived in Frisch's office and found Frisch alone.

"Alan, yes, we will be a few minutes before the other Admission

Committee members gather with us...I see you have a book by Bornekamm."

"Yes, David. *Jesus of Nazareth*. I have been slugging through it. Bornekamm seems to bear the integrity of a detached historian. (Smiling) Teutonic thoroughness."

David looked not at me but at his bookcase.

"They (not clarifying who 'they' were) approach theological history with a thoroughness which we (not clarifying) do not have."

I responded, my not judging it necessary to know of a professor's prejudices.

"I have for some time been curious about the life of Jesus, the man, as taught."

"The man...?"

Committee members began rolling in and the first was Classtick. I had not met him or any of the others who entered the office but the one who followed I knew well—beloved Registrar Bobby Hensworth. I smiled at her but she did not reciprocate. None of the Committee shook my hand when introduced. Each member was dressed in what appeared a uniform of tired jacket and scuffed shoes.

I sat down next to a wall of books with Bobby to my rear left, near the office door and just outside my vision. Classtick was to my right and facing me were 3 more Admissions Committee members, 2 with arms folded. Behind his big desk sat Dr. David Frisch. It became clear Frisch now spoke from a position of power and his eyes were not to meet mine.

"Alan, thank you for coming in today. We wanted to talk to you about our decision."

Decision? Anxious, I interjected.

"Well David, thank you, too. I want to read something to the group, since I know there was some misconception about the apparent capriciousness with which I dove into the United Church last year. My entrance was not at all cavalier but was the culmination of a lifetime dig into my spirituality and its fit in the world."

Two front professors shifted and Classtick blew air through his nostrils for all to hear.

"I don't think there is a need for you to read anything to us. We have no concerns in that area."

"But, David. You thought Regis Waters had just met me last year when I joined Clair Park Church and entered Emmanuel. I want to read to you to the contrary and on the roots of my thinking."

"We know of your relationship with Clair Park and Dr. Waters."

"Know only recently, David, in the midst of shaping your assessment. And of my beginn..."

"No need, Alan."

"I feel there is a need, David, if the group is to assess me and my sincerity fairly."

The 3 heads in front swung to Frisch.

"Is it short? We are all busy before Christmas break."

"Yes."

I read my short story and so bared myself to all. When finished, I lowered my head in shyness and some shame at being exposed.

Professor #1 of the front 3, spoke for the first time.

"What are we expected to take from this showing off of your ability to craft words?"

In my openness, I could not fathom this twist of my motives. In the ensuing silence, Classtick took his turn.

"So you've been charging around this week, getting all kinds of important people to phone on your behalf and influence our decision."

I turned to my right to get direct eye contact with Classtick.

"I would respectfully suggest to you that saying my conversations with 2 old friends Regis Waters and Brian Alexandra is 'getting all kinds of important people to phone on my behalf' is not a responsible use of language, particularly since…"

"O.K., O.K."

Classtick wriggled in his chair and moved to put his rear end at a kind of farting angle to my face. Frisch went next.

"Your finances, Alan, are of a concern. You suddenly can fund yourself when less than a week ago before being turned down, you could not."

I then came to realize why Bobby had been insistent upon my emphasizing restored finances. I turned back to eye Bobby but her eyes held fast on Frisch.

"My financial strife remains. I have in fact been nanny to my..."

"Father, Alan not nanny..."

"Sorry, David. I simply meant..."

"Some of us here," Frisch's head panned the room as if he were once again lecturing. "have been fathers to children and have seen our roles not as burdensome toil but as a part of the joy of father-hood!"

"But David, I did not mean..."

Bobby interrupted.

"We don't fund nannies."

I did not turn my body to Bobby, just my head, but my eyes caught her skulk. Classtick seized again the silence.

"Does the United Church really need the kind of business skills that successfully extract sums of money out of Emmanuel for personal use? We're not in that kind of business."

I suddenly sensed the prejudice that had been building before what I had thought to be my day in court. Classtick crossed his arms and assumed the defiant position. I grew less steady.

"Then perhaps it would help the Committee to know that I have given my remaining business clothes to 3 Toronto street people, this autumn. Directly, one-on-one."

Two seconds silence.

"Imagine the guilt you must have built up to do that," Frisch said.

"Guilt, Da…?"

"We in this Church operate as a team, in the tradition of Christian teamwork where chemistry with team members is vital. Not solo in acts of flashy heroism."

"Hero…?" I grew less steady still. "I was in a serious car accident 5 years ago and I have had much time since to…"

"We know of your car accident, Alan," Frisch said. "I gave 2 hours to your detective. We should have known of it last year. And Central Trust's turning you down for a job. It too has gone into our formulation."

"*My* detective? Central trust *didn't*. I don't *have* a detective… Formulation?"

Bobby seemed buoyed.

"We're not a social agency."

Before I could think, I spoke and in so doing, injured myself in front of all.

"True. But if one scrapes around every crevice of Emmanuel, one may find a smattering of Christianity."

The 6 sensed victory. Frisch stoked the momentum.

"Last year, Alan, we took you in at the last minute, only on the sound recommendation of people like Dr. Waters."

"But you didn't even receive Dr. Waters' recommendation until after I had been accepted. And David, you have not read that recommendation even now."

Professor David Frisch held.

"And this year you are once again asking us to make enormous concessions to wedge you in at a time when our professors, some of whom have been imposed upon by you, are complaining that they are overworked."

"I came last January, not December to talk to Emmanuel and had then been persuaded by professors like Emmanuel's Paul

Schweppes to join the school. And I was accepted again for this September. And my marks, which you understand to be weak, are..."

"Not an issue" Frisch declared.

"But I understood there to be confusion ..."

"Professor Cushet is locating that mark," Bobby said.

"And people you know have spoken well of me. My own minister, Ian Godfrey..."

Front Professors 2 and 3 spoke for the first time but in gibes to themselves.

"Ah yes, Lord Godfrey from the mighty Clair Park."

Classtick jumped in over the sarcasm.

"Namedropping."

"Name...? He's my minister."

"Waters, Alexandra..."

"They're my friends!"

The group's power suddenly reached full force and Frisch seized control.

"And there is the issue of your getting sick. Your detective..."

"The flu, David. And I *have* no detective!"

"And, *why* you got sick. And your resultant impositions on a young, female professor."

"Impos...David, a 3-day extension."

"If it *were* that."

"It was!"

"We don't have the mark."

"We're getting it," Bobby said.

"And will you get sick again and impose upon our beleaguered professors more?" Frisch asked. "Or will your car accident make for further illnesses?"

"David, you had not even known of my car accident."

"But we should have. A legal case, am I right?"

"Yes, David but ..."

"Alan, all we are saying is that if you go through the normal channels for acceptance into Emmanuel for next September, we will look at your application as we would any other."

"Any other? All you are say…David, your main inputs are concoctions of…"

Classtick charged. "Do you hear what we are saying? Do you listen ever?"

I looked at Frisch, Classtick and the front 3.

"Yes."

All rose from their chairs to escape. I tried to shake each hand, but before I could reach Bobby, she slunk out. Frisch stuck to his desk and his eyes never met mine.

I was out of Emmanuel and onto its sidewalk. I began to move across the University of Toronto but paused in front of Emmanuel's parent college, Victoria. Etched into its front was a weathered school creed, "The truth shall make you free."

I did not know then that weeks later Professor Cushet would submit my "unfinished" good grade or that more weeks later, Professor Cushet would protest the Committee's abuse of her joking about her husband's being jealous of my home phone calls. Or that months later, David Frisch would spend more hours with the opposing legal team, discussing the legitimacy of my car accident and thinking the legal opposition to be working for me. All I knew then was that the University of Toronto's Emmanuel College, revered body for imparting the principles of truth and love as embodied in The United Church of Canada, had spat me out.

# VALUES

By the beginning of March 1987, Maria's mother determined that my wife and sons could no longer fit into her house and Maria came back home. Before her return, she went to a marital lawyer who advised her that not only was she ineligible upon divorce to share in any proceeds from my brain injury lawsuit but that I could be eligible for support from Maria. Maria then said that she "...shoulda married for money. At least that way, I'd have something outa this marriage. This way I'm stuck." Maria took to sleeping in the TV room.

I landed a job that 1987, the first one in a year and a half, helping fired people get jobs. I was to earn 2/5ths of the pay that I had earned 2 years earlier at Blimiss Hope or 3/5ths of the salary I received 4 years earlier at the Ministry of Food. I was not scheduled to start for 2 months until the end of May. I, therefore had another chance to care full-time for James and Robert.

I would take my sons to Queen's Park to feed the squirrels, Varsity Stadium to play track and field, children's concerts at Roy Thompson Hall, the fantasyland of Harris water works, Black Creek Pioneer Village, Riverdale Farm, Toronto Island, Ecology Park, the Science Center, the museum, art gallery, zoo, the library often and the playground every day.

"Insulation, Daddy, like we have in our roof?"

"Actually insolation, James darling. I pointed to the April sky. " You see, our sun..."

"You mean Mr. Golden Sun, Daddy?"

"Yes, James. Our golden sun sends down its rays..."

"Its, Daddy? Not his?"

"Yes, James. Our sun is not really alive, except in our imaginations. Our sun is a huge ball of burning gas..."

"Gas, Daddy? Like you showed us in the pipe in the basement?"

"A combination of such gases I believe, James but I'm not sure what combination."

"You're not sure, Daddy?"

"Yes James, I'm not."

James halted his dancing on our home's back deck and looked 10 feet over to his dad. He then ran across the deck, leapt into my kneeling body and squeezed me around my whip-lashed neck. I didn't care about the pain.

"You know many things, Daddy. I love learning from you. You are the gentlest teacher I have ever known."

Robert, 19 months old, eyed us from the sand box and charged over to give his dad a hug. There the 3 of us embraced in the 50° Fahrenheit on an April day.

"Daddy, will we have time to build something today?"

"Yes, James. After we eat some lunch. I think we'll have milk, a banana each..."

"Munkees, Daddy?"

"Monkey style if you wish, Robert."

"May we make Monkey sounds too?"

"Yes, James. A banana each, carrots..."

"May we have whole carrots, Daddy so that we can do Churchills?"

"Well, Robert may have a small one...one hard-boiled egg each and some raisins."

James looked into my eyes with admonishment.

"Are you going to have a coffee, Daddy?"

"Tea, James. Earl Grey."

James looked down at me with the sternness of Milton and crooked his index finger to my nose.

"Tea has caffeine too, Daddy."

"Thank you, James. I'm trying to cut down."

My son James squeezed me again and Robert followed.

"Yes, I understand it's difficult with addictions, Daddy. I have the same problem with *Sesame Street* when you're playing with Robert. You're doing well with your addiction, Daddy. Just don't let your body think of it."

"Thank you, James. It's those turtles I worry more about when you're watching TV."

"I know, Daddy. You told me it's bad to hurt even bad people, sorry, misdirected people."

We sat down to lunch in the kitchen. The radio was tuned to classical music on CBC-FM. James was munching, when stopped by a familiar sound.

"Mozart!"

"Yes, James."

"Was he ever sad the way Chopin was?"

"Yes, in fact he died younger than Chopin."

"Died? Mozart is dead?"

"He died a long time ago."

"How long ago, Daddy?"

"About 200 years ago, James. Please finish your lunch."

Robert sat listening, while as always, eating everything on his plate.

"That was *before* old fashioned days! It must have been the old, *old* fashioned days!"

"One could think so, James, but please don't let me interrupt your eating the carrot."

"That's O.K., Daddy. I'm thirsty anyway. Daddy, was Mozart sick like Chopin?"

"He became sick differently, James."

"He didn't have tooberkoolosis? Oh...Sorry, Daddy. Oh, now there's a mess."

I grabbed a dishcloth and paper towels from the counter, and in the process of leaping up from the table, fetching and cleaning, I tried to resume the broken conversation.

"Not tuberculosis, James. Some other serious virus, I believe."

James had recovered his composure and was working again at his food while Robert sat patiently with an emptied cup and plate.

"But why, Daddy have I not heard sad Mozart music? Did he not have a sad period like Mr. Chopin?"

"He did, James, though I think it was short."

"May we go again to the Science Center, Daddy? Or the museum? I want to go to the Planetarium to play star guessing games."

"It's sunny, James and according to the radio, it is going to warm up to 60°. I think we should take your wagon to the fire station and the library but before we do that, we should put on our rubber boots, since I'll have to ask you boys to get out of the wagon when we go through the spring mud, way up high in Eglinton Park."

North one long block and through the park we wagoned on our way to North Toronto's fire station. There, 2 fire fighters permitted James and Robert to sit behind the steering wheel of a Hook 'n Ladder. While the fire fighters supervised my sons, they pushed buttons, flashed lights and sounded sirens. One fire fighter slid down the pole twice.

The North Toronto library was just 3 minutes away. When we arrived, I suggested to James and Robert that they select one book each for looking at in the children's section and one for taking home. After I helped 16-month-old Robert select a picture book, James began fussing over what story to get, but finally chose a short story by Hans Christian Andersen entitled *The Nightingale*. James insisted on reading to me the entire tale there.

I sat down on a reading bench and cradled Robert in my left arm while James plopped onto my lap and began reading aloud, working through new words using the phonetics I had taught him.

Except for 7 words, 3 year-old James read to me the entire 12-minute book.

At the end of James' reading, Robert selected his sole choice for takeout, a depiction of spider webs and how they are made. Once again, James turned fraught with Robert's decisiveness, but eventually settled on a book of 100 favorite nursery rhymes.

On the wagon home, it was now 4:30 p.m. and the clouds were beginning to spit. As we arrived at Eglinton Park's huge hill, James was in the wagon's front and started to hum a Raffi song, with Robert following suit. Then, with my 2 sons in the wide-wheeled wagon, I began the trudge up the "way-up-high" hill. Suddenly, the wagon overturned, tossing James' and Robert's blonde heads into a puddle of mud. Both boys were unhurt but covered in mud and they started to cry. After a fast check on them, I sat myself down in the puddle and to James' and Robert's delight, covered my face in mud and began singing.

"Mud, mud, glorious mud. Nothing quite like it for cooling the blood..."

Both boys laughed and started singing with me, all the while splashing and kicking in the puddle. Within minutes, the wet and muddy 3 of us were off again, my wagoning them over the hillcrest and down through the trees to the traffic lights, one block north of our home.

Inside the house, the 3 of us bathed, then piggy-backed into the playroom. James fixed himself on *Sesame Street* while Robert and I tried to build with Lego blocks. By 6:00 p.m., Maria had not arrived home, so I treated my sons to the only thing I knew how to cook other than eggs, macaroni. I topped it off with raw broccoli and 2 wild mushrooms. We drank cranberry juice, which to the boys' delight, I managed to spill.

We then adjourned to the living room where we danced to Peter, Paul and Mary. As always post-accident, I quickly became dizzy and had to beg off a ring around a rosy. Instead, we played

"Chinese Circus" and I became with my badly healed clavicle, the foundation for a 3-person rectangle.

"Oh, Daddy, we forgot!" Both boys jumped down.

"Forget what, James?"

"Insolation. What is it?"

"What little I understand, James is that rays from our sun are re-radiated from the ground, giving us our day's heat. At night, when the sun is shining on the other side of the world..."

"On Japan, where the Yoshimaras live?"

"On Japan, among other countries. Our ground radiates only the heat that has been stored during daylight, and the ground releases the heat slowly over an ever cooler night. I think bright colors such as silver feel hot in the sun because they re-radiate our sun's heat, whereas black soil feels cool because it is absorbing much of the sun. The ground's heating, if I remember from Grade 10 Science, is called solar insolation."

James began scampering around the room and Robert followed as best he could. James then thrust his arms up to the sky beyond the ceiling and eased them down to the floor.

"So the sun's rays swoop down, warm up the ground and keep us *warm*."

"I believe so, James."

"That's really interesting! Thank you, Daddy."


## Writing

After Maria got home, I went down to my basement cubby-hole and tried a bit of writing.

# The Trees of North Toronto

A stroll through the streets of North Toronto is one of life's little vacations that can restore the spiritual energy needed to cope in our now big, fast city. Pushing through the city's pollution are occasional breaths of fresh air, and on the side streets, there are fun-to-watch squirrels. Near Lascelles and Anderson are 2 couples of cardinals and blue jays, and the sound of birdsong is still in the air. Trees mature and once strong, have long blanketed North Toronto and are a main reason that the birds, squirrels, bits of fresh air and general quiet still bless us. Trees are also a main reason why we walk on cool streets, protected from the sun's mid-day brightness. Trees are beautiful too in their own right. Some, like the giant silver maples, seem to radiate the majesty of their many years. It's fun to pause and look at the thousands of shapes.

Some give off vigor. Or did. Their strength is being sapped. Drought. Rock salt. Acid rain. All 3 have ravaged North Toronto's trees. Some are dead and some are dying. Few are healthy. Before the year 2000, before the year 1995, North Toronto if left unchecked, could be a white-hot wasteland with no shade, no birds, no squirrels, no coolness but for the artificial cold emanating from energy-eating air conditioners.

Please plant trees now. Water your old ones. Trim them. Give city hall no rest on the damage of rock salt. Give the Canadian and Ontario Governments no rest on acid rain. Only then will we or our children in North Toronto, have any hope of continuing to enjoy the strolls through these streets of the past 60 years.

My published gift to North Toronto for letting me live here.

Alan J Cooper

ALAN J COOPER

266

Shortly after I wrote the note, it was published and then began a trickle of little writings I would do and see printed. With James and Robert, I exercised language. J and R would talk at 11 months, carry on conversations by month 17, read and spell before the age of 2 and before 3, write short stories such as "The Trees of North Toronto."

April 29ht, 1987

Dear Mommy,

I just thought htat you would like a nice letter from me to cheer you up on your hard day.

Daddy took us to the Toronto zoo today and the Rooge Valley where we hl threw stones into a polooted river.

Daddy takes good care of us so dont worry Mommy.

I love you Mommy.

XO XO

J

O

H

N

## The Politics of Death

Other than pouring through job ads in libraries, by May of 1987 I had not read a newspaper in 18 months and had not watched a newscast since 1985. But as I partially came back to life in 1987 and viewed again the 10 o'clock news, I found myself immersed in an issue—the question of capital punishment was looming anew. The concept of a government's sanctioning the pre-determined killing of a human being repulsed me. Nightly after reading to J and R, I was swamping myself in debates on state-stamped people killing. That spring, I heard a plea from a mother of an 11 year-old girl who had been raped and murdered. The mother's plea was for freedom from capital punishment and contained more understanding than I had heard from anyone.

I could not help seeing the huge gap between the United States and other countries. American Justices who showed "liberal" attitudes were swarmed out of their jobs by politicians who lived by polls. Though no study had ever shown capital punishment capable of reducing crime, U.S. politicians leapt forward to underscore their tough stand. At any moment in America, 2000 people were on death row and some for 10 years or more. A few were mentally retarded, and some were youths who had been children when they had killed but were later determined to be no longer juveniles. Many were Blacks who had murdered Whites. Some had been represented by law students. Each execution cost the U.S. taxpayers 4–5 times the cost of imprisoning a person for life.

Ignorance and anger, a deadly combination. Deadlier still, because in 1987, much of our world continued to look to leader United States for direction. Cooler heads prevailed in Canada and it joined Europe, Australia, New Zealand and hundreds of millions of other people in condemning capital punishment.

## With James and Robert Again
## on a Day in May, 1987

"A red one! Daddy, it's an old English subway train with windows that open! Now we can have fresh breezes!"

"Yes James, sweetheart. Please don't jump up and down on the platform and please hold onto my hand firmly...Thank you. Robert, are you ready to get on when the train stops?"

"Yes, Daddy, ut aft ee let t' peep loff first."

"Sorry, Robert, of course."

"Daddy, do you think we will get a seat?"

"I think so, James, since it's 10:00 a.m. and we'll be heading north away from downtown."

"So we'll be able to read the advernssmnts ?"

"Yes, James."

"N' see th' colors?"

"Yes, Robert sweetheart."

"You prefer these older English cars, don't you Daddy? I do, too. They have more character, even if they are a little wobblier than the new silver ones."

"I do."

Robert was studying the shapes and colors of a cumulus-of-fair weather cloud on a Salvation Army advertisement.

"Sss art, Daddy?"

"Of a sort, Robert."

Robert looked puzzled at my answer and James tried to help.

"Is it art or science, Daddy?"

"I have to say, James, that I don't entirely know the answer to your question."

Robert locked his right arm in my left and lodged his head under my left shoulder.

"Try, Daddy."

"Thank you, Robert...I see 2 differences between a work of art and science. The first is that the artist is pulling apart the world but also putting it back together in the same work, whether in pictures, words or notes of music." While seeing my sons' looks of puzzlement, I tried to make arm gestures. "The second is that if we watch the artist at work, we don't necessarily follow his or her thinking."

"Like you with your camera, Daddy?"

"Yes, James. In those 2 areas, science seems to fall short. Without the help of art, the work of science seems to be only prejudiced analysis, bent by the scientist's mind, his or her ever obsolete tools and the use of buzz words."

"Like bees?"

"Sorry, Robert. I too am being prejudiced in trying to explain to you."

"That's alright, Daddy, you're trying very hard. I love you, Daddy."

Unconditional love. I grew confident.

"The scientist too often, Robert..."

"Tub, Daddy."

"Excuse me, Tub, I forgot the name you've given yourself ...too often is concerned with describing facts when those so-called facts are really impressions coming from seeing, hearing, touching and smelling." I pointed to my eyes, ears, finger and nose. "What lies behind, we cannot see, hear, touch or smell. A scientist has to keep in mind her human limitations on what she knows before she starts on her work."

"You don't like scientists, Daddy?"

"On the contrary, James, I do and I feel they should keep going, but I am concerned about any thinking that locks a scientist into a focus on how she is looking at something rather than what she is looking at." I pretended to use a camera. "We seem to be trying to look at things that wriggle away from us to a vast unknown…" I swept both arms around. "…each time we close in to see and describe them."

"York Mills! We have only 3 more stops to go before we get a chance to go on a bus."

"Thank you, James. No, J and R, I respect science and the scientist who is open but…"

James turned and looked through my glasses to my eyes.

"Daddy, I don't completely understand you."

I had been talking in mega-bites as brain injured people often do. I swung around my arm and placed it on James' left shoulder, then looked into my son's soft brown eyes.

"James, *I* don't completely understand me."

James smiled slightly as if in reassurance of himself, Robert and me.

"Finch station!"

Robert pulled back my left arm and grasped my left hand with his right.

Off the 3 of us went on a bus atop Toronto's northern edge, and shortly after 11:00 a.m., we reached Black Creek Pioneer Village, a re-creation of a village north of Toronto 200 years ago. The tinsmith's shop, the mill, the schoolhouse, the farm, the wooden sidewalks, the hay wagon ride, the porridge, the cider, the fudge, were all fun. We departed at 4:00 p.m., went counter-traffic until 5:20 and arrived home to my dull supper at a 5:45. Maria was home by 6:20 with another supper and fed our sons a second time.

At midnight, I adjourned to my cellar table, its one light and my locked attaché. I opened it and placed the day's page back into what in essence had become my extended left brain-lobe—my protected black book. I checked each detail of the day to ensure I had crossed off each needed act and then as done to this day, I stroked a vertical black line down the full page, eyeing as the marker scrolled down, each scribble, word, letter and tick to ensure I had missed nothing. I turned the page to see what was written for tomorrow and carry forward from the previous days, the details I had to have: (10:00 a.m.) James' music lesson C/F; (11:30 a.m.) Ontario Place; Yitzi's deli; two 8 oz. milks, green beans, corn...; streetcar from King Station, no transfer; (5:00 p.m.) Sesame, build with T... Tomorrow's page was totally blacked in.

I put it in my buttoned rear pocket and checked all other pockets to ensure cash, keys and cards were buttoned in. Then I checked all pockets again, closed the attaché, locked it and checked the lock twice.

At 1:00 a.m., I made my way up from the cellar to the top floor and went to the bathroom, brushed my teeth and started back to the master bedroom. I saw James and Robert sleeping in the 2 others. I went to kiss them good-night, turned off all the lights and felt my way back to the master bedroom and former room of Mommy and Daddy. Then, with Maria asleep in the TV room on the far corner of the house, I laid down the closed-pocketed safari pants and safari jacket beside the former marital bed. Fatherhood shift was to start at 7:00 a.m. and I lay down at 1:15, falling asleep about 4:00.

## Letters

Though with me all day, James and Robert were eager to write to their dad and we had a game we had invented, called "Boomerang Letters."

May 16, 1987

Dear James,

Thank you for your loving letter. I have tacked it to the wall in front of my cellar desk, so that I can remind myself when doing my late-night black book work, of your gift.

Yes, I promise to help you search for your missing diary key and I will also keep my promise to share in our street's firecracker celebration on upcoming Victoria Day. Please tell Robert, my promise.

James, I didn't know one could not safely eat rhubarb leaves, that only the stem was edible. Thank you for ensuring our family's safety on that point. Thank you too for your helping me understand a sundial. Your hand-drawn circle in the sand box and its circumference girthed by the numbers 1 to 12, along with the shifting shadow on different sections of the circle, enlightened me, (if you'll pardon my pun).

James, your letters are helping me grow. Please write again soon.

I love you and will love you forever.

Unconditionally.
Love,
X O,
*Daddy*

May 16, 1987

Dear Robert,

Thank you for your love-felt drawing. I have tacked it onto the wall in front of my cellar desk, so that I can enjoy a visual vacation each night from my black book work.

Robert, please use your imagination and tell yourself what you see in the next page's picture.

Is what you think you see what you see, Robert? Is what you see what you want to see? Is what you see what others see? Is what you see what others want you to see?

Please feel free to see, Robert. I love you and will love you, forever.

Unconditionally.
Love,
X O,
*Daddy*

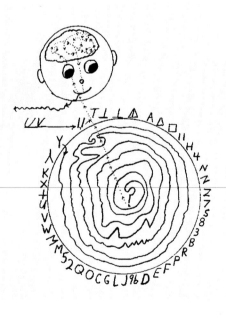

April and May of 1987 were an untamed Eden for James, Robert and me. Yes J and R did occasionally quarrel and sometimes scrap, and Maria was no help with her frequent poor-mouthing in front of them. I would have to counter when Maria would come home from work and say to James and Robert,

"We are not really able to live in this area. We're too poor."

I would see the helplessness in our little sons' eyes as their mother threatened the stability of their world and I would rush in to rescue.

"No we're not…We don't make as much money as other people in the neighborhood, but our nice house is almost paid for." J and R's faces would brighten and their fear slip away. "We started with more, so we're giving our friends a chance to catch up."

I did not know how to counter the odd shout of "Fuck!" by Maria in front of our toddlers.

Only twice did I raise my voice to James and Robert and both times to halt danger. J and R responded in kind and the rough stuff stayed confined to tumbling during our hikes. The orders of the day were tours of fire and police stations, outings, learning new words, meeting other children, ravines, swimming pools, libraries, tries on the piano, singing, reading, drawing, running, puddles, parks, playgrounds. The orders of each week were outings, provincial parks, national parks, the odd Bed 'n Breakfast. There also were scrapes, cuts, bruises, Robert's broken wrist, Sick Children's Hospital, shots, my psychiatrist. But there was also confidence—James', Robert's and spits of mine—my trying to work with what was left, after cognitive, sensual and motor function damage.

## The Yolanta Poison That Was To Come

The thought that God is a big king revealed in a time too long ago to comprehend, puts us all on stage under that lord's scrutiny. We reduce ourselves to slaves that obey or rebel, with the lights of human experience dulled. When things go wrong, we do not feel the freedom that we were first given and wonder why our god has tolerated such badness.

Moral copouts have been solidified by centuries of driven in perversion. For most of history, children have been told, out of some fear of god, to conform to the image of their parents and their parental extension, the adult. The growth of that child is thus shunted—spiritually, intellectually and physically—and long before puberty, perhaps before the age of 3, the child becomes static. The son/daughter does what the mother/father did and the father/mother does what the grandparents did. People stay focused backwards, barely tapping into their talents, surviving day-to-day in fear of an ever-watchful, tyrannical god.

For creativity to grow in a person or group, the brain's right side needs freedom to take risks. I think we live in a world where millions have been emotionally truncated pre-puberty—followers cannot discern, because they have not been allowed to develop critical thinking or grow their conscience. Early on, they have been given a religious paint-by-number set with no opportunity to exercise any sense of right or wrong. To that under-developed group conscience, society's answer has been in the short term, an overdosing of police and punishment, and in the long term, the lie to sustain suppression. The definition of "discipline" has been restricted to punishment, control, correcting, chastising, subduing or thrashing. Never a notion of "discipline" as meaning autonomy.

Can not autonomy evolve through physical, intellectual and

moral growth? Can not autonomy's purpose be to nourish sound conduct and actions by both supported self-learning and the relentless exercising and re-evaluation of such learning? Children who grow up in a home where discipline is understood as self-discipline, have better esteem, and their language development is years ahead of learners from one-liner environments.

It is not, I suggest, a parental purpose to mold our children or inculcate fear into them. Instead of our blaming, say god, I feel we need to grasp the role of personal responsibility as a first step in building our children and actualizing ourselves as parents. I think we need to understand that our sole tool of control is our own behavior and that such behavior makes little room for showmanship—when face becomes the priority, the rest of life becomes slavery to that face and its god of twisted theatre.

— • —

Yolanta had been raised in old Poland by aunts and as was the custom, taken away as a baby from her own mother, not to return until the age of 5. Yolanta would never for a moment let the world forget that fact or throughout every long day that she was the world's best mother. Yola slept with Maria's brother Constantine until his teenaged years but when Constantine entered university and his mother found it increasingly difficult to drive him to and from school, he found among his peers a car-driving female replacement. When she became his girlfriend, mother Yolanta screamed at Constantine in a jealous rage, "Fuck her, fuck her, that is all she is good for!" and then with her hard index finger stabbing at her own breastbone, decreed, "*I* am the woman for you!"

Husbands in Yolanta's world were egg fertilizers and nothing more. She cut up her poor husband at every turn and included his spiritual castration as part of her daily list to Maria. Yola talked of how her husband wanted to have sex and how sex was her wifely duty but that he was dirty and foul. She told Maria that she, Yolanta, wanted to be diagnosed with cancer, so she could be rid of her husband. Lucky for Yola, she got her wish and more when her daily mocked husband died of liver cancer.

Yolanta's own mother, Babcia, was condemned to hell for 50 years, never allowed to learn English, never allowed to read Polish books or magazines other than her Bible, never allowed to watch Polish TV programs or listen to them on the radio, never allowed to listen to music or speak to friends, kept fed but dehydrated, having a huge cyst build up inside her to the point where it poisoned her, having her elderly pension funds seized and her little mail pre-read, never allowed to voice an opinion and kept in fear of expressing anything not first sanctioned by Yolanta. Babcia was given less freedom than a hamster who spends each day in a cage, running on a tiny treadmill.

Babcia was a sweet lady with a good heart. She and I hugged often, and told each other "Ja ciebie kocham (I love you)". I took her to concerts, Polish movies and a vacation to Florida. Yola acquiesced, to keep intact her cover-up.

## Yolanta

I was to start a new job and Maria pretended to search for a new nanny but actually asked her mother to take care of J and R. Yola came in late May, at the end of my children's spring.

On the Friday when I was to register for my new job, Yolanta arrived at 8:25. To James' and Robert's plea to play, she hand-held them north the 150 yards to Eglinton Park and there, 30 minutes after breakfast, force-fed them massive sandwiches from her big bag. J and R wanted to go to their playground but Yolanta held them back from their exercise routines. She clutched their arms and shouted warnings, and blocked them from climbing trees. She filled them with fear of dog "shit," a word they had never heard and "catastrophe" if they fell. She grabbed them away from shrubs and said the shrubs had bees and dangerous spiders. Food, she saw as a tool for slavery but exercise, like socialization, she saw as a foil.

At the end of my first workday, Maria was yet to arrive home and I asked Yolanta not to leave the back door unlocked when she was out of the house. That was all. But 3 months earlier, Yola had trapped me inside her own house, and with James in my arms and my being inside their bolted back door, I had been stuck one stair below Yola. From her higher position, she had begun banging my nose with her index finger, all the while yelling, "You are (jab) jealous, you are (jab) jealous." In response, I had freed my right hand enough to slap her cheek, to get her to stop. Maria had heard Yolanta's scream and had come dashing to take her side. Constantine had also emerged, had grabbed my collar and threatened. I had done what I could do to shelter James, who had been hugging me ever more closely. When I had finally managed to escape, James had then taken his little hand, rested it on my left cheek and had given my eyes a loving look. James was not yet 3.

Maria arrived home on my first new job day and Yolanta seized the chance to declare in front of toddlers James and Robert that she was doing us a favor. She further shouted that I was treating her like shit and she was not coming back on Monday. Yolanta then slammed the front door and departed in front of my 2 shocked sons. Maria made no mention of Yola's foul language in front of our children and asked no questions about what had happened. Instead, she whined in front of James and Robert to a husband who had just started his first job in a year and a half, "I hope you're staying home, starting Monday."

I fell for Maria's blackmail and raced out the door to catch a charging Yolanta. As I started to apologize to her on the sidewalk of busy Eglinton Avenue and ask her to come back on Monday, she pulled from her purse the August 1982 letter that I had written to her 5 years earlier. She brandished it across my nose in the same way she had been hitting my nose 3 months earlier, and then while gritting her teeth and almost singing, she gloated, "I've got your letter, 'ha 'ha 'ha, and you're nothing but shit." She pointed a finger at me and bared her teeth. "No real man could do what you're doing, looking after children, but *you* can't do anything else. I will have *my* grandchildren. You are only with Maria for the money and I will bring them up as they should be, and you will be nothing." She curled her finger back to her chest. "I am their granny and know what's best for them. You know nothing 'ha 'ha 'ha, and I granny *know* what's best. Maria is now a big shot and will soon drive a *big* Mercedes." Her arms stretched out to the sky. "And *you* are nothing." Her finger uncurled and she jabbed into my chest. "*I've* got them now and you are just shit 'ha 'ha 'ha!"

Yola came back on Monday.

---

## Maria Gets Fired

Constructive dismissal was the formal description but no matter how it was worded, Maria got fired in June of 1987. The report by her staff was scathing and delineated many of the traits I had experienced for years. Despite her boss then trying to fake a head office position for Maria with no staff, it would have been only a matter of months before she would have been gone. I then gave Maria free relocation counseling, and through a wrongful dismissal lawyer, she managed to get some sort of severance. She then double dipped into unemployment insurance and cheated the government for a full year.

From the hour of her firing, Maria switched her professed religion from Roman Catholic to atheist. She then tried to renege on our marriage vow to have the children baptized Christian. My minister friend Regis Waters told her the United Church required only one parent's consent but she then told her parents that I was forcing the denomination on their grandchildren, making no mention of her turning atheist or being dismissed from work. Instead, she said she had taken her mother's advice and had chosen to stay home full-time with her children. When my Sunday school duties resumed in September, without one word to her parents, Maria wedged herself into United Church administration above my head.

Maria's father would later yell in front of James and Robert, what a bad father I was, and say that the children were always supposed to take the mother's religion. I would say nothing, but would reflect on Maria's complaints about her mother, on Yolanta's never hearing them and on Maria's sister saying her mother lied so much, she did not know that she *was* lying.

For the next 4 years, Maria would act as prime caregiver to James and Robert.

## Kawawaymog

"Round Lake" was English for "Lake Kawawaymog" or as we Whites would have it, "Kawawaymog Lake" was Cree for "Round Lake." The lake was an almost drinkable 6 square miles of water, minnows, baby catfish, ducklings, loons, hummingbirds, herons, frogs, turtles and bloodsuckers, all at 1,400 feet and 11 miles from electricity, just a river paddle away from the northwest side of Ontario's 3,000 square-mile Algonquin Park. It was the kind of lake that central Canada rarely experienced by 1987. Of Ontario's 1/4 million lakes, Round Lake was by then one of the few not devastated by acid rain. It sat high in Ontario, about 200 miles north of Toronto, far enough away to miss the poison pushed north from the United States industrial belt.

To appreciate a Canada that once was, you need to experience awakening to stillness, looking out of a shack window and peering through ancient birches to an unharmed lake whose only visible inhabitants were a mother duck and 9 ducklings. Then, to understand miles of drinkable water, you have to experience stumbling 30 feet down to a lake, falling into it and feeling the freshness hit your nude body.

James, Robert and Maria were shortly behind me, all nude too. J and R reckoned the shallow water to be the ultimate backyard pool and would not come out of the water. Breakfast had to be served on the 1,000-yard stretch of 20-foot wide beach. After breakfast, J and R varied their play between sand-castle villages and the 18-inch deep water that the lake offered for the first 200 feet offshore. I succumbed to the horseflies, moving back to the shack's screened porch, but my eyes held on James' and Robert's every move. Maria followed me and plopped herself onto the porch's other wooden chair, and then each of us took turns cutting back inside to put on our shirts and shorts and fetch a coffee from the small wood stove. We sat on the porch, sipping eye-openers as James and Robert played on the shore and splashed in the lake. On the shack porch, Maria and I found time to talk.

"Thank you, Alan, for bringing us this gift."

"You're more than welcome." Her cue to converse was all that my mega-bite brain needed. "I confess Maria, that I have never outgrown a childhood desire to write a definitively Canadian book, one non-American in style."

"Death of an Adverb?"

"I should not have made that comment. Not all Americans say 'Real good'. Sports maybe, but we can't keep bashing Americans. There are some highly literate ones."

"Twelve, you once said."

I grinned. Until then, I had not appreciated how much humor I had lost, post-brain change. I had become dead to a joke. I still knew laughter to be medicine but would not allow that a sense of humor could open doors to insight and balance, and give a chance to laugh at those things we love, while still loving them.

"Would it be fair to say that I am a touch heavy for a kick-off to 2 weeks in the wilderness?"

Maria leaned over and put her hand on my back. She kissed me on the right temple and I guessed that was her answer. I decided to go at it again.

"I would really like to get to the root of knowledge."

Maria allowed me the moment. "I didn't mean to belittle you, Alan. You would have made a precise scientist."

I managed a piece of composure, rare post-brain injury, and let the "would have" pass. "Doctor Fisher has told me that precision can backfire, locking a person into a state of precision-of-means with no goal left but precision for its own sake."

"But surely the answers to life require precision?"

"We only *extrapolate* that cells begin by starting with simple forms of life, then progressively more sophisticated ones."

"And so long as there remains a potential for the equilibrium we can see all around us..."

"We *think* we can see ..."

"... there seems no other way for life to go." Maria smiled. "Evolution *seems* to be the growth from the simple to the complex by a series of layers, but quantum physics underscores to us that all information which our mortal brains absorb is imperfect. As such, we must look upon all information with fresh doubt or we will open up not one door to the root of knowledge, but many doors to dogma."

"Can we mortals know nothing?"

Maria looked straight at me with a repressed grin when she said "mortals" and my tone turned apologetic.

"Maria, I think we can enjoy ever increasingly winning schools of thought, but I think it is for us to question, rather than follow without check what is purportedly known. Everything we do is based on judgment calls. I think we have witnessed the counter-concept under tyranny and the principles of cruel certainty, and I think we have seen that means-justified ends have destroyed those very ends in the process. The whole human spirit is betrayed. Supposedly perfect knowledge—dogma—closes our minds and turns us into bands of obsequious zealots."

"Mm...maybe."

I chose to ignore that I was losing Maria's listening and continued.

"Minds of the highest formal education or doctrine can be hurt by their own fear of questioning, and in attempting to find and build upon their mortal findings, their misreading can be made worse by the precision of their misdirected quest."

"So precision is bad."

"Maria, please. The need to know such perfection or to try to live in such perfection is frequently bred into us by a manipulative parent, usually mother, and the imprisoned child will often try to be perfect, as defined by what he sees as his main source of truth, say that mother. Perfectionists are made, not born."

"So, precision is bad."

I continued talking to myself. "Precision in some areas, perhaps photography, can be helpful, but preoccupation with precision in pursuing determinacy can produce intolerance, misdirected anger or worse, a heart attack, alcoholism, death or worse, a stroke."

"Daddy, come quickly!"

I stumbled down to an area just inshore from the beach and Maria followed. There, James and Robert had their eyes fastened on a stationary garter snake, whose mouth had the hands of one small young frog sticking out of each side.

"Is he eating him, Daddy?"

"Yes, Robert. Digesting him slowly right now, I would guess."

"Won't he choke, eating the frog all at once like that?"

"I don't think so, James. His mouth has acids that make the frog digestible."

"Is the frog hurting, Daddy?"

"I hope not, Robert but we should not interfere. It's a free country and the snake is as free to eat the frog as are we to eat chickens."

"I can see the frog inside. Why is the snake not afraid of us, Daddy?"

"James, I think his energy is being used to digest the frog."

— • —

And so it was for 16 days at Round Lake. Dozens of ducks passing daily. The occasional heron's soaring across the lake. A bull moose drinking at water's edge. Minnows and baby catfish. Frogs and toads bouncing along the beach and through the tall grass. Chipmunks circling the cabin for food. Nine mice inside the cabin. Red squirrels outside. One ambitious flying squirrel swimming from one side of the lake to the other. Down the beach off a swamp, big gray bloodsuckers that James liked to stick to his fingers. Turtles so numerous that one had difficulty not stepping on them. Clams by the thousands, trekking along the bed of shallow water. Bull frogs among the lily pads, their croaks counter-pointing with high pitched crickets, and alto loons calling aloud each evening.

— • —

Evenings led to nights and, with children asleep, Maria and I would look out from the porch over the sky's trillions of constellations. With nighttime sex a non-issue thanks to the traumatic brain injury, Maria and I would sit listening to the frog-led symphony, eyeing the odd firefly and looking at the stars coming down to touch the horizon.

"Maria, I pray what we are seeing, hearing and breathing will be here for James and Robert and other children, for thousands of years to come."

"Is it possible, Alan?"

"I don't know, Maria. I think freedom is becoming equated with the profit motive. Unbridled capitalism behaves like electricity—always taking the shortest route."

"I have heard this defended by people who claim that self-gratifying behavior is always the best option for optimizing the well-being of the most. Was Adam Smith right?"

"Smith, like the Bible, seems more quoted than read. Adam Smith was not the intellectual champion of self-interest. He saw in it, not virtue but danger. He tried to rationalize how the drive could be tied to social good and believed that fair competition held self-interest in check. Smith, I think would view modern man as one who has created governments that paralyze the 'invisible hand' with collectives, unwarranted aid and bureaucratic plans."

"As the Soviet Union has shown us fail?"

"As all governments of all countries have us shown fail. Modern so-called free enterprise is dominated not by thousands of check-countercheck little producers as perhaps it once was. It is driven by a small number of massive corporations and trade union monopolies, and favors are dished out in line with prejudices as if they cost nothing."

We were communicating. I did not and perhaps could not, stop to think that what I kept finding wrong with Maria was all post-injury, as were all clashes with her family. Maybe my not giving Maria the benefit of the doubt, post-injury had more to do with what Doctor Fisher had tried to tell her, "He can't help it! His personality is changed."

— • —

The second night at Round Lake still found my need to talk.

"... My brain is damaged, Maria."

"Yes, but the pre-damage foundation abounds with information."

"Maria, *your* foundation abounds with kindness. I love you."

I kissed her with my brain-dead lips and got all I could ask for in a kiss.

"We are watching the Soviet Union fall apart but how about Canada?" she asked. "If free trade comes to pass, will we become Americans with their extremes of wealth and poverty?"

"The social conscience does appear here more developed and there are safety nets that some Americans label socialist, but let's be fair. We've taken James and Robert to Point Pelee, Ontario where we have read of the massacre of virgin trees in only 10 years."

"But Alan, that massacre was 100 years ago."

"True, but Alberta's selling timber rights on a parcel of land bigger than Britain is today. Thousand year-old redwoods being buzz-sawed down in Canada is today. Not all Americans think 'liberal' a dirty word. Some don't believe in guns or capital punishment.

Maria, I don't know where Canada will go. I like its unwillingness to live with a massive portion of its people in an abject underclass. I like its controls on guns, lower crime, lower litigiousness and its making illegal, the striking of children in public. I love Canada."

— • —


The next Round lake evening saw me pontificating again.

"No one's perfect, Maria."

"Except you say, God?"

"No one."

"Including God?"

"God, as our son James says, must be very tired, working for billions of years to help us."

"Can we not have truth?"

"Absolute truth?"

"In some things? Wealthy people seem to have it all figured out."

"I respectfully submit that those rich of whom you speak cannot know, for they do not plumb such depths in their thinking. Absolutism is a finite limitation imposed upon the human mind by its inability to go beyond its humanness and grasp those things that go beyond those limits."

— • —

Night 4 and my rambling mega-bites from an injured brain took the floor again.

"Alan, you promised once you would tell me of a man named Servetus."

"A 24-year-old Spanish doctor who saw through Jean Cauvin."

"Jean Cauvin?"

"His real name. He changed it to James Calvin as part of his marketing himself in Geneva. When Cauvin achieved power, Servetus wrote to him from Spain, pseudonymous letters, criticizing his messages and exposing Cauvin's scam. The tragic flaw of Servetus then drove him closer to Geneva and he began dropping the pseudonym. Cauvin paid his critic Servetus the ultimate compliment by having him killed."

"Sounds like someone I know."

Again, a rare discretion, post-injury, caught me in check and I let the issue drop.

Next evening, I snatched once more the stage. Maria asked my thoughts on prayer.

"We may feel something from it but we don't know, in fact we can't, but keep on praying to a being we believe beyond ourselves. I confess I pray."

"To your imperfect God?"

"Yes, imperfect. So-called divine creation is for me a quick fix to the question 'What was here first?' And the fix comes to us translated from generation after generation of interpretation. Language and liturgy should not evolve into worshipped traditions, memorized, and regurgitated. Language and liturgy should instead be seen as part of a system of models which led institutions of the past. Our task should be to study the old models, glean from them the guiding principles and see the bells and whistles as just that.

## Genuine Canadian Hosers

The following day brought terror to Round Lake. Into the crown land, 1000 yards west of our family, rammed a 4-wheel drive van, full of men in their early 20s. They were loud and sounded drunk upon their noon arrival, and their van crushed all in its path. The young men sat down at the end of the long beach and began guzzling beer, hurling empty bottles against some of the lake's rocks above the surface. Glass exploded into the air and scattered all across the water.

James and Robert stayed in my arms, off the beach and in the cabin porch. We could not quite see the hosers but listened with horror, with the nearest police station over 50 miles away.

"Why are they destroying nature that way, Daddy? I don't understand."

"Nor do I, Robert. I don't think I can."

"Will they hurt us, Daddy?"

Dusk came and the hosers began howling that the "fuckin'

muskitas" were too much. They crushed their way back over the swamp to the dirt road and departed, drunk.

"J and R, I'm afraid you'll have to stay away from the lily pads and bloodsuckers. You may cut your feet badly if you go down the beach to the swamp."

"For the rest of our time here, Daddy?"

---

## There Was No Time When

It was too late. With help from the hosers, my fire was reignited. On that still summer evening with James and Robert asleep, without any prompt, I began.

"I don't believe for a moment, Maria, that there are good and bad people. Some seem born deranged and if that derangement is true, it is not their fault. Some come from brutal childhoods and get misdirected. Many now in these 1980s live brain injured and their acts often bear no sense to a structured world. Those born, bred or made impaired are brothers and sisters of us all, and we owe to them tolerance and compassion."

Maria nodded.

"Wars are testimonials to people's misdirection. Prisons are monuments to peoples' desire to shut out of sight, those souls who cannot find for the moment, any productive reason for being. We owe all living things a chance to make a fruitful contribution. Jails are costly and to anyone looking on from another planet, must appear comical. We don't see ants killing or hurting one another for something to do—they're too busy being productive. We don't see healthy dogs doing anything other than trying to help and be friends. We don't see whales often, but when we do, we usually see something positive.

If we human beings are so damn smart, then why are we wearing trinkets or dickering with guns over diamonds? We live on this planet right now in danger of losing its trees, drinkable water and oxygen, but when someone of huge help comes along, be he Dostoevsky, Maimonides, Jimmy Carter or Gorbachev, we go out of our way to find in him those failings that we all could have. We house prisoners for $70,000 per year in walls of concrete. Revenge has blinded us. Given half a chance, those imprisoned could feel the rehabilitating effects of contributing something to us all."

My broken brain fragmented further when fatigued.

"Maria, today's toleration of conventional painting alarms me more than the alarm that conventionalists had 100 years ago, when they exiled the works of impressionists."

Maria too became alarmed. She stood up and stared down at me. She had witnessed me before, building into such self-presumed vision. I spouted on.

"Maria, you're a social worker. Did you know that Americans created in 1924, because of a supposed Red scare, the Jameson-Reed Act which cut Jewish immigration? Did you know that we Canadians closed our door to Jews in 1933 and opened them only slightly again in 1948? That we turned back boats of Jews fleeing from fascist-dominated Europe, sending them back across the Atlantic to certain death?"

I got worse and soon was left to torture the night alone in the stillness of Round Lake.

## Blake

Nearing 9:00 at night on our final day at Lake Kawawaymog, my eyes could not leave a patch of cloud, silhouetted in the southwest sky. Behind the cloud was a pinkish color, coming from a sinking sun.

"Maria, I want to take a photograph of the cloud, the tall pines to the side and a hint of the lake."

"You will have to love mosquitoes."

With our old Leica and fast lens, I tried the photo. The moon was full but the fast lens still took a total second. I was stippled in fly bites but got the shot.

"Blake's clarity, Alan?"

Maria smiled at me, a smile I had long dared not look at.

On our last night, with James and Robert asleep in the 60° Fahrenheit and air whishing in through the open screens, Maria and I did the near impossible and for a few seconds, made love.

## On the Drive, 200 Miles Back to Toronto

"Maria, if I am a racist by my so saying, then so be it. I have never met a New Zealander I did not like and I am not sure why. New Zealanders seem to have cultivated out of a land blessed by remoteness, some group conscience. Icelandic people tell me they have a sense of responsibility derived from remoteness but New Zealanders have not. Are their doors closed? I think instead their windows are open. Iceland I would love to photograph but New Zealand I would love to go to with you, James and Robert, and hike across its hills, listening where we can to its people."

God, I was full of bombast but that's the way it was. I wanted to believe that my wish to go to New Zealand stemmed not from a want to find a pure land but from some lust for freedom. In the rear seats of our old Volvo, James and Robert were sound asleep and I would not stop but blurted further onto an unrelated tangent, finding a catharsis in words, places and knowledge all known to me, pre-injury.

"I'm an Ontario boy. Algonquin Park. Point Pelee ... The

1,000 Islands ... Temagami's ancient trees ... Tobermory's under-water park. Powwows on Manitoulin Island ... The northern ridge of Lake Superior. Lake of the Woods ... Ottawa. Historic Kingston. Prince Edward County. Mennonite country. Niagara-on-the-lake. Stratford ... Kleinburg's Group of Seven ... Ward's Island. The Toronto zoo, museum, art gallery. Toronto's mosaic. And U. of T.'s Hart House."

# SEPTEMBER 1987

The heat lessened and I felt myself in gentler weather, finding solace counseling others in my new junior job. Up to that point almost 6 years after my brain injury, I had given little thought to financial compensation for my broken brain. The lawyer for Maria and me was that Gordon Dour, a drinker who would later quit drinking. Dour had doubted me from the beginning. All specialists' medical reports, moreover, had been set up, funneled and filtered through the poisoned Dr. Steve Jensen. The only contributions Dour had made to Maria and me in the 6 years post-accident were to slap me with horrendous bills and to miss the statute of limitations cut-off date for filing a request for compensation to Maria.

Dour had to have a triple by-pass and the case was transferred to a snappy, young lawyer, Adam Stone. Stone wanted me seen again by a host of specialists—a neurosurgeon not connected with Flanders, a likewise unconnected endocrinologist and most important of all, without interference from Jensen, the Flanders' neuropsychologist, Gary Winter. Dr. Winter had, after Jensen's secret and vindictive input, sabotaged a battery of tests done on me in June of 1983.

Dr. Winter now in 1987 refused, and jacked up his fee to scare off Stone, but Stone said "yes" provided Winter himself did the tests. Winter knew that his assistant, Ellen Little, had with his backroom help, performed the sabotaged and unsigned 1983 battery.

I witnessed Dr. Winter's face change as he and I then went through the exhaustive 7-hour battery of neuropsychological testing. His face went from one of cynicism at the outset, through shock to shame. Using tests I had never been allowed to have, Winter found the multiple brain deficits and their permanency.

"In hindsight, Mr. Cooper, I'm glad you came in," was all he would first say upon the test's completion. He sent his report to Stone, confirming my permanent brain damage, contradicting the first one he had been reluctant to release and had finally released unsigned. Winter made no mention of the first test's false claims that I had fallen down drunk and sustained several head injuries, but as a camouflage of his earlier sanctioned lies, Winter made much in his 1987 report of an emotional overlay which I purportedly had, out of proportion to my cognitive impairments. He seemed to know little of the diffuse nature of my broader brain injury, and would not confirm where he had sourced his "overlay" information. He merely said he had taken it from his old notes.

— • —

A neurosurgeon Clive Day, not from Flanders Hospital, also found the many areas of brain deficit, in fact more—his 1987 CT scan showed not only the hematoma to my left frontal lobe but also the permanent swelling of key ventricles in the back of my brain. The Dr. Day-ordered CT scan also showed that the whole brain had been shaken and torn.

Dr. Winter and Dr. Day confirmed to me both the permanency of my brain damage and the high scores in my remaining brain. Each told me I would never again perform at my previous executive levels and each told me of the predictable addictions I had experienced post brain injury, saying my combatants to addiction had also been injured. Each further told me of my personality being rewired to greater self-centeredness, anger, sour humor, indecisiveness and sporadic volatility. They had seen such cases before.

My cry, now, was not because of new facts revealed to me, but because medical specialists now free to inspect without Jensen, had found what I had felt but could not express, for 6 years.

## St. Andrew Hospital's Head Neurosurgeon, Dr. Day's Report, November 2, 1987

Neurosurgeon/neurologist/psychiatrist Clive Day's report was pages of small type, confirming much of what I had thought. When I read it, I was reminded of my taking hormone shots. They had been administered by the endocrinologist who had discovered both decreased testosterone levels and below-norm levels of sexual release hormones, both resulting in decreased libido and potency. The Day report substantiated areas unknown to laypeople, medical generalists and neo-specialists. Here is what it said.

> His basic intelligence appeared to be considerably above average. There was no formal thought disorder and sensorium was clear...He was able to read a newspaper paragraph (in front of Dr. Day) but he frequently slurred the speech and he misread several words...He did not grasp the meaning (and said that when reading, he highlighted in yellow highlighter pen key points, then collated them into a précis, then high-lighted the précis, filed it in succinctly entitled files, then cross-referenced the titles to his permanently-with-him black book)... Sense of smell was diminished to 4 test odors and he could detect them only in an indistinct manner...The face was considerably spastic with a snout reflex and there was a left palmo-mental reflex...Dr. Michael Fisher examined him 78 times psychiatrically and described the details of his personal history, exceptional school record, athletic and leadership skills and other abilities, such as public oratory, vocal and instrumental music, during his lower and higher education years...He had, from all the evidence, developed transient diabetes insipidus as well as depression...Personality testing had been done in December of 1984 and a diagnosis of narcissistic personality and incipient psychosis, requiring

immediate emergency treatment and mind-altering drugs was recommended. His superior intelligence had been noted at that time, though he'd had difficulty defining words, and problem-solving had been poor.

At the time of the accident of December 27th 1981, he suffered a closed head injury with concussion followed by confusion, agitated behavior with post-traumatic amnesia of over 24 hours duration. A CT scan 3 days later revealed left frontal lobe contusion with an intracerebral hematoma of about one centimeter diameter surrounded by edema. He also suffered a fracture of the left clavicle as well as musculoskeletal strain involving predominantly the neck and shoulder and a laceration about the left eye. Symptoms of increased thirst and urination (polydipsia and polyuria), speech and memory difficulties, numbness of the upper extremities and mouth, loss of taste and smell, impaired balance, insomnia, depression and irritability, impotence, developed after the accident and he has received out-patient psychiatric care since October 1982; post-firing in January 1985, he began drinking heavily with increased bouts at times until November. He encountered extreme difficulties in trying to return to his high level executive work and he has not, since January 1985, been able to continue with this. His continuing symptoms are those of forgetfulness, difficulty with new learning, slow and hesitant speech, difficulty with word finding, with misnaming and mispronunciation. His impairment is such that he requires copious note-taking, indexing and his writing has changed. He has neck pain, impairment of coordination, numbness of the lips and palate, diminished taste sensation, diminished energy, occasional dizziness, loss of libido, depression, anxiety, irritability and associated difficulties. My examination reveals hesitant and slurred speech, misnaming, reading impairment, memory difficulties and abnormal facial reflexes (spastic face with pout reflex) and a left palmo-mental reflex. There is mild incoordination on heel-to-shin testing and sense of smell is diminished with diminished sensation of the inner aspects of the lips, palate and tongue. Mental status examination revealed a serious, worried, somewhat pedantic patient with slowness of speech, who describes considerable depression and anxiety.

A further finding during my examination was that of diminished sensation over the palate and inner aspect of the lip and anterior of the tongue to pinprick.

He does have limitation of neck movement on rotation to the left with local muscle tenderness. I understand that cervical x-rays are within normal limits. He appears to have suffered a relatively severe cervical strain at the time of the accident. He has received unusually prolonged physiotherapy and in my opinion, this could now be discontinued. He should receive gentle massage to the neck muscles and he should attempt to move his neck regularly through a full range of movement short of significant pain. He will probably be left with residual neck symptoms as a result of the accident and musculoskeletal strain.

He describes a complete loss of smell and taste for several months following the accident and there has been a partial return. The sense of taste is largely mediated through the sense of smell (olfactory nerve) and my examination reveals diminished smell sensation to multiple test odors. This is on the basis of damage to the first cranial nerve (olfactory nerve) at the time of the accident and brain injury. This diminution of smell and taste sensation is of a permanent type.

He describes diminished sensation of the lips, palate, tongue and mouth since the accident and there is some reduction on testing. This symptom is somewhat unusual and it could be on the basis of trigeminal nerve injury involving elements of the second and third division, at the time of the accident without any abnormality of facial sensation. Regardless of the exact basis of this sensory disturbance, the changes are of a permanent type, as a residuum of the accident and closed head injury.

His history does indicate polydipsia and polyuria which

developed immediately after the accident. Extensive endocrino-logical investigation 2 years later did not reveal any continuing abnormality but it is reasonable to conclude that he suffered post-traumatic and somewhat prolonged polydipsia and polyuria on the basis of hypothalamic injury as a result of the accident. This appears to have subsided and the residual increased urination that he describes as on a far lesser scale is probably relatable to anxiety.

He did suffer concussion with cerebral contusion (bruising) and a hematoma (blood clot) within the left frontal lobe of his dominant hemisphere. A recent follow-up CT scan revealed mild ventricular enlargement involving especially the lateral and third ventricles, confirming that he has suffered post-traumatic cerebral atrophy of a more generalized type, following the accident, in addition to localized frontal lobe injury. Symptoms of memory and speech impairment, difficulty with learning and a loss of his former superior abilities involving general intelligence, creativity, energy, capacity for wit and articulate speech and associated functions are on the basis of permanent brain damage and significant intellectual impairment. His motor coordination has also been permanently impaired as a result of the brain injury, on the basis of either cerebral or cerebellar damage such that he is no longer capable of his former sports activities. He has also developed organic type personality change with diminished energy, loss of interest, irritability, anxiety, social withdrawal attributable to the brain injury; there is also an associated depression and a significant component of the emotional symptoms appear to be of a reactive type, arising out of his awareness of his diminished abilities and out of his continuing difficulties and frustrations.

As a result of the accident and injuries, he was completely disabled over the next weeks and he returned to part-time work in early February 1982 and then to full-time work. His work appears to have required a high level of intellectual, administrative and associated abilities and the effects of the brain injury interfered with this in a substantial manner. He found it difficult to cope with his work and the intellectual, emotional and personality changes attributable to the brain injury did substantially interfere with his judgment and actions over the next months and years. His altered behavior and irritability appear to have substantially contributed to marital breakdown, and symptoms of insomnia and associated difficulties appear to have led to heavy drinking and eventual alcoholism such that he has since joined Alcoholics Anonymous. Because of these intellectual, personality and emotional changes, he was not able to persist in his former type executive work and he was repeatedly fired.

The residual impairments of intelligence, memory, speech and the personality and emotional changes are such that in my opinion, he will no longer be able to function at an executive level and he appears to be prepared to accept this. His capacity for sustained work at a lower level has not been proven as yet. A significant degree of depression and anxiety will probably continue as a permanent emotional effect of the accident and residual impairments. Some patients of superior ability and occupational status and who have suffered permanent brain damage are able to adjust to a career at a substantially lower level involving routine, repetitive, non-stressful activities and it is hoped this will occur here. He will probably require long term psychiatric treatment over the next 2 to 3 years. He will remain vulnerable to emotional illness in the future and will continue to require psychiatric treatment. As a result of the brain damage, he remains at risk for the occurrence of post-traumatic epilepsy in the future and I would estimate this likelihood to be at about the 5 % level.

Yours sincerely,
Dr. Clive Day

## Late Fall of '87

Lawyer Dour's replacement, Stone, was hot to trot on what he felt to be a rock solid case but I was not. I felt no hate for the cognitively challenged Barry Lewis who had hit me. His car was not his own but that of his estranged wife, and Lewis did not even know if he were married. I guess I should have hated his wife's Regal Insurance, the facility insurance company that regularly charged exorbitant premiums to people with bad driving records. Unbeknownst to Regal's hired lawyer, Gauze—reputedly Toronto's best for handling brain injury claims—Regal had employed a detective to spy on my every movement across those 6 years. Regal's CEO, Mr. Shooter seemed worthy of his name.

In November 1987, Stone pressured a reluctant me to document the nasty goings-on of Regal's detective work. Opposing lawyer Gauze had promised such goings-on would not happen, because this type of detective work would further expose the cold truth of my car accident and related brain damage.

Stone also pressured me to describe in detail the ugliness of the 6 years post-brain injury, dredging up the awful facts and forcing me to live through them again. I had not the wish, nor did I feel the ability, to recite the details. I knew they would not be confused or blurred, because my memory of them was not confused or blurred. My post-accident memory of those events was of a different sort, episodic, and stored in large impressions. My brain's bank retained key post-accident incidents, because those post-accident events were of such magnitude as to have changed my life. I had also written the incidents down on innumerable pads of 8 1/2" x 11" paper and had kept them meticulously filed, for whatever conscious reason I did not know.

## Something Was Rotten …
## G.P. Dr. Steve Jensen

After Stone sent me Day's clinical report, Stone again pressed me to write of my last 6 years' experience. I refused until November 10th 1987, when I received from Stone a report by Dr. Steve Jensen. Jensen was the G.P. who had told Maria that he was doing all he could to help but that neurosurgeon Mark Schwantz "hated Alan's guts and between Alan and Dr. Schwantz, there had been a total breakdown in doctor-patient relationship." There had been no such breakdown, at all.

Jensen had pressured me to leave the Food Ministry, saying that I needed to get back to doing some real work "away from all those useless silly servants." Jensen had also pushed me to get my hearing checked post-accident, knowing full well of my previous hearing impairment. The hearing specialist, Dr. Fent, had been unable to find my old file but I had insisted on relaying my earlier impairment. Jensen had later chastised me, when I had reported back that I had told the specialist of being checked years earlier by him.

Jensen had urged me to go to a second Flanders neuropsychiatrist, after Jensen had discovered that neurosurgeon Schwantz had bypassed him and written directly to my lawyer Dour. It was Jensen who had prejudiced neuropsychologist Dr. Gary Winter, before Dr. Winter had greeted me on the phone with extreme hostility about his doing a battery of neuropsychological tests.

I had begun sensing by 1983-84 the prejudiced Jensen input, when I had met the second neurosurgeon at Flanders and in the first 10 minutes, he had echoed Jensen's lecture that I should settle the lawsuit as soon as possible "since it was the cause of my anxiety." Years later, after I had abandoned G.P. Dr. Jensen, he had telephoned me to say that his lawyer brother was a close neighbor of mine and had been keeping an eye on me. Whether there was a bribe laundered through Dr. Jensen's lawyer brother, I do not know nor do I know of any other Jensen motive. Perhaps the opposing hired psychiatrist Dr. Malthrop had tricked all professionals into thinking at the start that he and the opposing legal side had been working for me, while I had still been in intensive care.

At one point in a 1983 check-up on me, G.P. Dr. Jensen had paused and whispered that my pupils were of 2 different sizes, indicating he had said a severe brain injury, but he had then followed with a quick note that my ribcage was asymmetrical and had abandoned the pupil size issue.

In November 1987, Jensen finally dropped his mask and revealed in writing to Stone what he had hypocritically hidden for 6 years— his poisoning of all inputs to and outputs from, Flanders Hospital and other specialists. G.P. Jensen's lying letter about me to Stone re-ignited an indignation that I had for reasons of survival, shelved into the recesses of my mind. Before I assented to Stone's request for my flushing out all of the 6 years post-accident, I had to respond to the lying letter by G.P. Dr. Steve Jensen.

---

Mr. Adam Stone:

November 14, 1987

RE: DR JENSEN'S REPORT TO YOU, NOVEMBER 7 1987

Mr. Jensen's report is a wildly distorted mix of 1/2-truths, 1/4-truths and outright untruths. It seems designed to paint as negative a picture of Alan Cooper as is possible. It betrays Dr. Jensen's hypocrisy in the final sentence, "… so I trust this brief factual account will assist Alan in his endeavor to seek compensation."

It is a fact that Dr. Jensen had said he doubted there was anything wrong with me as a result of the car accident, that I was trying to capitalize on a lawsuit and for the sake of my health, I should "take the first offer." Dr. Jensen had also told me that if the other side wanted to win the lawsuit, "All it would have to do is put me in the witness box, since my personality would turn off everybody in the courtroom."

Dr. Jensen's malevolent thoughts and behavior for at least a year after the accident, in fact for all of 1982 and 1983, were unthinkable to me. I had not understood Dr. Jensen's summarily dismissing all psychiatrists as "bullshit artists for the weak-filled" when I had told Dr. Jensen about my beginning to see Dr. Fisher. By contrast, neuropsychologist Dr. Winter told me this autumn of 1987 that I was to be commended for having sought out and continued with a psychiatrist, after the type of brain injury I had sustained.

SPECIFIC COMMENTS ON FALSEHOODS IN DR. JENSEN'S REPORT

1. I did not advise Dr. Jensen "...in 1983 (or at any other time) that an out-of-court settlement had been reached."

2. I did have a motor vehicle accident (MVA) in September 1969. I did not, as Dr. Jensen states, have a head injury nor did I have any head injury problems beyond being momentarily knocked out. The injury was to a transverse lumbar in my back.

3. I did not have a "...peptic ulcer due primarily to excessive alcohol intake and prostatitis." I never had a peptic ulcer reported to me at all. It was esophagitis caused by a hiatus hernia that I had sustained at the age of 16 in gymnastics in high school (a virtual carbon copy of the same affliction and circumstances that my 83-year-old father has had since he sustained a hiatus hernia at the age of 16 in high school gymnastics).

Alcohol had never been earlier mentioned to me by my G.P. nor did I drink excessively pre-injury. In fact, like most of my working colleagues, I got drunk 3–4 times a year at Marketing/Sales social blowouts. Coffee had been the main problem in aggravating my esophagitis caused by the hernia. My prostatitis was diagnosed pre-marriage in 1974 as being caused by pre-marital "feast or famine" type sexual intercourse.

4.   Jensen was not the one as he so claims, instrumental in arranging my "… transfer from North Bay to Flanders Hospital." Maria and North Bay G.P. Dr. Laird were.

5.   G.P. Jensen is, as has been indirectly confirmed to me by Dr. Gary Winter, and I began to suspect with horror in 1983, the medical doctor who negatively prejudiced every specialist he talked to, before I met them. That upfront prejudice now makes clear why nueropsychologist Dr. Winter had been so negative on the phone to me when I had tried in 1983 to set up neuropsychological tests with him, why he had tried to talk me out of having the tests done, why Dr. Winter had not administered the tests, why his assistant Ellen Little was constantly on the phone throughout the tests and wanted me out of her office not to hear, why Ms. Little herself was hostile to me and even tried to talk me out of doing the tests on the day I arrived for them, why the results of the tests bore some outrageous untruths about my then drinking and falling down drunk and sustaining head injuries, why the test report was so long in its wait for completion, why the test report was not signed by either Dr. Winter or Ms. Little and why the long-awaited report finally appeared to be written in such way as to be sabotaged so that it could not be used by my lawyer in court.

In fact, Dr. Jensen later told me that neurosurgeon Dr. Mark Schwantz had told Dr. Jensen the report was written in such a way so as not to be any good to my lawyer. Why, because of all the aforementioned acts, my lawyer felt it necessary to repeat a battery of psychological tests with Dr. Kellerman, who told me at the outset that he could not understand why he, Dr. Kellerman was being asked to repeat on me tests that his "...highly respected colleague Gary Winter (had) already carried out. (Was I) not happy with Gary Winter's results?" was Dr. Kellerman's prejudiced question to me.

Concerning my neurosurgeon Dr. Schwantz, with whom I had always seemed to have a normal doctor-patient relationship, Dr. Jensen told Maria in 1982 that Dr. Schwantz "hated Alan's guts" and that between Alan and Dr. Schwantz, "The relationship had experienced a complete client-patient breakdown." At that time, when Maria had seen Dr. Jensen to discuss Alan's post-accident handicaps and severe depression, Jensen had spent the bulk of the time talking and had concluded with the cutting comment to an upset Maria, "Well, Napoleon had his Josephine."

6. I set up, at Jensen's urging and logistical help, a second neurological opinion by Dr. Maul at Flanders. Jensen seemed particularly anxious to have me see Dr. Maul after Jensen heard from me that my lawyer had received a satisfactory report (which I had not seen) from Dr. Schwantz. When I saw Dr. Maul who'd had by then the prejudices of Jensen as well as the malevolently produced neuropsychological report, Dr. Maul told me in the first 10 minutes that I was obviously doing well in my job. He furthered that I should settle the lawsuit as soon as possible for the sake of my own health, since litigious greed and related anxiety were seriously affecting my health.

Later, when I saw Sunnybrook endocrinologist Dr. Fuller, Fuller told me that Dr. Maul had told Dr. Fuller "...that (my) problems were anxiety related."

7. Dr. Steve Jensen poisoned the thinking of the specialists before I walked into the specialists' offices. His poison, whose strain runs so rampantly through his November 10, 1987 report to you, prejudiced at very least the following doctors:

Dentist Dr. Will
(Whom I saw about my
'dead' lips and palate,
but after his hour 'briefing'
by Jensen.)

Psychologist Winter

Neurosurgeon Maul

Assistant
Little

Psychologist
Kellerman

Endocrinologist
Fuller

8.   Dr. Jensen is writing outrageous falsehoods in saying that the following "...traits had been present at times prior to the accident"

A.     Depression
B.     Alcoholism
C.     Impotency
D.     Indecisiveness
E.     Loss of Intellectual Function

A. Depression; B. Alcoholism. In May 1982 I marched into Dr. Jensen's office and told him I had been drunk 4 times in April. He looked at me with moral condemnation and asked if "my lady friend" had forced me to "come clean to him." When I said "No," Dr. Jensen said he liked "...to get into it on the weekends" but kept off it for the most part during the week. Jensen told me that he didn't believe in addiction programs like the Donwood Center and that the only solution for me was my own will power. Jensen went on to tell me that "all alcoholics are cheap," and he often recommended to them that they buy "more expensive stuff," to drain their supply. Dr. Jensen then quipped about the new and severe memory, recall and word-finding difficulties I'd been having post-accident—"That's the alcohol." Dr. Jensen then did not listen when I said I had only started drinking post-accident in April, coincident with my beginning to feel the brain damage permanent, and that I had drunk only 4 times.

After that May '82 meeting with Jensen, I stopped drinking entirely for over 2 months until I began in August my quasi-medicinal use of 750 ml of red wine with 750 ml. of water, before going off to sleep for 6–7 hours every night.

I saw Jensen again at the end of 1982 and he then said that while most people don't say they're alcoholics until long after developing the illness if at all, I had been premature in saying I was one, based on my non-difficulty in stopping completely and moderating thereafter. Dr. Steve Jensen admitted to not believing earlier my getting drunk only the 4 times in April, because he expressed surprise at my not having done the kind of liver damage that would have required years of abuse.

C. Impotence. It's false to say that I'd had this problem pre-accident. Prostatitis yes, but that was quickly eradicated. Impotence no. I complained to Jensen of it in 1982 and he asked me in rough tone if I got "piss hards" (later, I found out that the proper term is "nocturnal erections"). When I said I wasn't sure, post-accident, Jensen did not listen and sharply replied, "Well, if you get a piss hard, there's nothing wrong."

D. Jensen is false in saying my indecisiveness was a major problem pre-accident. And he would not have known.

E. Loss of intellectual function, pre-accident. Jensen is making another false statement. Again, 100% so.

9. Dr. Steve Jensen has tried to contact me at least twice since I fired him in 1983—once, when he reached me at Blimiss Hope and he said he'd been visiting his brother, a neighbor of mine, and had not seen me for a long time; the second time occurred in 1986 when Jensen reached my wife and asked Maria who my new G.P. was, so that Jensen could transfer his file and give the new G.P. relevant input on Alan.

SUMMARY

Dr. Steve Jensen, with initiative and malice of intent, has attempted to paint as bad a picture as he can of his patient Alan Cooper as input to every medical specialist. Had it not been for Dr. Steve Jensen, Dr. Gary Winter would in all likelihood have found Alan Cooper's permanent brain damage over 5 years ago, Dr. Kellerman's report and tests would never have been done and I would not have been put through either the extreme anxiety around a job change (which Dr. Winter now confirms I can not do as a result of the brain injury) or the horrendous torture of almost 2 years of exhaustive work at Blimiss Hope, the subsequent firing and despair which set in, January of 1985 and has remained to a greater or lesser degree, ever since.

'Dr.' Jensen has exhibited both real and extreme cruelty in his viciousness, continued premeditation, self-righteousness and blind prejudice. He has almost completely destroyed a human life as well the lives of his loved ones.

*Alan J Cooper*

## I Tried to Write to Stone

From November 14 to December 27, 1987, I wrote an 81-page document. The last of the 81 pages read as follows.

As I complete this note, it is approaching the 44th day that I have been trying to write. I am plagued by bad recall, with my having to leave blank spaces to fill in later from my mountains of post-accident notes. This note itself is one that I could have produced pre-accident in only a few days, not 7 weeks.

I guess I'm a far cry from the person who in 1968 was invited by University of Toronto religious studies professor Marty Freeman to attend Harvard for a year on scholarship and study various Judeo-Christian religions, leading into the profession of church minister or rabbi in a denomination of my choice. Or the Alan Cooper who through his own initiative, wrote a fiction novel on architecture and sang full-time in the exhaustive timetable of the Mendelssohn Choir, right up to the time of the car accident. I had even begun work on a second novel in the year preceding the car accident, the first having been really a self-test to see if I could write one.

The car accident and brain injury stopped all that with a giant thud. My balance is now so bad that if I did one ring around a rosy with my 2 toddlers, I would get dizzy for minutes. The brain damage is more extensive, as confirmed by Saint Andrew Hospital's neuropsychiatrist Dr. Day, who saw me this autumn. (Because of my poor recall, I forgot to tell Dr. Day of my differently sized pupils post-car accident or my viscous saliva post-car accident, still existing to this moment.)

Maria and I have never been allowed to heal but instead, we have been attacked with lies and half-truths, particularly those from G.P. Dr. Steve Jensen.

I have to fight to keep any kind of faith in humankind and I have now seen so much ugly human behavior that I have depression rushing in and shrouding my mind 4 or 5 times per week. But I will be damned before I let these misdirected people complete the destruction of Alan Cooper, begun by the December 27, 1981 car accident. I love my wife and I love my children deeply, and I won't let anyone further destroy their loving husband and father.

*Alan J Cooper*
December 27, 1987

## A Point of Clarity With Stone in His Office

Alan: "Adam, as you are aware from your notes and talks with partner Gordon Dour, I was forced to undergo yet another battery of neuro-psychological tests for the Central Trust job. As you know, Central Trust probed me about my car accident and insisted on seeing the results of any neurological tests but your partner Mr. Dour refused. Central Trust then made a job offer to me, conditional upon a battery that it volunteered to fund.

Central Trust found a psychologist to do a quick job on me. As you know, finding *psychologists* to work for money these days is easy, because the Ontario Government has not allowed their bills to be 100% covered by subsidized health as it has *psychiatrists*.

I met Dr. Pin one evening in July of 1986 and was forthright with him about my perceived deficiencies. After 20 minutes, Pin replied, 'Well, I don't want to stop your getting this job.' Pin then studiously avoided giving me tests where I told him my cognitive deficiencies would surface. As for personality testing, Pin himself filled in the multiple choice answer cards, while I gave quick answers. The parody was completed and I departed in 2 hours. Dr. Pin wanted to go home after what he described as a hard day and Central Trust wanted the results the next day, so that I could start work the week after. Adam, neither you nor I nor Mr. Dour were ever informed of Dr. Pin's test results. We only know Central Trust offered me the job. I did not query Central Trust nor did Mr. Dour."

Lawyer Adam Stone looked at me, shrugged a response

and assured me that if the Dr. Pin tests surfaced, they would be dismissed "as another aberration."

Stone then chose not to furnish opposing lawyer Gauze with either the fact of Dr. Pin's tests or the results, which no one but Pin and Central Trust had ever seen. The issue was dropped.

# FORCED TO GO TO COURT

Stone stood proud. He had taken my 81-page note to Jensen and returned beaming. In Stone's law firm lobby, he shouted out when greeting me, "Jensen has come around." Stone did not think to realize that with all the Jensen-prejudiced tests now in, the worst possible scenario was to have it appear that Jensen was now supporting Alan. Litigation lawyer Adam Stone fell for the bait hook, line and sinker.

By happenstance, I was helping via free career counseling, to secure a job for Tommy Naples, a childhood friend who had gone on to become both a psychologist and lawyer. Tommy got wind of my case and saw Stone of his own volition. Tommy then told me that my lawyer Stone had a weak understanding of traumatic brain injuries.

While still refusing to admit liability, late on Friday January 13th 1988, the opposition's Gauze offered Stone a sum without legal costs of $200,000. It was less than Stone had spent to that moment and was offered late in the eyes of the law, in fact less than one workday before the 10:00 a.m. start of trial in an Ontario Supreme Court on Monday, January 16th.

Thanks to Maria's false description of the car accident, Stone's predecessor Dour had never bothered to find out how the car accident had actually happened. Opposing lawyer Gauze, whom Dour said had a nose for finding weak spots, had smelled an opportunity not to admit liability. Only in month 2 of the trial and after thousands spent by Stone to track down accident reports and witnesses, would my description of the accident prove 100% right and Maria's 100% wrong. Gauze would then admit liability.

Regal Insurance and opposing lawyer Gauze claimed I was malingering for money but the idea was preposterous. When I heard it, I had difficulty not believing it to be the standard statement of Gauze the hardened lawyer who knew otherwise. Stone told me that Regal Insurance and Gauze had spent vast quantities of money to ensure that Regal's impressive win-loss record would remain intact and that no person of residual intelligence could substantiate a claim of permanent brain damage. The issue was critical to the entire insurance industry, because if it could be shown that brain-injured people could still be intelligent but non-uniformly so, actuaries would have determined that there was no telling where future claims in North America could go.

Nanette Carter was an Ontario Supreme Court Judge who had been a real estate lawyer but whose father had been a senator and Stone told me she got her job through patronage. Adam Stone was the fast-tongued man who had confided to others, his own previous personality problems with the Judge, but did not tell me about them until he relayed the Judge's question as to why I had not finished my MBA. Stone then did not listen to my saying I had never been enrolled in an MBA. The opposition's Gauze was a man of empathetic age with 60ish Carter and knew how to milk her prejudices. As Gauze may have guessed, Judge Carter's mind could not grasp the nuances of inconsistent intelligence contained within a brain, still bright but broken. My lawyer Stone's plan was to have me thoroughly despised by the court, then won back when my bad behavior was contextualized in terms of a brain injury. Stone won on the having-me-despised half.

The personal injury trial began January 16th 1988 and lasted 6 months until June. Stone told me that credibility not truth, was the issue. At one point outside the courtroom, the other side's psychiatrist Malthrop said to me "Sorry, but it's my job." I started to lecture him about truth and the Hippocratic oath but opposing lawyer Gauze whisked him away.

From scribblings on scrap paper while I sat on the back benches of a Canadian court, I will try to pull together some sense of that 1988 trial.

Wild driver Barry Lewis still did not know how the accident had happened and kept referring to a 3rd lane that did not exist. In my testimony to my lawyer Stone, I could not retrieve the word "slogged" and misused the word "jogged" to describe my movement at Round Lake. The opposition's Gauze zeroed in on what he described as my inept hiding of my post-accident ability to jog. Given his brain injury expertise, Gauze had to know of my word retrieval problem but chose instead to label my misused "jog" as a Freudian slip that supposedly unveiled the real truth of my post-accident athletics. Judge Carter looked to be fooled and as Gauze intended, I became inflamed.

Gauze's cross-examination of me kicked off with the Supreme Court Judge saying how much she was looking forward to it. Opposing lawyer Gauze focused for 10 days on the troubled childhood stories I had written post-brain injury. Blow by blow, Gauze tried to extract his wished-for meaning from each word, sentence and piece of foul language to a morally literal Judge. Gauze dwelt on the sweet story of my first date as an 8 year-old, something of which Judge Carter visibly did not approve.

The Judge took time to lecture me on my lack of co-operation with her fellow senior Mr. Gauze and she castigated me on my roundabout answers. My lawyer Stone never intervened to inform the Judge that my mega-bite responding was a textbook sign of a left lobe brain injury. Nor did he ever interject to explain my somber childhood stories, the way Dr. Day did to Stone as classic symptoms of a left frontal lobe injury. Not once did lawyer Stone try to contextualize my pre-accident short stories and their happy contrast to those written post-brain injury by a rearranged mind.

Then came my supposed "skating." Gauze was quick to subpoena a Lord Advertising employee who had seen me trying to teach my son James to skate. Suddenly, Gauze appeared to convince Judge Carter of the "fact" that Alan Cooper, who'd said he could no longer perform athletics post-accident but for walking and swimming, was jogging and skating post-accident and thus lying. Stone said nothing and in silence I seethed.

Dr. Steve Jensen, who had repeatedly instructed me to get the "other side" to pay for my childhood "cynical lip," knew about my pre-accident high-frequency hearing deficiency, because I had told him. As tested post-accident, my hearing was worse; a testing otolaryngologist had told me that the increased deficiency could very well be a result of the accident. That information, too, had been forwarded to my G.P. Doctor Jensen, but Jensen had pushed me to make hearing an issue, presumably because he knew that its earlier deficiency would damage my credibility. I had not suspected anything and had followed Dr. Jensen's advice. Opposing lawyer Gauze seized upon hearing and my pre-accident deficiency, claiming I had reported it to no one, with my supposed cover-up being further proof of my malingering.

Gauze snatched onto my Grade 12 Latin story and dismissed my translation feat as impossible. He talked of my temporary psychic impotence in front of Maria just after we met, a fact I had reported to Flanders endocrinologist Dr. Fuller, who had dismissed the issue as a normal reaction for many males. Neither Gauze nor Stone acknowledged the repeatedly low scores that Dr. Fuller had discovered when testing my testosterone and sexual release hormone levels, or of the upward change in them after I had begun hormone shots. To the judge's comment that there must have been frequency of sexual intercourse to produce 2 babies, no-one said anything to illuminate her, while I just shook my head.

The opposition's Gauze did single out endocrinologist Dr. Fuller's finding no diabetes insipidus 2 years post-accident, but Gauze did not tell the court two facts. First, Dr. Fuller herself had suspected earlier transient diabetes insipidus and secondly, neurosurgeon Schwantz had suggested to me, "You may have diabetes insipidus" during his first 12 months testing. Stone again said nothing. Gauze then stretched credibility to its limit by referring to my 85 year-old father's totally different diabetes as one that I had purportedly concealed.

Gauze continued with reference to my reported dizziness. He had his Dr. Malthrop say that such dizziness was indicative of a more diffuse brain injury, and therefore, impossible for me to have. For months post-accident, I'd had to stagger bowlegged and while my dizziness had improved until about month 10, I was still too dizzy to skate as per pre-accident or ski or ride a 10-speed bicycle or perform gymnastics. To this day, I cannot put on trousers and socks without first being seated. However, at month 24, when tested at Flanders for dizziness, former gymnast Alan Cooper had fallen within some sort of testing norm.

No mention whatsoever was made of my loss of music or Mendelssohn Choir, and like so much else, my lawyer Adam Stone had no grasp of it.

Gauze sermonized on my further hiding information from the court when he spoke of my "head injury" in a 1969 car accident. In 1969 I had been temporarily knocked out, but a brain injury had never been an issue in that accident—the issue had been a breakage of a transverse lumbar in my lower back. Stone left the matter untouched.

Gauze finished his cross-examination with a lying accusation that I had dominated innocent Maria and had seduced her into leaving her Catholic Church, the same creed as known-to-be-a-pillar Supreme Court Judge Nanette Carter. The Judge scowled.

Maria's composition was such that her ring of verisimilitudes prompted the Judge to ask me what I could possibly have against Maria's mother if she had produced such a nice daughter. I protected Maria and said nothing of her firing, switch to atheism, lies to her parents about my religion being forced on our children, her agreeing with my critical letter to her mother or her description of the car accident, wrong in every detail. Instead of my indicating to the Judge that my personality was changed, my changed personality led me to say that there had been marriage problems before the accident.

Weeks into the trial, Gauze spoke via his richly paid psychiatrist Dr. Malthrop of my supposed alcoholism pre-accident. Knowing that Her Ladyship's late husband had died of alcoholism and had left her with 5 children, Gauze falsely painted Alan Cooper as a chronic drunk of 25 years from age 15 to age 40 by the time of the 1988 trial. To Stone's proof with photos of my ripped ventricles across the brain—damage Gauze and his Dr. Malthrop could then not deny as they had earlier in the trial—Gauze and Malthrop attributed the damage to my falsely purported 25 years of alcoholism and drug abuse.

Gauze presented psychologists to state that my cognitive abilities were still something to be envied and that my recall of numbers and visual memory were excellent. The psychologists knew such information to be only marginally relevant and relayed by me before their tests, but Gauze was evidently confident Judge Carter would be sucked in.

Maria's mother Yola made the blatant lie that I had ridiculed her ethnicity and religion.

"We were so proud of him...I am ashamed to say he is the father of my grandchildren," she told the court.

The impact on Her Ladyship was staggering and Stone again made no move.

To Stone's description of my pre-accident relationship with my own mother as excellent—he cited my arranging a surprise 65th birthday party for her, with all her friends present at her church—Gauze retorted, "Where is Mrs. Cooper now to support these claims?"

More horrifying to me than any of Gauze's contrivances were

his actions in private with a court reporter during many recesses. With all absent but I, Gauze regularly sauntered to the desk of the court reporter to "make clarifications" on what had been transcribed. A multitude of times across the 6-month trial, Gauze repeated this act. I began frantically taking notes of key sentences said in court but when I confronted Adam Stone with Gauze's transgressions, Stone looked at me as if I were paranoid as the other side had accused. He snapped that senior lawyer Gauze was a man of known honor, that such thoughts of mine were preposterous, such actions unthinkable and therefore, impossible.

But the greatest horror of all in the 6 month trial was Gauze's presentation of the hidden battery of "neuropsychological" tests done for Central Trust by hack shrink Dr. Pin. When a stunned Judge began to confront Stone with the issue of concealed evidence, Stone jack-in-the-boxed to his feet and began ranting, his stonewalling Her Ladyship with a barrage of doublespeak in defense of his integrity. When Judge Carter tried to probe Stone's knowing, he shouted at her "Look here!" and the Judge stumbled for words, went speechless and withdrew to compose. I was blackened by my lawyer to save himself.

Canada's 1988 July 1st birthday was coming and along with it, summer vacations. Stone stayed both insensitive to his bad chemistry with the Supreme Court Judge and clueless as to how his stonewalling had both intimidated M'Lady Carter and humiliated her in front of all. Judge Carter closed, by saying the issues were complex and she faced a challenge. Stone was made to feel he had won and the trial ended.

## Behavior

I took again that July of 1988, Maria, James and Robert to Round Lake. James and Robert loved its naturalness and Maria hated its dirt. Daytime would keep me alive with the life of my young sons, but nights would allow time for me to catch up with smoldering rage.

I had read that a high intellect, left free to inquire, can generate further hunger for that intellect to know. Such hunger can enhance integrity, keeping it at a level of honesty beyond the limits of those who practice the crafts of street smarts. If one person's range of honesty were 60–90% and another only 30–65%, there stood little chance of the latter's being able to see the difference, only that both were not 100% honest. The slim chance of communicating within the 60–65% overlap could then be made worse by any self-protection in the lower 30–65% person, thus moving communication worlds apart.

From a village payphone, I reached my AA sponsor, James Camden. He was a senior lawyer from old Toronto money, and had by coincidence been M'Lady's late husband's drinking buddy. Camden had served as an infantry captain at age 18 in World War II and had a kind of militarism about him that served well his life's denial. He had also been prejudiced about me by a fellow lawyer and bi-sexual alcoholic, Bryan Parrot who had tried to put the moves on me. When I had refused, Parrot had gone to Camden to say I was malingering.

My post-trial rage was further proof to Camden that I was being driven by greed and fuelled by alcoholic thinking. He said he just happened to have bumped into opposing lawyer Gauze who told Camden that Cooper was bright but Stone was brilliant. Camden added that as a lawyer, he was 120% sure I had won. But before the trial, he had said to me he was 120% sure I had no brain damage, and if I lost, I was just "…to accept it."

I pondered how people in their parochialism could stay stuck in the comfort of their own parishes. Dour in his poker mind, Stone in his verbal tap dance, Maria in her sycophantry, the Supreme Court Judge in her paint-by-numbers thinking, Regis Waters in his wish to hear and think the best, Doctor Fisher with his focus on childhood and my AA sponsor Camden in his role of reformed alcoholic, denier and old army captain.

And I wondered about these people's thoughts on alcohol. My earlier lawyer Dour had his health collapse from it and brother die of it, G.P. Dr. Jensen said he liked to get into it on weekends but managed during the week to keep it under control. My psychiatrist Dr. Fisher wanted it banned. Stone himself jogged to avoid what he called excessive drinking. Sponsor Camden was a self-declared expert after his own decades of alcoholism. Maria's father, cousins and uncles drank heavily as a matter of course. Blimiss Hope's Gene Darling was an alcoholic as was his cow Judi Jones, and they had both commented often on my not drinking much at all during my 2 years at Blimiss Hope. Cork had been fired from the Ministry of Food for it, and Regis Waters had a long history of helping alcoholics in his churches and university. My local church minister Godfrey had a brother whose career had ended because of alcohol. The husband of Supreme Court Judge Carter had been my AA sponsor's drinking buddy and was dead from alcoholism, leaving her alone with a handful of children.

A key strategy used by Gauze and shrink Malthrop had been adopting G.P. Dr. Jensen's lie of "my compulsive behavior fuelled by greed, anxiety and alcoholism." It appeared watertight—when earlier I had met with neurosurgeon Dr. Maul and he had said at the outset that I should settle as soon as possible "for the sake of my health," I had gone into quiet but visible torment. Maul had not seen the real reason, that I was permanently brain injured, but only his Jensen-fed one that I was malingering and consumed with greed. The angrier I got at this misunderstanding, the more so-called experts, like neurologist Dr. Maul, had been confirmed in their prejudice. When later I had reported taking a photo of a detective lurking outside my house before he had taken off in his car, my lawyer Dour had said I was paranoid and had said again I should not run my life by lawsuits.

An even more toxic strategy had been Dr. Malthrop's misrepresentation to Flanders Hospital, to job recruiters, to Professor Frisch and others that he and Gauze's side had been working and trying to maximize money for me. I had been put in an impossible Catch-22—the more frustration and indignation I had showed, the more my rage had confirmed people's prejudice. That in turn had fuelled more rage in me and in turn more prejudice. Any explanation that I had tried to give calmly had been seen as my being too clever, so others had perceived me as analytically crafty and certainly not brain injured.

Often those people trying to help had made things worse. Dr. Fisher had not known of G.P. Dr. Jensen and had not appreciated the fraudulency of the first neurological tests. Dr. Fisher had, therefore tried to offset Dour's disbelief of my permanent neurological damage by telling him I had permanent *psychological* damage. Dr. Fisher had added that I was "entitled to that belief" and had assured Dour "It was not my fault I'd had a delicate skull pre-accident." Dr. Fisher also had not recalled all that I had told him. For me to be perceived as recalling neurological symptoms, when in reality they would still be present, but not have the learned Dr. Fisher remember them, would do huge damage. My lawyer Stone would make credibility worse, when the symptoms I had written to Dr. Fisher would be coached by Stone as written instead to my wife.

Regis Waters, too, had spouted forth in his own parochial construct, and in trying to help, had further damaged my credibility. He had praised my ultra-liberal Protestant theology to a Judge known to be a staunch Roman Catholic. More damaging had been Reg's saying that Alan could do anything he put his mind to.

Stewart MacCallum, my old Deputy in the Ministry, had been called upon to testify on my behalf but 2 complications had emerged. The first was Stew's own alcoholism. He could still articulate but had been in withdrawal and reckless of voice as his court appearance had approached noon. The second had been that my old Ministry boss, Willy Cork, had got to Stewart and Stew was if nothing else, sensitive. Cork had heard of my trial and had been scheduled to testify against me, but my denigration of Cork in court had made Gauze change his mind. When Cork had then heard he wasn't to testify but Stewart was, Cork had overridden his own knowledge of my impotence and had fabricated another false story, one in which I, Alan Cooper, had supposedly fornicated Stewart's #1 girlfriend. Stew had pretended not to care when confronting me jokingly but had not believed me.

Stewart had then done much in court to confirm a notion that the Judge had often probed, that of my supposed disloyalty, as if pre-accident I had been a charlatan who had left jobs constantly to go to the highest bidder. It was an unfounded notion. In reality, I had worked for many years for each employer and I had resisted the pull of recruiters; however, Cork had circulated this charlatan notion around the Ministry and beyond, and the Judge's mindset had mirrored Cork's poison-painted picture. One would have thought that Cork and the Judge had known each other from church.

For my part I had done as I did always, protect. I had not nodded my head to the Judge when she had looked to me for confirmation that Stone had hidden Pin's tests. I had kept my word during the trial and to my wife's frustration, had not discussed it at home. I had not revealed Maria's 100% false "reality" of the accident when Stone had told me in court that Maria had a much "different version of reality" around my drinking. I had not told about Maria's getting dismissed, turning atheist, trying to stop our children's baptisms and telling her parents that she decided to stay home with the children, while secretly suing her employer and cheating on unemployment. I had not told the Judge of Maria's letting her Catholic parents think I had forced my church upon Maria, when the Judge had asked me how Maria's mother could be so bad as to have turned out such a nice girl as Maria.

No, I had protected and taken the rap. I did the same by refusing to tell the Judge that Maria had taken her rich sister's cash to go to the best marital lawyer in Toronto, only to learn that any proceeds I got from the car accident would not be due to her in divorce. I did the same by protecting Darling in 1984 in front of his boss. I did the same with Blimiss Hope subordinates who had sabotaged me to advance themselves, but later needed my help. I did the same with pregnant Jo-Anne in 1967 when people all around had accused me of corrupting innocent her. I had done the same at all times as a child to protect my mother, when she had wrongly accused me and I, the loyal puppy had safeguarded her and taken the blame.

During the night at Round Lake, I lay alone in the shack's second bedroom, reflecting on Maria's father. Like his own mother, the poor man would die of liver cancer because he would refuse out of fear, to get his colon checked. Fear had been his driving force, and when not swallowing wads of Valium or drinking on weekends, the man had seeped in fear.

I remember inviting Maria's father over one Friday night to play chess. I had to make up with him, for the years he had wanted me to exert what he saw as my manhood and get drunk with him, but I had refused. I had driven him from his home across Toronto's Gardiner Expressway, and he had been awestruck by cars being on the road and people on the streets. He had simply assumed that after work, other people did as he did and bolted their doors. Other than his rise at dawn to a factory job, he had never been out at night and as I had walked him to the subway that evening for his return home, he had asked me if I were afraid. He had then seen people on the sidewalk, muttered "Oh, oh!" and had stopped and stood aside until they had passed. The women who had walked by, had triggered his quiet "Heh, heh." He had presumed them all to be street walkers. He had carried a shoehorn in his pants, so he could avoid embarrassment: he had kept his shoe laces tied because his wife had not been there to tie or untie his laces.

The poor man had little outlet in his life. He didn't have sex from a wife, because she slept with her son Constantine. The son was so overprotected that he was driven to and from school, never allowed outside "where he might get bitten by a squirrel," and force fed. As Maria's sister said, he was unable at 18 to pour himself a glass of milk. If Constantine were out of the room, his father would do checks on him to ensure "Con was safe and not sweating." His parents encouraged him to cheat at chess and everything else, "because he was only a boy." For his first 10 years of life, Constantine had been labeled "a baby."

I did not fit into any category of Maria's mother. Yola's lies and her husband's alcohol had been used to force a fit. They had not liked it when I did not eat or drink enough, and Maria would have been chastised for my being too skinny "because I had an Angleck mother." I was musical and drank wine "but that was because of Maria." I had manners "but that was because I was English."

My in-laws thought me weird and could not imagine how I as a bachelor had kept myself fed. They could not even imagine why I had lived away from home, but their racism against my being 'Angleck' had fed their final determination. They were racists against Canadians, Ukrainians, Germans, Lithuanians, English, Jews, Arabs, Blacks, Pakistanis, anyone not of their circle. They determined that Scots and Irish were English. Maria's parents survived in their tiny world of fear, superstition, religion, over-mothering and the omnipresent lie.

At first, Maria's parents had found me fascinating and their prejudices had stayed submerged. Without Maria's foreknowledge, I had given them a special Made in Poland crystal gift on the 35th anniversary of their World War II trauma, and Yolanta had orchestrated the group's crying response. I had studied Polish and sponsored Constantine's Catholic confirmation. I had made friends with Maria's sister and husband, and had hosted them often. I had done favors for them all, and every one of them had heaped praises on me. Yes, Maria had complained to me at every turn about Yolanta's interference and bad mothering, but the issue had never hit the surface before my August 1982 letter. Maria had been master of telling her mother all that her mother wanted to hear.

Prior to my marrying Maria, her mother had invited dinner guests to sniff me out, and one such family had been Mr. and Mrs. Petrone. Over dinner, while Maria's father had been ramming me with straight vodka, followed by his homemade wine and Yola's huge dinner, Mrs. Petrone had started her inspection by asking what nationality I was. I had replied, "Canadian."

"But what background?"

"Well, Canadian for over 200 years."

"You mean you're Indian?"

"No, White."

"There *were* no Whites back then."

I had politely explained that I was what she might call a Wasp and Mrs. Petrone had then given me the judgmental question.

"You mean there is no Catholic background in you at all?"

I should have left the table, but being polite, I had talked about my famous Irish Canadian grandmother. Mrs. Petrone had begun to show her disapproval, but Yola's tongue had intervened, followed by Maria's father with his booze. It had been one night of many in which I would have to endure the relentless racism and endless alcohol from Maria's family and friends. Not once did I inject ethnicity into any argument and I shocked all with my tolerance and open-mindedness.

— • —

My Round Lake torment drifted and landed on my now being married to Maria. She had not accepted marital therapist Doctor Fisher's diagnosis about her anxiety going through her breast milk, making both James and Robert colicky. Dr. Fisher had seen straight through her and told her so, when she had tried to quash his learning about her teenaged brother sleeping with his mother. Her solution had been to switch shrinks. Maria had teased her fat new shrink, Freedberg, whose wild fantasies of him and her, she had relayed to me. Maria had manipulated his diagnoses. She had spilled to her sister my intimate meetings with Dr. Fisher and had set up her sister to see Dr. Fisher for help with her own newlywed bag of wet noodles.

Maria had used her mother's false diagnosis on toddler Robert about why he had often been sick and had ignored his pediatrician's calls that Robert had not had a bowel movement for 4 days. My wife Maria had used again her mother's misdiagnosis to label Robert's chronic eye infection a nervous twitch, and toddler Robert had gone on for a year before I had quietly snuck him to an eye doctor.

In the stillness of night at Round Lake, in bed alone, I raged.

Social conscience. Judge Carter had heard nothing of my long years of social responsibility and strict ethics, and my lawyer Stone had known none of it to tell her. When the Judge had kept calling into question my job loyalty, Stone had been too busy checking his own script to hear or see Judge Carter, just as he had been when the Judge had sent him a knowing comment and smile on St. Patrick's Day. And as for the "headhunter" recruiters, Stone had one of them testify that I had always refused headhunters but Judge

Carter seemed not to have listened. Toronto headhunters had then picked up through Stone that "I was permanently brain injured and an alcoholic."

My 28-page loving letter to my mother written in July '78 before my accident had not been found nor my toddler photo showing my pre-accident pupils of then equal size. I had both the letter and photo somewhere but had not been asked to produce them. Little else had been found of my pre-accident kindnesses or demonstrated love to both Maria's and my families. Much of the reliance for retrieving such support had been left to Maria, Yolanta and my mother.

Stone had been pushing for a $1.8 million award and had indirectly turned down half that sum, after Gauze had seen the Dr. Day-assessed CT scan. Stone had then stayed on his roll until trial end, never sensing how badly Judge Carter had been deceived by false facts. Stone had kept saying that if we lost, we would appeal and he never once referred to the niceties of the appeal process and how restricted it was to points of law. Stone had considered preposterous, the notion of a complete mistrial in which the Supreme Court Judge had radically wrong facts as supposed evidence in front of her. Preposterous as my talk of Gauze's altering transcripts or of psychiatrist Malthrop having misrepresented himself as working for me, or my wife's understanding of "reality" regarding the actual accident or my supposed history of drinking as a youth, or of G.P. Dr. Steve Jensen having poisoned key specialists.

The peace of Round Lake in July 1988 was not with me. I tried to summon something to fight the indignation, and swam mile after mile, but my mind held onto thoughts that for almost 1/2 a year, a system had crushed truth. Finally, at night, alone under a coal oil lamp, I wrote.

Dear Mr. Stone:

RE:     **COOPER VS. LEWIS**
        Round Lake. July, 1988

As touched on in June, I believe that Judge Carter has not been given full clear facts.

## 1. DR. PIN'S NEURO-PSYCHOLOGICAL TESTS

As you know, your law firm has known about my tests with Dr. Pin, since before I took them. They were done because your partner Mr. Dour would not release to Central Trust, results of neuro-psychological tests done on me. I have never tried to hide these tests as Madam Carter queried, and as opposing Mr. Gauze stated outright. Nor have I malingeringly tried to suppress the results, an act which Mr. Gauze emphasized in court. Nor have I ever known until all heard in court, the results of Dr. Pin's tests. I was not told by Dr. Pin, prospective employer Central Trust or anyone else.

And Pin's cognitive tests themselves—I was open and candid in telling Dr. Pin upfront of my areas of cognitive deficiency, and Dr. Pin chose to test me in virtually none of those areas. As to Dr. Pin's saying I had an I.Q. over 150, no point was made of the medical plausibility of a high I.Q. in tandem with other brain damage.

And Dr. Pin's personality tests—I did not take home the almost 600 questions but raced through the 600 questions that night in under 60 minutes with a Dr. Pin anxious to rush to completion. Technically, much of the 600 question test (MMPI?) I did not even do myself—Dr. Pin did the vast bulk of the answers on the answer sheet and at one point when he found he was off 2 full points with the answer sheet (498 not 496?), Dr. Pin quickly made corrections on his own.

When you and I, Adam discussed all these circumstances pre-trial, you dismissed the tests as an aberration that could quickly be dismissed in court. I believe Judge Carter does not at all have a grasp of these Dr. Pin circumstances and I believe the same circumstances are critical to her assessing me.

## 2. MY IRRATIONAL POST-ACCIDENT LETTERS IN JULY AND SEPT 1983

Quite the contrary to what Mr. Gauze stated in summary, I did not affirm that these letters are factual. They contain fragments of truth of my pre-accident life, the positives denigrated by Mr. Gauze and his experts as boastful lies, the negatives highlighted by Gauze and group as hard facts. All fragments were written by me, a person with a wildly changed personality from the December 27, 1981 brain damage. It is extraordinarily difficult for me even now to see those fragments in any objective light, because I am judging both them and my brain-crashed personality with the same changed personality. Dr. Fisher viewed both letters as such and told my wife,

"He (Alan) can't help it. His personality is changed (by the brain injury)."

I don't understand my changed personality but I do think the following approximation.

|  |  |  |  |  |  |  | Satisfactory |  |  | Outstanding |
|---|---|---|---|---|---|---|---|---|---|---|
| 0 | 1 | 2 | 3 | 4 | 5 | 6 | 7 | 8 | 9 | 10 |
| Unacceptable |  |  |  |  | Marginal |  | Very Good |  |  | Impossible |

| My Personality Relationship | Pre 12.27.81 Accident | Post 12.27.81 Accident |
|---|---|---|
| 1. With my wife | 9 | 6 |
| 2. With my parents | 8 | 1 |
| 3. With my wife's parents | 8 | 0 |
| 4. With my friends, associates, both in quality and quantity | 9 | 1 |
| 5. With my outlook on life | 9 | 2 |

I could not retrieve these facts to oralize them, nor did you.

### 3.  MY STORIES PRE- VS. POST-ACCIDENT

Gauze asked Judge Carter to focus on my post-accident short stories submitted to the court. But Gauze was ever so careful not to ask me for any of my pre-accident short stories, except for the one happy story I wrote about my first date when I was 8 years of age, (the intent, as you confirmed to me, to cast moral turpitude in front of Judge Carter on my dating at such a young age). My post-accident short stories are written from the same deranged personality that wrote the "schizophrenic" letters of July 1983 and September 1983. And are potentially damningly misleading.

As for other writings, I wrote a book pre-accident and was collating notes for a second at the time of the accident. I have not, quite to the contrary of what the deluded second psychologist Dr. Kellerman said, written 2 novels post-accident and have not been able to hold and retain my thoughts even enough to pick up on the second novel, begun pre-accident. I am concerned that the way the evidence was put in, the Judge may think I wrote or completed 2 novels after the accident.

And Gauze's talk of my wordsmithing, which Gauze told the Judge is superb and belies word difficulties and articulation problems, is again a totally misleading message left with the Court. Given as I have oft repeated, a long open-ended amount of time, I can search through my large pre-accident knowledge and former command of English, to find words to express myself on paper, when I can't do it orally.

### 4.  MY POST-ACCIDENT IMPAIRMENT TO LEARN (ACADEMICS)

Opposing Gauze, in his oralized summary said that my 1986 academic successes at Emmanuel College proved out my ability post-accident to perform well academically, thus belying my learning-to-absorb-new-information plus recall difficulties. Books and notes require many readings and high-lighting, before I can absorb them at all into memory. Even then, I don't recall them quickly or completely and take hours and days to recall bits of the information. This confusion was again not clarified for the Judge.

The courses I took at Emmanuel were oriented not to exams and tests but to essay-writing, an area where given an enormous excess of time, I can still function. But the 4 months January-April 1986 saw me working on these courses for 90 hours per week, trying to do courses which I could do pre-accident in 1/2 the time. I had received 20 years ago in 1967–68, the University of Toronto's award for the highest undergraduate mark in Religious Studies.

## 5. MY BLACK BOOK

(a) Mr. Gauze said in his summary that Dr. Fisher had told me to wean myself off what Gauze and his Dr. Malthrop painted as my "childhood-compulsive" need for my black book. But Dr. Fisher made that weaning comment to me in one of my first visits to him, before he had formulated any kind of diag-nosis. And even then only as the suggestion, "Have you con-sidered?" Dr. Fisher now completely supports my black book system and has for years. And psychologist Winter and neuro-surgeon Day have very much encouraged me to use such a black book. My life would be chaos without it.

(b) Gauze communicated before the court that I had deep-sixed my black books pre-accident to hide my "pre-accident similarly excessive use of them." Again, 100% false. Each calendar year pre-accident, I would receive my new black book in the normal October period of the year, transfer all names, addresses and financial information to the new one in about November and discard the old one in December. How would I have known, come the Dec. 27th 1981 accident that

I would need my 1981 black book, having discarded it almost one month earlier?

Why did I not answer Gauze in cross-examination this way? Because I can't retrieve information quickly post-accident, getting me into difficulty early at Blimiss Hope.

## 6. MY 1982 (LATER EXTINGUISHED) FEELINGS OF FULL RECOVERY WHEN RESPONDING TO JOB APPROACHES FROM MARKETING FIRMS AND BLIMISS HOPE

I was told via Maria by Dr. Mark Schwantz that I would have a full recovery in 3 months. Then he changed his diagnosis to a full recovery in 6 months, then 12 months. Then he changed to "maybe never a full recovery." Then he changed it to never.

Before my scheduled joining of the new company on August 1st 1982, my 6 months for recovery had run out and I began to suspect that I would never have a full recovery. Dr. Schwantz told me of this strong possibility himself in that summer of 1982 and I began to appreciate that I could not do at the new company, the old marketing job I had done so well in the past. And that I would quickly be unemployed in a city away from Toronto, relying only on Maria's inadequate-for-expenses salary at her new job.

In the second 6 months of 1982, after I went back to my old Ministry position, my job was still difficult for me. Rumors of my brain damage were rampant and painfully real for all to see, and Mr. Cork was trying to make both my work and personal life as difficult as he could. Cork even told me to take the earliest job exit to save my reputation, despite what he described as my obvious-to-all brain damage.

And, while my recovery had essentially stopped by then, I still clung to the newly revised prognosis by neurosurgeon Schwantz of a possible full recovery in 12 months.

My solid pre-accident reputation had directed Blimiss

Hope to seek me out, not me it. And I had expected to recover my full intellect, including memory and word finding by the 12 months post-accident, on or near the end of 1982. I was offered and accepted the job at Blimiss Hope in month 13, still not able to express my memory difficulties and still without any battery of neuro-psychological tests to gauge or categorize any of my shortcomings.

I am unhappy that both the progression from an expected full recovery in 3, then 6, then 12 months, then never, and the various job possibilities during the period post-accident were presented in such a way as to question integrity.

## 7. OBSERVERS' FEEDBACK ON ABSORPTION OF NEW INFORMATION DIFFICULTY

In response to Mr. Gauze's claim that no one layperson defined my exact "difficulty in absorbing new information" problem, such lay definition is unreasonable to expect. Defining that dysfunction involves a scientific categorization, which falls in the domain of highly skilled neurologists and neuropsychologists, many of whom have demonstrated to me now that they do not test for my exact problems. But on the more layperson-like description "bad memory," I had enormous feedback, especially after I went to the new work environment of Blimiss Hope.

## 8. COULD I NOW COMPLETE EMMANUEL AND BECOME A CHURCH MINISTER?

Gauze is again false in his carte blanche statements. I would have an almost impossible time with the next courses on such things as Old and New Testament where I would have to absorb lectures, notes and books and then be tested on the information within them. Even if some pieces eventually got into memory, my recall and sorting of them would still be poor, a neurological malfunction that Gauze flatly denied in existence, his saying that my problem of absorbing and recalling new information was the only problem. Moreover, as a minister, I would never remember people's names. When I teach Sunday school, I can not recall people's names and have called children and parents by their wrong names, dozens of times.

## 9. PUPILS OF DIFFERENT SIZES; MENDELSSOHN CHOIR AND SINGING GONE

The court has no Mendelssohn knowledge or the "different-sized pupils", despite being in my 1983 letter, used in other parts by opposing Gauze to show me to be a malingerer.

## 10. ABSORBING NEW INFORMATION NOT THE ONLY MEMORY PROBLEM

Mr. Gauze has again left the Court with information 100% false or very misleading. My most obvious problem may be neurologically impaired ability to absorb new information but many times during the day, I call people by their wrong names, even people I know well such as my 2 children or close friends such as Regis Waters. My spelling, once excellent, is slow and mixed up and I often get my syntax reversed. I often use the wrong words in sentences; e.g. "This shower sure is black" when I mean "hot". I often ramble in sentences and am circuitous and verbose, all of which is regularly fed back to me by Dr. Fisher. And I often mix up consonant blends or double-slur them, and am told frequently post-injury that I "speak with a dry mouth."

In fact, I do speak with a dry mouth—my lips have been numb since the accident as has my palate. My saliva has been "3-in-1 oil" viscous, my mouth now feels parched and numb 100% of the time, and I can no longer whistle.

When I write, I now make enormous corrections to mis-placed word consonants ("lpease" instead of "please", "rpy" instead of "pry") and to fix syntax. And my handwriting itself: pre-accident, my handwriting was smooth and artistic; post-accident, it is illegible. I have to hand print at all times, and even my printing is jagged and sporadic.

My right-hand knuckles since the injury are almost always bone dry. In the winter, they turn purple and my finger-and-toe extremities get cold very quickly.

## 11. GAUZE FALSELY STATES THAT RECALL IS NOT KEY TO AN EXECUTIVE JOB.

Mr. Gauze put forward in summary that no key executive decision is made on the spot or spur of the moment, where immediate recall is necessary. A 1/2 truth, for indeed no critical legal judgment is made on the spot either. But (and the identical situation holds true for my former executive functions) if you as a lawyer, Adam, needed to jump up in objection on a critical issue and began, "M'Lord...sorry M'Lady, I strongly object to what Mr. Gall...Mr. Gauze is putting forward. We know the lady, uh with the brown hair said Mr. Cooper was skating but we don't hear, I mean Mr. Cooper was jogging, sorry skating, or at least generically in that park I can't recall, oh Eglinton, but...,"

Imagine the fool you would appear in court? Such brain malfunction has happened many times to me as an executive, and its unpredictability has created enormous stress.

## 12. MR. GAUZE AND DR. KELLERMAN HAVE SAID BLIMISS HOPE PROBLEMS WERE OVER A YEAR IN SURFACING.

There were problems from the start. I believe there has not been due emphasis on the evidence showing that my problem existed from the beginning at Blimiss Hope. Gauze is, again, 100% false. Because my Blimiss Hope predecessor had been fired, I was given vast lead time in learning my job and had a direct report backup Guy Vacks during most of the first full year. Even my first (November 1984) presentation in New York was (contrary to what Gauze said in summary) minuscule and what few questions I had, I handled badly—I just could not remember the important details and could not then run to my mountains of documents and notes.

No. Despite my exhaustive hours even in year one of Blimiss Hope, I was having enormous difficulty with new information and was, to the annoyance of boss and subordinates, continually trying to draw marketing arguments back into the abstract to rely on my pre-accident knowledge of marketing principles.

## 13. MR. GAUZE SUMMARIZED THAT BLIMISS HOPE'S KNOWING OF THE ACCIDENT, NOT THE ACCIDENT ITSELF, CAUSED MY AUTUMN 1984 FRENZY.

My extreme upset in autumn 1984 was caused by my need to hold on to my livelihood, while suddenly realizing that much of Blimiss Hope and the marketing community could daily see the results of my brain impairment, and had known since the accident.

My work hours became crushing throughout the autumn of 1984 and I didn't learn how much recruiters and the marketplace knew until after I got fired in January 1985. I then fell into total despair, thinking my situation hopeless and began drinking to coat the hopelessness.

## 14. MR. GAUZE SUMMARIZES THAT MY TOTAL MEMORY, INCLUDING MY VISUAL MEMORY, SCORES WELL.

I was upset by the failure to refute Gauze's allegation that I score well on "total memory" when the evidence of memory impairment was in front of the court. In the first place, I have not and do not complain of visual memory post-accident. I remember faces and buildings but I can't recall names or say, street signs. To lump visual memory into a total memory score is grossly misleading, but that is what is left with the Supreme Court and Madam Nanette Carter.

## 15. MR. GAUZE SUMMARIZED THAT I STARTED AN MBA AT THE UNIVERSITY OF TORONTO AND DID NOT COMPLETE IT.

Again 100% false. I was neither in nor enrolled to enter, an MBA. I started the Diploma Business Administration course and completed it with a high scholastic average.

## 16. MR. GAUZE SUMMARIZED THAT I "JOGGED" AT KAWAWAYMOG AND SLIPPED THE WORD OUT INADVERTENTLY.

Again 100% false. I did not jog. In fact, my using the wrong word "jog" is the very type of word misuse that my brain damage causes me to do each day. I was searching for a word to say "slogged" the 30 feet to the shoreline's edge.

## 17. MR. GAUZE SUMMARIZED MY "SUICIDE PLANNING" WITH REGIS WATERS IN 1986 AS ANOTHER EXAMPLE OF MY CONTRIVED MALINGERING.

Again 100% false. My 1985 funeral planning was never portrayed by me to anyone in that light, nor did I intend anyone to interpret it that way. It was done with all planning paid for as part of the executive compensation package at Blimiss Hope. And I was simply carrying out a planning act that I felt all responsible fathers should do.

## 18. GAUZE TALKED OF MY THWARTED TESTS WITH KULISKY, BECAUSE OF VALIUM/WINE.

False. The tests were virtually complete before the night-time, children's-dosage Valium and wine was mentioned by me. Psychologist Kulisky chose to abuse this information and shut down the tests to rush downstairs and see psychiatrist Hooker.

## 19. GAUZE HIGHLIGHTED MY CREATIVE WRITING COURSE, POST-ACCIDENT.

A 1/2 truth—I wrote nothing for it. I had done the identical course pre-accident. And I believe I said so in court.

## 20. GAUZE SUMMARIZES THAT THE JOB MARKETPLACE KNOWS OF MY CAR ACCIDENT'S EFFECTS AND I AM DOING WELL, REGARDLESS.

False. I am now in a much more junior non-marketing job. And potential employers, too numerous to recall, have fed back comments on my memory, black book dependency, obtuseness, circuitous verbosity and stumbling speech.

## 21. GAUZE'S MISREPRESENTATION OF ENDOCRINO-LOGICAL FINDINGS

Quite the contrary to Gauze's summarized communication that Flanders' endocrinologist found my post-accident testosterone levels abnormally low just once, Dr. Fuller found them low on several tests done across a year, and found that the testosterone level did temporarily improve with sexual hormone injection shots. Dr. Fuller, furthermore found not just testosterone to be low—she also found at least 2 other sex-related hormones abnormally low too, (luteinizing hormone? luteinizing release hormone?), each time she tested them before her administered shots.

And again quite the contrary to what Gauze communicated about my malingering and withholding key information to doctors, I told Dr. Fuller and her assistant Dr. Sand right up front about my one sexual "miss" with Maria pre-accident, as well as the pre-accident prostatitis and the post-accident wine/water night-time ritual, all of which Drs. Fuller/Sand dismissed as not directionally meaningful to their endocrinological diagnosis. Dr. Fuller told me by phone over 2 years after the Dec. 27 '81 car accident, that I did not then have diabetes insipidus but that I could quite probably have had it in the first year post-brain injury. As did neurosurgeon Dr. Schwantz in my first 6 months post-injury.

## 22. THE COURT HAS A RADICALLY WRONG UNDER STANDING OF MY POST-ACCIDENT ALCOHOL.

Mr. Gauze misled the court with the "revealing" that I had begun drinking to excess before 1985. Alcohol had nothing to do with my Blimiss Hope fiasco and workplace failure. The post-accident alcoholic condition was not active until despair set in after the Blimiss Hope firing and marketplace brain damage rumors.

Gauze has left the court with the grossly misleading impression that I drank "100 ounces of vodka" per day. False. The drinking of a fraction of that order happened only twice in 1985. When I said "100 ounces" to a doctor whose name I can't recall, she was quick to feed back to me that I was exaggerating (in fact bragging) and that such consumption was impossible for the impaired consumer to monitor.

Gauze's chief psychiatrist Malthrop said I had begun drinking at age 16. False. I did not drink through university years until my 21st birthday in final year.

And post-accident, excluding the Aug. 1982–Jan. 1985 wine/water night-time ritual and the 4 times abuse in April of '82, I drank to excess only for short periods in 1985 and 1986.The incorrect description in court is of my episode in 1985. In 1986 I was on Antabuse for 6 months, making drinking impossible; I was working 90 hours per week in Emmanuel College during the 4 months prior; I was job interviewing with the Canadian Government and Central Trust for 6 months; I logged accumulated swims of over 100 miles at the University of Toronto in 1986 and walked over 100 miles; I joined Clair Park Church in January 1986, faithfully took my children each Sunday and was invited in the spring of 1986 to teach Sunday school in the autumn of that year.

And contrary to what Gauze summarized was my direct disobedience of Drs. Fisher and Schwantz, Dr. Fisher admonished my drinking habits only in 1985 when they escalated out of control, not during the Aug.1982–January 1985 period when Dr. Fisher told me that my night-time water/wine consumption was "under control." And contrary to what Gauze said, the drinking was not done in combination with other sedatives. Dr. Schwantz was not concerned about my "liter of wine"; moreover, my "liter" of wine was actually a 3/4 liter bottle. I used then the terms liter and bottle interchangeably.

DTs (Delirium Tremens) 4 times is also false. It was by my own misdiagnosis in 1986 and told by Flanders Emergency doctor at that one time only, as my misdiagnosis.

And my 1 to 4 bottles of weight-restoring Guinness per day for 8 days—Gauze changed to "pack-a-day" in cross-examination, later a "case-a-day" in summary.

### 23. DRUG ABUSE

No. Dr. Fisher knows and reiterates that this is a distortion. But the court has a grossly exaggerated impression of my abusing drugs and combining them with alcohol.

### 24. ALCOHOL MAKING MY BRAIN DAMAGE WORSE?

Gauze is false. My neurological problems are the same before as after. This point was not made. When I started my 1985 excessive drinking, 3 full years had passed since the Dec. 27, 1981 car accident.

But with the grossly distorted impressions of my post-accident alcohol consumption before the Court, Gauze is claiming that alcohol, not the accident, has caused my brain damage, still in existence since Dec. 27, 1981.

### 25. WIFE LEAVING ME BECAUSE OF ALCOHOL?

Gauze is false. My wife left me as part of plans laid out by her mother after my 1982 letter to her and after my wife's having her mother's 2 planned grandchildren.

### 26. SEX WITH WIFE POST-ACCIDENT?

Mr. Gauze's summarized assertion is 90% false. Sex there

was, yes but rarely, 2–3 times per year versus frequently pre-accident.

## 27. BALANCE

My balance is still wobbly today and I would get dizzy were I to twirl my kids once as I tried to do in 1986. Very dizzy. The fact of my balance being much improved, post-accident in the 2 years up to the time I took the balance tests, seems not before the court. My balance was 100% pre-accident, 30% for 1–2 years post-accident and about 65% now. The otolaryngologist could not explain the problem but he did say that my worsened hearing post-accident could have been caused by the accident. In fact, the otolaryngologist Dr. Fent had no knowledge of the pre-accident hearing problems until I took the initiative, both to tell him and help him retrieve old files. I then told the hearing specialist Dr. Fent to inform Dr. Steve Jensen, whom I knew would be communicating to both legal sides about the car accident.

## 28. *SEVERE BRAIN INJURY VS. MILD-TO-MODERATE.

Gauze falsely summarized my brain injury as "mild-to-moderate." Even in final cross-examination, the court had the factually wrong understanding. The fact is:

| DAY 1 | 2 | 3 | 4 | 5 | 6 | 7* |
|-------|-----|-----|-----|-----|--------|--------|
| Dec. 27, 1981 | 28 | 29 | 30 | 31 | Jan. 1 | Jan. 2 |

January 2, 1982, when I still had amnesia and incoherence is not DAY 5, as the court understands for "MODERATE-TO-SEVERE;" January 2, 1982 is DAY 7 for "SEVERE."

## 29. PRE-ACCIDENT PRINCETON-BASED LAW TEST SCORES IN THE HIGH PERCENTILE; ALCOHOLISM POST-BRAIN INJURY STATISTICALLY SHOWN

The court has neither.

## 30. BAD MEMORY MARKETPLACE FEEDBACK

Gauze is 100% false. Dozens of people, as named by me to you, have fed back to me my bad memory, a key factor which triggered my known unemployability and consequent despair. The marketplace feedback occurred *before* the excessive drinking.

## 31. OTHER LEGAL SIDE FALSELY REPRESENTING ITSELF AS WORKING FOR ME

Headhunter Richard Fast had been under the impression from Gauze's and Regal Insurance's detective agency that it had been working for me. Mr. Fast had thus been left with the impression that I was malingering. A similar impression had been left from the detective's 2-hour interview with Emmanuel's David Frisch. Was this misrepresentation of the kind that caused Dr. Schwantz in Flanders Hospital to misunderstand how the car accident had happened? Was this type of misrepresentation done from the outset in Flanders Hospital by the other side's Dr. Malthrop, to alienate as many people as possible from an Alan Cooper whom he painted as malingering?

## 32. WHAT HAS TRIGGERED MY MEMORY NOW, JULY 1988?

What has triggered my memory now is the combination of Mr. Gauze's false summary and my notes, while he used 1/2 truths, 1/4truths, 1/16 truths and ZERO truths, all before the Supreme Court. And his summary is what the case has closed with. Even with my bad memory, his triggering of pivotal events/facts, because of their enormous and long-pounded-in effect on me, is there. And I feel enraged beyond belief that such distortions as Mr. Gauze has made are being allowed to sit, in judging me and my brain damage before Madam Justice Carter and the Ontario Supreme Court.

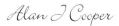

Back in Toronto, Dr. Fisher would stop my sending this letter, saying it would antagonize my lawyer Stone as I had done earlier lawyer Dour. Dr. Fisher would also stop my purported badgering Stone into settling with the opposition's Gauze, saying that Stone "refused to crawl." Dr. Fisher went on to give me the assurance that he had apparently been given—that I would be pleased with the final outcome of the trial.

# 9 MONTHS FROM THE CLOSE
# OF TRIAL TO JUDGMENT

After Round Lake of 1988, I continued family outings but was forced to stop taking Maria's grandmother anywhere—she fell victim to the lies told by Maria's mother, Yolanta, who was directing as much alienation from me as she could. Her husband returned to me old gifts of a framed photo and Irish knit cardigan, while her son Constantine returned bicycle and Burberry trench coat, all via Maria and the lie.

Work-wise, I counseled fired persons on how best to find another job. I found myself good at helping others, but clients said my memory was the worst they had seen. Deep-felt thank you letters did come in and I began to see myself as a wounded healer, but company accountant Barbara Crake took a disliking to me and altered not only every expense report but also my time sheets and bonus reports. Crake was performing criminal acts that cheated me out of thousands of dollars but I needed a job and was losing faith in legal systems. Other people at work were backstabbing but I felt no fight, only the smallness in which I found myself, post-brain injury.

Tuesday, March 13, 1989 halted it all. Ontario Supreme Court Judge Nanette Carter's ruling came down. Stone phoned to say Judge Carter "...had bought none of our arguments" and that the Judge had gone beyond the boundaries of condemnation, which opposing Gauze had hoped for and had accepted all of Gauze's distortions, while adding in her own.

I phoned Dr. Fisher and he began crying through the receiver. He gave me a prescription for Ativan and I took the first 2 milligrams at once. That night March 13th, 1989, despite the earlier 2 milligrams, I felt a fire building inside my chest and I broke 27 months of sobriety. Somehow, I still got to Dr. Fisher.

In the 2 weeks thereafter, I managed with the 6 milligrams of night-time Ativan to sleep. I took no Ativan during the day and I limited daytime drinking to a job-acceptable glass of wine. Night-time alcohol never really built to much: I sensed that the 11:00 p.m. Ativan was there for me for sleep and within 2 weeks, I weaned myself off the alcohol altogether.

I still had not seen the judgment. Stone feigned protecting me from the damage that reading it would do, and it was weeks before Maria and I finally saw Stone in his boardroom. Stone was then suddenly less sanguine on appeal than he had been throughout the 9 months post-trial, his emphasizing that the chances for appeal were limited to points of law and not as to how the evidence had gone in. Stone kept mentioning the name of Walter Chintak as the best appeal lawyer in Canada "…but of course Alan, you are free to choose whatever appeal lawyer you like." Stone knew I had no knowledge of appeal lawyers.

Medical reports had to be paid for and the doctors were clambering, according to Stone. It was up to me he said, to negotiate directly with them for reduced charges, since Stone said the doctors' charges of tens of thousands of dollars were done directly for me. It soon became evident that the doctors had been earlier guaranteed full payment by Stone.

Stone held onto the Supreme Court judgment and I still had not seen one word of it. Judge Carter's rationale was known only to Stone but he kept focusing my attention instead on what he called "appropriate next steps." It took another month of Stone's orchestration before I got to see the judgment.

On the day I received the judgment, Stone declared that time was of the essence and he needed a speedy reply. I wrote after work past midnight for a month.

April, 1989
Mr. Adam Stone

Dour, Stone & Smart
First Canadian Place
Toronto, Ontario

Mr. Stone: **RE: COOPER VS. LEWIS:
M'LADY CARTER'S JUDGMENT**

1.   The judgment is riddled with factual errors. I enclose corrections and clarifications.

2.   The judgment oozes prejudice of Alan Cooper as a lying, treacherous, money-greedy orchestrator of events, when Alan Cooper is in fact the naïve, truthful opposite. But once the tone is set by the Judge at the beginning of the judgment, all evidence she gleans from the mountain of evidence is selected to support her overriding prejudice, to the almost total exclusion of selecting any other.

3.   The Judge thinks I hid the Dr. Pin-Central Trust neuropsychological tests from the court, even from my own lawyer. My own lawyer Dour your partner, knew of them though neither he nor I knew of the results. Dour also knew the tests were not geared to my memory or neurological deficit problems, and he knew that Dr. Pin had conducted the tests in a sham-like way, holding the answer card himself to obtain favorable results. You, Mr. Stone did too. The Judge does not.

4.   The Judge clearly demonstrates a total lack of understanding of the symptoms of left frontal lobe injuries (e.g., bragging, lack of impulse control over nicotine, sugar, caffeine, alcohol, supposedly misinterpreted racial slurs, attacks by the injured against his parents and childhood, etc.).

5.   The Judge has no idea of Alan Cooper's G.P. Dr. Steve

Jensen's sabotaging the inputs of psychologists, neurosurgeons, endocrinologists, even dentists, before I ever met them.

*Alan J Cooper*

**NO: 1 • PAGE: 7**

**Judgment:** "The Hospital said his mental state improved quickly ..."

**Reality:** Hospital reported still incoherent on Jan. 2, 1982 which is day #7, indicating a *severe* brain injury.

**Comment:** This did not come out in court. Discussions of *mild* and *mild-to-severe* were attributed to Jan. 2, 1982 which was incorrectly calculated as day 5, not 7.

**NO: 2 • PAGE: 7**

**Judgment:** "He was discharged from hospital on January 4, 1982"

**Reality:** Discharged against neurosurgeon, Dr. Schwantz's advice, but done so on condition he would be in social worker wife's full-time care.

**Comment:** Doctors like my post-accident orthopedic Dr. England and others, expressed alarm at the unusually fast discharge for a severe brain injury.

**NO: 3 • PAGE: 7**

**Judgment:** "... For a minor neck injury as the symptoms seemed to have changed (from Jan. 13 to Feb. 10) and he was having some neck pain symptomatology."

**Reality:** The symptoms in fact had never changed. I simply could not articulate then Jan. 13 1982, given the more immediate shoulder pain. The neck problems were further corroborated by Physio Center Head, Gwen Peters.

**Comment:** No mention of my extreme dizziness or bowlegged walking, only of minor neck injury. Judge has only tiny fragment of the information.

**NO: 4 • PAGE: 7**

**Judgment:** "He returned to work in mid-February on a part-time schedule and by April 1982, was working full-time."

**Reality:**   I desperately wanted to quash workplace rumors and to show I could perform. And G.P. Jensen refused to give me medical leave. So I went back late, not mid-February and was having tremendous difficulty doing former work.

**Comment:**   People at work all around me witnessed my dizziness, slowness of speech and incoherence but I told them my healing could take up to 3 months, as per Dr. Schwantz's first diagnosis.

### NO: 5 • PAGE: 8

**Judgment:**   "His orthopedic Doctor England (noted) full range of movement in both (neck and shoulders)."

**Reality:**   That doctor in fact noted restricted, not full, range of movement.

**Comment:**   False input to Judge.

### NO: 6 • PAGE: 8

**Judgment:**   "Orthopedic Doctor England (said) neurologically, he was completely normal."

**Reality:**   Orthopedic Doctor England made no such statement. In fact, Dr. England expressed concern to my wife of a serious personality change which was confirmed to him by my wife.

**Comment:**   100% false evidence.

### NO: 7 • PAGE: 11

**Judgment:**   "...he enrolled in a two-year MBA program at the University of Toronto."

**Reality:**   False. I enrolled in a one-year Diploma of Business course which I completed.

**Comment:**   100% false evidence.

### NO: 8 • PAGE: 12

**Judgment:**   "He ... succumbed to their lures (the headhunters) to join a new company."

**Reality:**   False. No headhunter was involved and I wanted to quash Ministry rumors and re-prove myself in Canada's marketing world.

**Comment:**   100% false evidence. In fact, I never succumbed to the lures of the contingency headhunters or took a job via them.

**NO: 9 • PAGE: 13**

**Judgment:**  "Within two years, Cooper was promoted to Group Product Manager ..."

**Reality:**  The 2-year attainment is a record for Warner-Lambert where the normal period of progression is 7 years to Group Product Manager.

**Comment:**  Not brought out, Cooper's record high rate of success, prior to brain injury.

**NO: 10 • PAGE: 13**

**Judgment:**  "In July 1979, Cooper again succumbed to the lures of the head-hunters.

**Reality:**  Again totally false. No headhunter was involved at all.

**Comment:**  Second 100% false evidence on "lured by headhunters." I never took a job via a headhunter.

**NO: 11 • PAGE: 14**

**Judgment:**  "...and was able to return home after one week in hospital."

**Reality:**  False. Longer. Discharged against neurosurgeon, Dr. Schwantz's advice, but done on condition that I would be in wife's full-time care.

**Comment:**  Doctors like my post-accident orthopedic Dr. England and others, expressed alarm at the unusually fast discharge for a severe brain injury.

**NO: 12 • PAGE: 14**

**Judgment:**  "...back to work in middle of February."

**Reality:**  Late February, and my sick-leave pay had run out.

**NO: 13 • PAGE: 14**

**Judgment:**  "On April 1 1982, he was promoted ..."

**Reality:**  The promotion had been promised, pre-December 27, 1981 car accident. And, one of the key reasons I had gone back to work late February was to try to quell ugly rumors and prove I was still ready for the April 1, 1982 promotion.

**NO: 14 • PAGE: 14**

**Judgment:**  "... and expected to be fully recovered by summer."

**Reality:**    In fact, neurosurgeon Dr. Schwantz had changed his prognosis from a 3-month recovery to a 6-month recovery and I was banking my hopes on that.

**Comment:**    Judge has no understanding of changes in Dr. Schwantz's recovery forecast from 3 months to 6 to 12 to maybe never to never.

### NO: 15 • PAGE: 15

**Judgment:**    "He wanted to show everyone he was exactly the same as he had been before the accident."

**Reality:**    In fact, I was being pressured out of my existing job by rumors of how bad I was, post-accident.

### NO: 16 • PAGE: 15

**Judgment:**    "Blimiss Hope ... at an annual salary of $100,000."

**Reality:**    The salary was $68,000 plus car, and bonus if I earned it.

**Comment:**    False evidence.

### NO: 17 • PAGE: 16

**Judgment:**    "Stewart MacCallum... told Cooper he could take six months leave of absence and he returned in six weeks."

**Reality:**    False. Stewart MacCallum never offered the six months leave.

**Comment:**    100% false evidence.

### NO: 18 • PAGE: 17

**Judgment:**    "(Stewart MacCallum) said the Ministry would keep his job open for him for several months after he resigned."

**Reality:**    False. Never said.

**Comment:**    100% false evidence.

### NO: 19 • PAGE: 17

**Judgment:**    "(Stewart MacCallum) told (Cooper) that he could return, on condition he stay with the Ministry at least a year."

**Reality:**    False. Never put forward by Stewart MacCallum. And I said I could not make any commitments other than to do my very best. The response to me was that every week they got from me would be worth it.

**Comment**: False evidence.

## NO: 20 • PAGE: 17

**Judgment**: "That 1983 winter, Cooper was sought out by Blimiss and left."

**Reality**: After 8 months, where boss Willy Cork was sabotaging my work at every corner, even trying to get me fired, and the rumors of Alan's not having recovered after 6 months (July 1 '83) were rampant.

## NO: 21 • PAGE: 17

**Judgment**: I find it curious that he did not tell the doctor of the many symptoms he was complaining of at that time (Blimiss Hope doctor at hiring)…One can only conclude that Cooper was either deceiving that medical doctor or he was not suffering from those symptoms."

**Reality**: 100% false. I did tell the Blimiss Hope doctor who gave me some crude tests and he was satisfied. And I still fully expected to be recovered in 12 months or so, before Dr. Schwantz changed from 12 months to "perhaps never". And I still had no battery of neuro-psychological tests to quantify anything about me, so I was still very confused but hopeful. And the moment (July '83) I heard of problems from the tests, I told boss Darling at Blimiss Hope.

**Comment**: False evidence and badly prejudiced "only" conclusion by Judge. I told the Blimiss Hope doctor the truth as I then knew it. And later told the BH President the truth post-test as I knew it.

## NO: 22 • PAGE: 18

**Judgment**: "… things improved considerably when Alan took over the job at Blimiss Hope."

**Reality**: The expectations of me for the first year at Blimiss Hope were low, since my predecessor had been fired, but even after 16 months, my boss and peers were complaining, even cruelly joking publicly of my bad memory.

**Comment**: False evidence.

## NO: 23 • PAGE: 18

**Judgment**: "The following November he made a poor presentation at the head office in New York City and was placed on leave-of-absence."

**Reality:** In fact, I almost completely broke down and was forced to go to a psychiatrist, Dr. Hooker, and a psychologist, Dr. Kulisky, who tested me as pre-psychotic, requiring mind-altering drugs and probably hospitalization.

**Comment:** And all over the marketplace, the rumors were flying from peers, employees, recruiters and others that my bad memory from the car accident had caught up to the point where my not being able to handle such an executive job, had produced a nervous breakdown.

## NO: 24 • PAGE: 18

**Judgment:** "He was fired on Jan. 6, 1985."

**Reality:** And was offered long-term disability by Blimiss Hope, given my "severely imbalanced psychological state." I did not take the BH lawyer O'Hara's offer of Long Term Disability.

**Comment:** I refused the Long Term Disability offer because I wanted to work.

## NO: 25 • PAGE: 18

**Judgment:** "He joined the firm of Central Trust full-time after his tests with Dr. Pin showed there was nothing cognitively wrong with him."

**Reality:** False. I did not join the firm of Central Trust. Ever. And Dr. Pin's tests were distorted, as pointed out.

**Comment:** 100% false evidence.

## NO: 26 • PAGE: 18

**Judgment:** "...accepted a senior position with a senior Canadian Crown corporation ... and subsequently withdrew."

**Reality:** False. I was not offered the job. I did not withdraw.

**Comment:** 100% false evidence.

## NO: 27 • PAGE: 18

**Judgment:** "His drinking problems escalated and Maria left with the children.

**Reality:** False. My alcoholic annihilation began as a *result* of their leaving, not cause.

**Comment:** False evidence and based on Judge's own experiences with alcoholism.

**NO: 28 • PAGE: 18**

Judgment: "In January 1987 (he) stopped…joined (AA)."

Reality: False. The date was Dec. 11, 1986.

Comment: False evidence.

**NO: 29 • PAGE: 19**

Judgment: "He criticized (his wife's) ethnic background and her religion."

Reality: False. I criticized neither her ethnic background, nor her professed religion, the same as staunch Roman Catholic Nanette Carter. And the "Pollack" remark was made by Willy Cork, not I: I was quoting Cork disparagingly.

Comment: Maria's mother made the hearsay lie in court that I had criticized her ethnicity and same-as-Judge's religion.

**NO: 30 • PAGE: 19**

Judgment: "Regis Waters conceded that Cooper had turned strongly away from the business world because of the way he felt he had been treated at work."

Reality: 100% false. I had been spiritual as a child, had won an award for the highest mark in Religious studies in 1968 and had been approached in 1968–1969 to study divinity at Harvard shortly thereafter.

Comment: Totally wrong evidence.

**NO: 31 • PAGE: 29**

Judgment: "Dr. Mark Schwantz… was satisfied Cooper had recovered from the acute effect of his brain injury when he returned home on January 4, 1982."

Reality: No. Schwantz was very concerned with my leaving prematurely but my social worker wife guaranteed her own care.

Comment: Totally wrong evidence.

**NO: 32 • PAGE: 29**

Judgment: "…and (Cooper) knew he was in the hospital."

Reality: I repeatedly kept calling Flanders Hospital "Sick Children's."

Comment: Badly distorted evidence.

**Judgment:**   "Dr. Schwantz arranged for Cooper to see Dr. Winter."

**Reality:**   No. GP Jensen did and blackened Winter's thinking ahead of time with severe prejudice (i.e., malingering) so that Winter did not see me after his hostile phone call with me. Instead, I saw his assistant Ms. Little who first tried to talk me out of taking the tests at all, then wrote extreme falsehoods into the results to make them useless to any court assessment, as Dr. Schwantz sadly later admitted.

**Comment:**   Key false evidence.

**Judgment:**   "Dr. Fuller and Dr. Chan... each concluded that Alan Cooper did not have diabetes insipidus."

**Reality:**   Fuller first saw me 2 years after the injury, after my excess urination had partly subsided. Dr. Chan was 5 1/2 years post-injury. Whether there was transient diabetes insipidus in 1983 was never properly answered. Also, no mention in court of the low testosterone levels and luteinizing hormone (sex drive hormones), found by Fuller in more than one series of tests to be low and her giving me hormone injections over a period of time.

Dr. Fuller also made repeated reference to Dr. Maul's thinking my problems were anxiety-related, based on one very hostile 40-minute session with him, when in the first 10 minutes it had become painfully apparent that Dr. Maul had his mind made up before he met me, based on G.P. Steve Jensen's extremely prejudicial input. (Jensen had insisted that I see Maul, once Jensen had heard that my then lawyer Dour had received a supportive document from Dr. Schwantz.)

**Comment:**   Complete misunderstanding of endocrinological findings.

**Judgment:**   "Was seeing Dr. Michael Fisher for psychic impotence."

**Reality:**   False. Dr. Fuller found the hormonal damage in my testosterone and luteinizing hormones, on more than one series of tests across the next 12 months.

**Comment:**   Badly distorted evidence.

**NO: 36 • PAGE: 34**

Judgment: "(Dr. Jensen's) notes include gout."

Reality: No. There is a family predisposition towards gout but I've never had it.

Comment: Falsely hinting at decades of alcoholism.

**NO: 37 • PAGE: 34**

Judgment: "The (Jensen) notes... Cooper...has a history of diabetes."

Reality: No. There is some diabetes of the old-person type in family but not in Cooper himself. And diabetes insipidus bears no relation to the other diabetes.

Comment: Badly distorted evidence.

**NO: 38 • PAGE: 35**

Judgment: "On cross-examination, Dr. Jensen...history of diabetes in the family..."

Reality: 100% irrelevant to diabetes insipidus.

Comment: Grossly misleading.

**NO: 39 • PAGE: 35**

Judgment: "Alan wanted another neurological opinion and he arranged for him to be seen by Dr. Maul at Flanders Hospital."

Reality: No. Jensen pushed me to Maul, forced me to sign a paper of request, after Jensen heard that my lawyer had received a report from Dr. Schwantz. Jensen then prejudiced Maul's opinion pre-meeting, so that Maul told me in the first 10 minutes of seeing me that there was nothing wrong with me and that I should legally settle with the first offer from the other side as soon as possible. Maul then went on to prejudice Fuller, before I met her. All on Jensen's vicious, lengthy input. (Maul is in AA with me.)

Comment: Grossly misleading and prejudice upfront.

**NO: 40 • PAGE: 35**

Judgment: "...from a moderately severe brain injury."

Reality: It was severe. Day 7, Jan. 2, 1983 still incoherent.

Comment: 100% wrong critical evidence.

**NO: 41 • PAGE: 37**

**Judgment:**   "The brain injury was mild to moderate…"

**Reality:**      Wrong. Severe.

**Comment:**    100% wrong critical evidence.


**NO: 42 • PAGE: 38**

**Judgment:**   "(Dr. Malthrop) did not observe any evidence of poor memory and found (Cooper's) speech normal."

**Reality:**      Wrong. He never checked either.

**Comment:**    100% false evidence.


**NO: 43 • PAGE: 38**

**Judgment:**   "…had been promoted to his level of incompetence."

**Reality:**      Wrong. Pre-accident, I did jobs with consistent excellence and was recognized repeatedly for such.

**Comment:**    Gross, prejudiced distortion.


**NO: 44 • PAGE: 38**

**Judgment:**   "…incompetence due to…alcohol problems."

**Reality:**      Wrong. Alcohol not involved at all, relative to the Ministry or Blimiss Hope.

**Comment:**    Gross, prejudiced distortion.


**NO: 45 • PAGE: 39**

**Judgment:**   "(Dr. Malthrop believed) Cooper was devious and dishonest and the appropriate diagnosis was malingering."

**Reality:**      Malthrop is the devious and dishonest one and told me so outside the courtroom, apologizing to me but saying that was his (Malthrop's) job in this case.

**Comment:**    Maliciously prejudiced, wrong conclusion by M'Lady Carter.


**NO: 46 • PAGE: 39**

**Judgment:**   "Maul's Saturday Jan. 12, 1985 findings."

**Reality:**      Findings totally superficial and biased upfront by Dr. Jensen.

**Comment:**    Key evidence withheld.

**NO: 47 • PAGE: 41**

**Judgment:** "(Dr. Fisher) agreed that Alan Cooper was unhappy about the psychological testing performed by Dr. Winter in June 1983 and by Dr. Kellerman on April 12, 1984."

**Reality:** Dr. Winter's assistant, Ms. Little sabotaged the first set of tests and Dr. Schwantz knew that. And Dr. Kellerman told me he did not want to contradict any of the findings made by the exalted colleague of his, Dr. Winter, who is considered by many as Canada's best neuropsychologist.

**Comment:** Judge has no idea of the reasons why.


**NO: 48 • PAGE: 41**

**Judgment:** "(Kellerman) concluded...mild-to-moderate closed head injury."

**Reality:** 100% wrong and he did not know of pupil size or 7 days of incoherence in hospital.

**Comment:** It was severe and Kellerman had only prejudiced input, from Winter's sabotage.


**NO: 49 • PAGE: 42**

**Judgment:** "A year in the position of Vice-President Marketing struck Dr. Kellerman as quite an accomplishment and not characteristic of brain injury."

**Reality:** In fact, I was having all kinds of problems that first year at Blimiss Hope, with peers, boss, colleagues oralizing loudly about my bad memory and foul, anti-social humor (something I had not had pre-accident). But I, in fact, had in effect a year's reprieve, since the previous VP Marketing had been fired after only 18 months; i.e., many benefits of the doubt were being given to me in the first Blimiss Hope year.

**Comment:** Judge knew none of the Blimiss Hope first year problems nor did Kellerman, who doubted me at the outset, asking why I was unhappy with any tests initially done by his esteemed colleague Dr. Gary Winter.

**NO: 50 • PAGE: 42**

**Judgment**: "Dr. Kellerman...saw the black book (as) a positive sign rather than a negative one."

**Reality**: Ironically, I could not survive without it as both a U. of T. memory expert and later Dr. Winter, confirmed to me.


**NO: 51 • PAGE: 43**

**Judgment**: "Diffuse injury would be worse than what he had."

**Reality**: I *do* have diffuse injury and Dr. Day saw it even in the years-later CT scan photos.

**Comment**: 100% wrong key evidence.


**NO: 52 • PAGE: 43**

**Judgment**: "verbal similarity was...lower."

**Reality**: Of course. That's a problem area for me.


**NO: 53 • PAGE: 43**

**Judgment**: "...interpreting proverbs, Cooper did very well."

**Reality**: I wasn't interpreting but knew them pre-accident.

**Comment**: Judge does not understand new information to be the problem.


**NO: 54 • PAGE: 44**

**Judgment**: "...visual memory (very good)."

**Reality**: I never complained of visual memory.

**Comment**: Judge focusing on irrelevant point.


**NO: 55 • PAGE: 44**

**Judgment**: "...learn the 12 words in 6 or 7 tries. Cooper... twelfth try. As there was no other test finding he could relate to his performance, Dr. Kellerman concluded there was no pattern of deficit."

**Reality**: That's where the problem is! A key error in Kellerman's diagnosis. And Dr. Winter in the autumn of 1987 conducted a massive series of other neuro-psychological tests directly related to the primary problem and found a strong pattern of multiple deficits.

**Comment**: Misunderstood diagnosis.

**NO: 56 • PAGE: 45**

**Judgment:** "MMPI results totally non-functional and probably needed hospital-ization. But Kellerman changed his feeling when he saw the report of Dr. Pin."

**Reality:** Such bad MMPI results are typical of brain injury and Kellerman did not report them at all to me.

**Comment:** Critical misinformation.

**NO: 57 • PAGE: 46**

**Judgment:** "Dr. Pin...MMPI in the standard way and scored them in the stan-dardized way."

**Reality:** False. Dr. Pin did them sloppily and illegally, holding the answer card, and we breezed through them, getting off-track on the num-bering of the answer card at least once. Pin wanted to finish and go home.

**Comment:** Critical error in case.

**NO: 58 • PAGE: 46**

**Judgment:** Dr. Pin's assessment.

**Reality:** Never performed on me the word-pairing types, where I had had problems on all the other tests.

**Comment:** Critical error in case.

**NO: 59 • PAGE: 48**

**Judgment:** "Other than Cooper himself, no one appeared to be aware of Dr. Pin or his assessment prior to trial. This tended to highlight the assess-ment and led to adjournments, the recall of expert witnesses and lengthy delays."

**Reality:** False. I told my lawyer Gordon Dour of the tests before, during and after, though I knew not the results of them. Dour's partner, my new lawyer, Stone, also knew of the tests and knew they had not been geared to focus on my memory problem. In fact Adam Stone told me that Dr. Pin's tests if brought up in court, would be readily dis-missed as an aberration, given what they tested and how done.

**Comment:** Absolutely critical to Judge Carter's final very bad judgment.

**NO: 60 • PAGE: 49**

**Judgment:** "MMPI for Kellerman and Kulisky wildly erratic but not for Pin's."

**Reality:** Pin conducted the tests by coaching me and by keeping the answer card.

**Comment:** Critical to Judge Carter's very bad judgment.

**NO: 61 • PAGE: 49**

**Judgment:** "Once again, on Dr. Winter's examination in 1987, Mr. Cooper again produced an abnormal looking performance. It was Dr. Kellerman's opinion that this is only consistent with a person who is responding to this test in a manner in which he wishes to appear emotionally disturbed or non-disturbed, depending on the circumstances."

**Reality:** Pin had been holding the answer card, coaching me to "look good." With Winter, it was strictly orthodox. Even though by the time of Winter's 1987 report, I'd heard of Jensen's vicious oral feedback to Stone, and was once again livid with indignation. But I did not lie on or manipulate Winter's test, done subsequent to Pin. Also, Winter in 1987 did a huge range of specific memory tests which zeroed in on the problem(s), one(s) which no one else had done.

**Comment:** The court doesn't know these critical points.

**NO: 62 • PAGE: 52**

**Judgment:** "…tended to give answers that were verbose rather than simple."

**Reality:** That kind of verbosity (vs. my pre-accident precise communication) is a textbook sign of the kind of mega-bite rambling and verbosity, while trying to find the right words, characteristic of a left frontal lobe injury.

**Comment:** Judge is commenting on classic left frontal lobe brain injury symptoms but does not recognize them.

**NO: 63 • PAGE: 53**

**Judgment:** "His MMPI Profile reflected a great deal of psychopathology…His daily routine at his own office did not reflect psychopathology…

**Reality:** My office routine was not known to the doctor; in fact, my behavior was often just that of someone deeply emotionally disturbed.

**Comment:** Judge has no knowledge of my problems at work, whatsoever or of recalling that I had done poorly on the Rorschach when it was critical that I do well, to save my Blimiss Hope job.

**NO: 64**

**Judgment:** Knowing this test is easy to fake…Rorschach…people with frontal lobe damage give impoverished answers…not the case with Cooper."

**Reality:** I had already had the Rorschach 10 months earlier with Dr. Kulisky who described me as pre-psychotic.

**NO: 65 • PAGE: 54**

**Judgment:** "He has almost no energy left over to be very concerned about the needs of others…"

**Reality:** I have spent my life in work and beyond, doing social work/helping/giving to others.

**Comment:** Absolutely false values comment on me by Judge versus the opposite in reality.

**NO: 66 • PAGE: 55**

**Judgment:** "No confusion in the pronunciation of the words Massachusetts, Methodist and Episcopal in 1983 but in 1987."

**Reality:** False. Winter in 1987 refused to allow me to talk slowly, to camouflage my mispronunciation as I did in 1983 with his assistant Ms. Little.

**Comment:** Judge totally misunderstands from only partial evidence.

**NO: 67 • PAGE: 57**

**Judgment:** "Dr. Winter testified that… the most specific ability changes referable to brain injury were the difficulty in word finding, the difficulty in learning verbal material and some mild difficulty in delayed verbal recall."

**Reality:** Exactly, and only Winter tested them fully, Pin not at all in his infamous sham!

**Comment:** Crux of issue missed by Judge.

**Judgment:**   "Dr. Pin falloff to Winter's was motivational."

**Reality:**   No. Pin did the sham tests himself and did not concentrate on memory.

**Comment:**   Key pivotal point.

**Judgment:**   "Cooper certainly faked Dr. Kulisky's MMPI…"

**Reality:**   False. I was getting fired and I was desperately trying to appear normal to keep my job but still failed MMPI.

**Comment:**   Critical prejudice by Judge.

**Judgment:**   "Cooper's 1987 tests worse than 1983…Cooper was not trying as hard in 1987. He was not motivated."

**Reality:**   False. 1987 tests were different and 1983 was sabotaged by Little.

**Judgment:**   "Cooper shaping answers for Kellerman, Winter and Pin."

**Reality:**   100% false. Different tests and Pin fudged the tests.

**Comment:**   Critical misunderstanding by Judge.

**Judgment:**   "Dr. Pin was the only psychologist in a position to recommend him for a job and this explained why in 1986 he shaped his answers to produce a normal profile for Dr. Pin."

**Reality:**   100% false. With Kulisky, I was trying to save my Blimiss Hope job but my results were disastrous and I failed. Also, Pin fudged the tests.

**Comment:**   Critical misunderstanding by Judge.

**Judgment:**   "Psychologist Pin said I was doing homework to improve scores, hence the high Pin scores."

**Reality:**     Absolutely 100% false. All testing was done in 2 hours there. Pin is lying to protect himself.

**Comment:**     Critical false evidence.

## NO: 74 • PAGE: 61

**Judgment:**     Pin also claimed Cooper was also not candid on MMPI and WAISR.

**Reality:**     100% false. Pin is lying to protect himself and had told me I was honest in test.

**Comment:**     Critical false evidence.

## NO: 75 • PAGE: 64

**Judgment:**     Mr. Cooper told Dr. Clive Day he thought his sense of smell was normal.

**Reality:**     But that I had no way of being sure. Others (my wife) had found it below normal (e.g., in a stove-oven fire). As did Day.

**Comment:**     Judge wrongly implying I was making up my bad sense of smell.

## NO: 76 • PAGE: 65

**Judgment:**     Malthrop said I had tried squash only once, that I was not trying to rehabilitate myself.

**Reality:**     We know from other witnesses (e.g., James Cheapsake) that I tried many times. And, with swimming I was very much trying (on average up to 1 mile per day, as documented in Hart House).

## NO: 77 • PAGE: 66

**Judgment:**     "The photographically shown brain atrophy was…highly likely a consequence of alcohol in this particular patient."

**Reality:**     My alcohol consumption has been widely, wildly exaggerated: Pre-accident, one ounce at 17, none thereafter all through high school and university until age 21; 4 or 5 times per year for 10 years, like everyone in Warner-Lambert; Post-accident, 9 days of 4 bottles of Guinness in Jan.–Feb. 1982. Drunk 4 times in April '82; Aug. '82–Jan. '85 one 3/4-litre bottle of wine at night (without drugs); winter 1985 temporarily excessive in my post-firing period; nothing April–May–June 1985; sporadic in late '85; 3 weeks in total in all of 1986; nothing in all of 1987; nothing in 1988; nothing in 1989 until this Mar. 13 Supreme Court Judgment and still none.

**Comment:** Alcohol is probably based on Judge's own personal experiences with ex-husband. And her empirical knowledge of my drinking is 95% wrong. (See also #87).

### NO: 78 • PAGE: 69

**Judgment:** "Dr. Clive Day's opinion… Cooper temporary diabetes insipidus.

**Reality:** Of course. The thirst and urination were worst in the first 9 months as reported but I still urinate too much.

### NO: 79 • PAGE: 72

**Judgment:** "Cooper misused 'hypothalamic disturbance'."

**Reality:** Dr. Schwantz told me that I had probably had it, during the first 9 months post-accident.

**Comment:** Bad Judge misinterpretation.

### NO: 80 • PAGE: 72

**Judgment:** Diabetes in family not known.

**Reality:** A completely different kind. I told Drs. Schwantz and Fuller who said it is not relevant.

**Comment:** Judge using irrelevant material.

### NO: 81 • PAGE: 72

**Judgment:** Increased drinking (water) and urination prior to the accident.

**Reality:** Prostatitis. And I told endocrinologist Dr. Fuller who said it was not directly relevant.

**Comment:** Another critical Judge misunderstanding.

### NO: 82 • PAGE: 73

**Judgment:** "He conceded no compelling evidence of hypothalamic disorder.

**Reality:** Nine months post-accident of extreme amounts of water and urination, and Fuller's low hormone results.

**Comment:** Hypothalamic disorder had been suggested by doctors, not me.

**NO: 83 • PAGE:** 73

**Judgment:** And Stewart MacCallum wanted to keep him on, after he resigned the second time.

**Reality:** False. I was never asked to stay on.

**Comment:** False evidence.


**NO: 84 • PAGE:** 73

**Judgment:** Stewart MacCallum counseled against Blimiss Hope.

**Reality:** False. He did not.

**Comment:** False evidence.


**NO: 85 • PAGE:** 73

**Judgment:** Job work for first year at Blimiss Hope satisfactory.

**Reality:** False.

**Comment:** Key misunderstanding.


**NO: 86 • PAGE:** 73

**Judgment:** Cooper did not tell Dr. Day of the irreconcilable differences in marketing between Cooper and Blimiss Hope's Darling.

**Reality:** That difference was a concocted-by-lawyers-O'Hara-and-Shin "release story" given to me by Blimiss Hope upon his firing me.

**Comment:** Judge misunderstanding.


**NO: 87 • PAGE:** 73

**Judgment:** "Cooper did not tell Dr. Day he had been consuming large quantities of (alcohol) in February 1985."

**Reality:** I did tell Dr. Day, and he said short-term alcohol abuse does not bring on the type of brain damage or pre-alcohol problems I had.

**Comment:** Critically missed point on alcohol.


**NO: 88 • PAGE:** 74

**Judgment:** "Cooper didn't tell Day of Central Trust's psych. testing through Dr. Pin."

**Reality:** I had already told my lawyers Dour and Stone who briefed Dr. Day.

**Comment:** Critical misunderstanding to Judge by Stone.

**NO:** 89 • **PAGE:** 74

**Judgment:**   "Cooper didn't tell of 9-hours long 1969 knock out."

**Reality:**   Hospital confirmed less than 1 hour; no lasting effect. I had told Gauze's querying neurosurgeon and he had himself confirmed not relevant. I had a back (lumbar) injury.

**Comment:**   Critically wrong evidence.


**NO:** 90 • **PAGE:** 74

**Judgment:**   "Cooper didn't talk of childhood frustrations."

**Reality:**   Classic complaint signs of left frontal lobe injury, as confirmed by Drs. Clive Day and Michael Fisher.

**Comment:**   Critical misinterpretation by Judge.


**NO:** 91 • **PAGE:** 76

**Judgment:**   "Dr. Maul found nothing."

**Reality:**   Jensen prejudiced upfront.

**Comment:**   Not known to Judge.


**NO:** 92 • **PAGE:** 77

**Judgment:**   "The swings in Cooper's marks and moods… (Dr. Pin)…were only consistent with a person who is responding to the test in the manner he chooses depending on the circumstances."

**Reality:**   False. Why fail Dr. Kulisky when at stake was my job? Also Pin fudged the tests and lied in court to self-protect.

**Comment:**   Critical, false evidence.


**NO:** 93 • **PAGE:** 78

**Judgment:**   "Cooper has rather poor social judgment and exaggerates."

**Reality:**   Classic textbook signs of left frontal lobe injury as confirmed by Dr. Clive Day.

**Comment:**   Critical misunderstanding by Judge.


**NO:** 94 • **PAGE:** 78

**Judgment:**   "Cooper can be extremely devious."

**Reality:**   40 years of philanthropy, high honesty, and help to others prove that false.

**Comment:** Judge has eyes and ears closed to what little truth is getting through to her.


**NO: 95 • PAGE: 78**

**Judgment:** "Cooper's so-called 'love letters' saturated with exaggeration."

**Reality:** Classic left frontal lobe injury symptoms, as confirmed by both Drs. Clive Day and Michael Fisher.

**Comment:** Critical misinterpretation.


**NO: 96 • PAGE: 78–79**

**Judgment:** "Cooper's 'the Brain,' musical ability, 100% on some school tests gross exaggerations."

**Reality:** All true.

**Comment:** Judge choosing to believe nothing I say.


**NO: 97 • PAGE: 79**

**Judgment:** "Cooper told Fisher he had an MBA."

**Reality:** I did not. Ever.

**Comment:** 100% wrong fact again.


**NO: 98 • PAGE: 79**

**Judgment:** "Cooper had not told Fisher of Blimiss Hope firing or problems at Warner-Lambert."

**Reality:** I had, in every tiny detail. Dr. Fisher was a day-to-day part of each and every step of the process.

**Comment:** 100% False.


**NO: 99 • PAGE: 79**

**Judgment:** I find it curious that Cooper never mentioned to M.D.'s he consulted post-accident, depression, anxiety, insomnia, hearing, impotency (6 months in 1982), fatigue, polyuria, and polydipsia."

**Reality:** I had 100% to Fisher, Fuller, Schwantz, etc. And they had all dismissed as of no real relevance to my main bad memory cause.

**Comment:** 100% wrong critical facts again by Judge.

**NO:** 100 • **PAGE:** 79

**Judgment:**   Balance.

**Reality:**   Exceptionally bad for first 9 months.

**Comment:**   Judge has no knowledge.


**NO:** 101 • **PAGE:** 79

**Judgment:**   Diabetes insipidus.

**Reality:**   Schwantz told me that.

**Comment:**   Judge has no knowledge.


**NO:** 102 • **PAGE:** 79

**Judgment:**   Hearing.

**Reality:**   Jensen knew of my old problem and pushed me to get it checked again.

**Comment:**   Critical evidence not known by Judge.


**NO:** 103 • **PAGE:** 79

**Judgment:**   Loss of smell.

**Reality:**   I was not concocting it. Wife told me; Schwantz tested. Dr. Day confirmed.

**Comment:**   100% false evidence to Judge.


**NO:** 104 • **PAGE:** 80

**Judgment:**   Balance tested in the norm.

**Reality:**   That was 2 years later after much of my first 9 months dizziness was restored. And I can still not do ring around a rosy to this day: I get head-spinning and semi-nauseous right after.

**Comment:**   Complete misunderstanding by Judge.


**NO:** 105 • **PAGE:** 80

**Judgment:**   "Gauze's neurosurgeon, Emblem, said Cooper not trying to get himself back in shape."

**Reality:**   With initially disastrous balance, I chose swimming and was doing one mile per day in 1982, 1/2 of 1983, part of 1984, all of 1985, part of 1986, part of 1987.

**Comment:**   Factually wrong evidence.

**NO: 106 • PAGE: 80–81**

**Judgment:**    Hearing: Past History.

**Reality:**    Jensen knew of it and pushed me to get it checked again and report back to him. I volunteered to him that I had a past history and I retrieved the records with the hospital. The otolaryngologist told me the slight worsening could be the result of the car accident.

**Comment:**    Critically wrong evidence.


**NO: 107 • PAGE: 81**

**Judgment:**    "Malthrop tested Cooper for linguistic French and Cooper refused."

**Reality:**    Malthrop did not. And I volunteered to prove my French in court but was stopped by the Judge.

**Comment:**    More false evidence given.


**NO: 108 • PAGE: 82**

**Judgment:**    His diction is not impaired.

**Reality:**    It was of an elocutionist's before. And it is impaired. I make 20 mistakes at work daily, despite talking much more slowly, as the evidence frequently points out.

**Comment:**    Critically wrong evidence.


**NO: 109 • PAGE: 82**

**Judgment:**    "Cooper must have 'understood' diabetes insipidus, diminished smell, appetite, libido."

**Reality:**    100% false. All information was diagnosed to me by Doctors Schwantz and Fuller.

**Comment:**    Critically wrong evidence.


**NO: 110 • PAGE: 83**

**Judgment:**    "(Cooper) set the merry-go-round in motion."

**Reality:**    100% false. No.

**Comment:**    Absolutely critical to Ms. Carter's overall judgment.


**NO: 111 • PAGE: 83**

**Judgment:**    Put to rest by Fuller in 1984.

**Reality:** My thirst and urination were less, 2 years later but still high. And Fuller did find hormonal/libido problems.

**Comment:** Wrong interpretation of evidence.


**NO:** 112 • **PAGE:** 83

**Judgment:** Dr. Pin's tests known to him.

**Reality:** No. Central Trust never told me results.

**Comment:** False Judge assumption.


**NO:** 113 • **PAGE:** 84

**Judgment:** "I find it very unusual that Alan Cooper did not report this testing (Pin's) to anyone."

**Reality:** I did. To Stone, and his predecessor Dour already knew about it.

**Comment:** CRITICAL, PIVOTAL POINT OF CASE.


**NO:** 114 • **PAGE:** 85

**Judgment:** "No personality change."

**Reality:** The "love letters" to Maria, and stories, prove there is.

**Comment:** Critical misunderstanding by Judge on personality.


**NO:** 115 • **PAGE:** 86

**Judgment:** Promoted in April 1982.

**Reality:** Done prior to accident.

**Comment:** Wrong evidence.


**NO:** 116 • **PAGE:** 87

**Judgment:** "No problems at Blimiss Hope in Year 1."

**Reality:** False.

**Comment:** Judge has no knowledge.


**NO:** 117 • **PAGE:** 88

**Judgment:** "Heavy drinking at Blimiss Hope."

**Reality:** No. Only the 3/4 litre of wine at night, Aug. '82–Jan. '85.

**Comment:** Wrong evidence.

**NO:** 118 • **PAGE:** 88

**Judgment:** "Problems with family, friends and colleagues were alcohol related."

**Reality:** Absolutely false. Maria and her mother heard of Judge's husband's alcoholism.

**Comment:** False evidence for Judge's prejudiced conclusion.

**NO:** 119 • **PAGE:** 89

**Judgment:** "Little care for wife."

**Reality:** Pre-maternity, delivered both babies, wisdom teeth, help, etc. Maria protected herself again.

**Comment:** Critically false information on Alan as person. May be Judge's prejudice from own personal experiences.

**NO:** 120 • **PAGE:** Page 46

**Judgment:** "Dr. Pin testified that Cooper also stated that he felt he was between a rock and a hard place, i.e., do poorly for litigation, do well for job, in psych tests."

**Reality:** 100% false. Pin made that comment to me and I made no comment in return. Dr. Pin is again lying to disguise his professional negligence.

**Comment:** Absolutely false and critical to the overall judgment.

*Alan J Cooper*

April 30, 1989

## Written in Rage

There is more in my notes but my reading of the trial has pushed my brain circuits close to another crash as predicted by Dr. Day. Until today 15 years later, I have dared not look again at the Ontario Supreme Court Judgment of M'Lady Nanette Carter.

I feel I should not alter this MEMO OF RECORD as written then. Editing it would lend less than a true picture of my mental state at the time of its writing. Instead I will try to sketch the events that followed April of 1989.

After multiple midnights of writing, I mailed the rebuttal to Stone and then took again my 6 milligrams of Ativan. No-one but I knew the trial's truth and in the days and years ahead, I would learn it would stay that way. Next night, I took once more to writing. I wasn't sure what, but I sensed my writing would reach some yet-to-be-known world of understanding. I wrote:

"I won't see it but I feel certain that Gauze, Her Ladyship and the powers that run Regal Insurance will all fall into a Hell-on-Earth. I may even be asked to pull them out, but I cannot presume such grandeur, for such presumptuousness betrays an arrogance I feel I should try to stop. If someone asks, I will help them, for helping them will not only help them but also humankind, my family and me. I fear, though that Supreme Court Judge Nanette Carter, Gauze and the facility-insurance company's rulers will devour themselves one day...How on earth in Canada can this injustice be really happening?"

## Appeal

Though opposing lawyer Gauze had delivered his pre-trial offer only hours before the trial start, Judge Carter waived some statutory clause that stated Gauze should have allowed Stone 3 days before court to respond. In addition, Carter awarded Gauze, his law firm Timpson Cable and its client, facility insurance company Regal, all costs.

Gauze must have known that my lawyer had already spent more than Gauze's offer when he had made it; with no admission of liability, Gauze had wanted court.

Stone's costs, undocumented and unsupported, were trumped up by a numbers-dumb Stone to an eye-grabbing and easy-to-grasp $500,000. Given the limit of driver Barry Lewis's liability coverage—$500,000 on his wife's insurance—their lawyer Gauze's costs had also swelled. I was led to believe that all costs were to be paid by me. Lord advertising also wanted its costs for my earlier lawyer Dour's going after it over breach of my contract.

Stone again counseled me to see Walter Chintak, "the best appeal lawyer in Canada." A week before I met him, I personally delivered to his office, my hand-scribbled notes from the trial, as well as my post-trial letter of concern to Stone, the one Dr. Fisher had stopped a year earlier. I did not know yet about Stone's close association with Chintak.

Shortly after I arrived to see Chintak in his office at 10:00 a.m. May 1, 1989, he began with "Let me be perfectly clear. Adam Stone is a very dear…and I will not in any way help your…". I was shaken by Chintak's presumption and told him so, but he evidently believed me to be a manipulative liar. He repeated his portentous "Let me be perfectly clear" message and then he handed me a letter, which confirmed his clarity.

Chintak stated to me that the chances of a successful appeal were remote, because Ontario's and Canada's appeal courts were reluctant to overturn judgments, particularly Supreme Court ones that dealt with credibility. The rationale was that the appeal judges had not been at the original trial and thus could not make a full and proper judgment of my credibility or lack thereof.

I left Toronto's core of lawyers and walked north the 6 miles home. I then went into my basement office, took my mug, filled it with water from the laundry room tap and sat back down on my office chair. I looked at the photos of James, Robert and Maria on the wall in front of me, and I wrote:

"Stone knows that I am permanently brain damaged. His doctors all know. Opposing Gauze knows. Gauze's law firm Timpson Cable knows. Regal Insurance may know through Gauze, because such truth would heighten Timpson Cable's reputation as Canada's #1 law firm for handling brain injuries. Gauze's doctors all know. But I, Alan Cooper, am a condemned, manipulative, devious liar as determined by Canada's largest province's Supreme Court and will soon be penniless...What next?"

Stone's assistant lawyer phoned to ask how my meeting with appeal lawyer Chintak had gone. To my astonishment, Stone's assistant added that she had re-read the judgment and thought it a good one. Stone's articling student echoed the assistant's view that the Judge had dealt well with gray areas. There seemed no stop to the spread of misinformation from lies first set in place by G.P. Dr. Jensen, my wife and opposing Doctor Malthrop.

# DR. FISHER

It was almost 2:00 p.m., May 1, 1989. I had taken the day off and had a 3 o'clock appointment with psychotherapist Michael Fisher. His office was a 3-mile walk to the southwest. Along the way, I stopped at a delicatessen and had an egg and watercress sandwich, with a 10 oz. can of grapefruit juice. At 2:55 p.m., I reached Dr. Fisher's office and went immediately to his washroom to urinate, and then put my mouth around the cold tap for water.

At 3:00 p.m. I entered Dr. Fisher's office, sat down 5 feet opposite him and with eye contact direct as it could be, spoke and shared thoughts.

"Dr. Fisher, there can be no appeal."

Psychotherapist Dr. Michael Fisher sat motionless in front of me.

When he spoke next, he chose the kind of tangential talk that often accompanies people at a loss for words at funerals.

"And how is your cousin Peter related to you, Alan?"

"...My father's mother, the one who died of diabetes, the day Pearl Harbor was bombed. She was the Irish rabble-rouser who married my staunch Wasp grandfather. A young Roman Catholic female in small city Ontario in the 19th century. "

"Peter Brawn—it must be 20 years ago—was one of the brightest psychiatric residents I ever had...It's in your genes."

"She's in Mount Pleasant Cemetery. Papa took me there often. He took me everywhere. A retired Vice President of Domtar, still years later wearing a 3-piece suit and a fresh white handkerchief, pressed each day. He was honest, generous and practiced what he preached. Yes, self-righteous but he really was more honest than others, Dr. Fisher, and he did not approve of dishonest people. Or of cowardice—he gave a very hard time to a male survivor of the Titanic. Papa was an athlete, too, a champion lacrosse player. When Papa was 65, he beat his track star son in a race."

"You strongly identify with him, Alan. Where was he born?"

"Kingsville, Ontario in that south-western part of Canada which actually dips 50 miles south of Detroit. Born in 1876. His father Arthur Cooper died in Seattle in 1914. You were curious, Dr. Fisher—I have a copy here of the death certificate. Papa's father was born in England in 1838, the son of Samuel Cooper. His mother's maiden name was Nichols and she was descended partly from Scotland."

"Not a Loyalist?"

"It gets murky there, with part of the family tracing to some aide to George Washington and parts tracing to Benjamin Franklin."

"You are related to Benjamin Franklin, Alan?"

"There is such concern in my immediate family about sex and legitimacy that no one has ever fully explained to me, why the name Franklin appears as the second name of the first male child in every generation. My son's name is James Franklin Cooper."

"What about your mother's side?"

"The Nestlea side is clearer. A Nestlea was given 1,000 acres west of Toronto in Stratford where the Shakespearean theatre now is. That Nestlea ancestor had helped defend Canada against the Americans in the War of 1812. His earlier family had emigrated in the late 1700s from the United States…Delaware. Near the end of the 1900s, one descendant went north to an area about 150 miles north of Toronto. There his granddaughter, my mother, was born. She became a one-room country schoolmarm."

"And going back to this Papa whom you loved so much, how did he start life?"

"He had a fight with his mother when he was 17, and then hitchhiked that summer of 1893, out west to Saskatchewan to trim wheat fields. Some time around the end of the summer, he went to the Chicago World's Fair, where he was later fond of telling me that he had spent the loneliest time of his life. Then, unlike his brothers and sisters who moved to the United States, he came back to Canada. At age 20 in early 1895, Papa married Mary Clara Emily, a Roman Catholic girl from Barrie, 50 miles north of Toronto. They moved north another 30 miles to a little village called Longford, where Papa became postmaster and started a general store. The village is long gone but the shell of a store is still there. Papa's brothers became very wealthy businesspeople in the United States, one being founder of the Southern Pacific Railway and another Vice President of NBC and co-inventor of the transistor with Marconi."

"Really!" Dr. Fisher had been listening professionally but perked at the transistor part.

"And this young Roman Catholic bride of a 19th century Wasp as you call him, did she live happily ever after as a Protestant in small town Canada?"

"Hardly. She started her own church, had it built of stone. It is still there, near that huge new casino in Rama."

"A Roman Catholic church?"

"No, her own. She was her own person. I guess I come by it honestly. Alfred Lord Tennyson is in her family's past as well as some grand master Shriner."

"A Shriner? Roman Catholic?"

"It gets mixed up there, too. I'm not sure how English blood gets mixed in with the Irish. Again, my family won't talk. I do know, though, that my grandmother was a poet, elocutionist and visual artist. Her oils and water colors were all over the walls of my North Toronto home. One of her sons, my uncle, William Cooper, had a talent she recognized early in his childhood, and instead of being scolded for playing with girls and dressing up dolls, he was nurtured to go as a teenager to Toronto and take dress designing at Central Technical School. After that, Uncle William went to New York and after World War I at the age of 20 in 1920, became one of the greatest dress designers in New York and Paris. He lived with Eva Gardner for 11 years and I think he was bi-sexual—I guess I always *have* accepted homosexuality. Decades later, when he moved to Los Angeles, he had an extremely private house which became the Beatles' secret hideaway in the 1960s. My dad actually talked to their manager, Brian Epstein, when phoning to wish his brother a happy birthday, on August 24th. My family didn't believe my father after he got off the line, because he was such a blowhard. Only a month later did we see Uncle William's house on the front of some grocery checkout newspaper that my mother bought."

Dr. Fisher sat silent, leaving us both to live in the pause. He knew I always had an agenda and he peered down at my black book, closed on my lap. I opened it to the day.

"Dr. Fisher, Moses was a prophet, not a King, divine medium or sovereign legislator, is that not true?"

"Yes, Alan. And Jewish writers described his human weaknesses."

"Do not Jews yearn for a stable and peaceful society where the welfare of the soul and body come first?"

"I would like to think we all do, Alan."

"Were Jews seized for *Judenhetze*, for apocalypse, because of their relentless appeal for ethical justice?"

"Some so say, Alan. I don't know." Dr. Fisher began halfsmiling.

"Jesus was a learned Jew, was he not, Dr. Fisher?"

"I believe so, Alan."

"But did he not believe that elaborate, formal learning was unnecessary, that in law for example, the spirit and not the letter constituted the essence?"

Dr. Fisher gave me a warm, kind smile. His voice that followed was that of an aged baritone.

"Much of your mind is still intact, Alan. You are permanently brain damaged, to be sure, but we need to continue building on the success of those parts left."

"Did you dodge the question, Dr. Fisher?"

He laughed and shook his head. "I don't think so, Alan."

"Didn't Jesus believe that, not man's obedience to the Torah but the grace of God to people of faith, made men and women keep Moses' Commandments?"

"I cannot say, Alan."

"You cannot?"

"Because I do not truly know, nor I suspect does anyone."

"Is not Jesus' thinking much the same as that of Maimonides?"

Dr. Fisher smiled reassuringly. "You still have your curiosity, Alan. Your damaged brain still wants to delve deeply for underlying answers."

"Dr. Fisher, were not Spinoza and Rabbi Nieto much like Plato or Göthe or Seattle in their love of nature and love itself?"

"I sincerely hope so, Alan."

"Dr. Fisher, tomorrow my friend Regis Waters is treating me to breakfast at the university. He is your age and a Gentile. Much of your thinking seems like his."

"A very fine gentleman, from what I recall."

"As are you, Dr. Fisher...Dr. Fisher, when if ever did Christianity embrace anti-Semitism as ideology?"

"I have read that Pope Gregory the Great took the feeling into doctrine around the Christian calendar year 600 A.D. but I would be very interested in your friend's answer, should you ask him tomorrow."

"Dr. Fisher, I love him and I love you. I feel a deep friendship for you both."

"It is good, Alan, to love friends but do not be overpowered by us. We are human."

"Dr. Fisher, it is my understanding that in 13th-century Barcelona, a series of healthy intellectual debates began between Christians and Jews, the last debate occurring some time around 1413 or 1414. I have been led to understand that there was great difficulty in discussing the key point of ideological division, because the Christians and Jews present could not agree on what that key point was."

I heard again the voice of a papa bear.

"You have a good mind, Alan, and are an honorable person."

"Thank you, Dr. Fisher. For you to know and recognize that means a great deal to me."

"Your friend, Regis Waters, undoubtedly recognizes it, too."

I was rekindling.

"Mendelssohn saw the 'miracle' as folly, is that not true?"

"I believe so, Alan."

"Dr. Fisher, my sense of injustice is never allowed to sleep."

"It will sleep tonight, Alan if you swim a mile today."

"I will, Dr. Fisher. Swimming is in the black book."

"Is Wednesday, May 9th good for you for our next appointment?"

"Dr. Fisher, I can't pay your total bill to Mr. Stone."

"Is 8:00 a.m. all right?"

I walked the 2 miles to the university pool and stopped along the way for 2 bananas. I swam a mile, drank a jug of tap water and walked the 5 miles home. Then I fell asleep on the bed at 8:00 p.m. until 4:00 the following morning. At 8:00 a.m., I went to work.

## To That End, I Believe One Should Do All One Can

Canada's medical-legal system and key people within it had produced a Soviet scale scam, and no one knew but I. My family was threatened with financial ruin, but brain injury or not, I had to provide and protect. For her part, Maria was urging me to sell the house and ditch all money in the Bahamas.

I began to tear apart my thinking, trying with a shattered brain to gather, sort, collate, prioritize and communicate answers to unresolved questions.

I went to my giant Clair Park Church near Toronto's Avenue Road and St. Clair, and asked if I could borrow its 1,000-seat sanctuary. I arranged and had publicized across Toronto, my speaking on an October, 1984 day. I felt I could still help others.

# FROM A PULPIT IN OCTOBER 1989

"Welcome to you all and a deep thank you for coming...

Were not people created good, for good? We are the products of billions of years of genes taking the high road, selecting the better way, and for such searching by our basic makeup, does not logic dictate we must be at our cores, good? Unless our source is in the business of creating badness and the only evidence I have seen of that is Canada's mosquito.

But we human beings can be perverse, horribly so. Each of us has seen perversity, greed, callousness and some have witnessed unutterable degrees of inhumanity. Why? Does not herein the logic of fundamental goodness break down? The answer, I believe is contained in the complex world of the human mind. People were created, I believe, free, and rooted in each mind is a driving need to stay free. Freedom of the mind or spirit, I suggest is part of God's hope for us and outweighs any wish of God to shelter us from harm.

So, here we are—human beings, each with a brain of intellect, emotions and motor drives, set free to tackle life. And how we can then do it to ourselves and those around us. This century alone contains some of the most brutal representations of how low minds can go, of how mixed up minds can get. Some of you believe this century proves that billions of years of genetic selection has not been for the better purpose but for survival of the nastiest. I suggest not. We tend too often, I feel, to expect progress to be linear, but perhaps our growth is more like that of an ellipse, inching ahead like the incoming tide—we move forward, we draw back, we press further forward, we regress. The regression can be demoralizing if we do not understand that when we move forward, we can move a tiny point ahead of where we were previously in history.

Think of issues in Canada today and how our thinking has evolved across this maligned century—on our treatment of aboriginal peoples, workers' rights and support systems, on alcoholism, child beatings, rape, women's rights, homosexuality and capital punishment. There do remain issues in need of our wisdom and compassion. How many have not known someone who has left life on Earth from AIDS? What one of us has not been riveted by stories about sexual abuse of children? These stories hurt us and so they should, enough for us to act, because these issues need our acts of wisdom and compassion. But before we act, we will need to have exhausted information around the issue and to have developed an awareness of its importance relative to others, so to have prioritized it within our conscience. Unfortunately, often before penetrating our conscience, the issue will have become critical, but the symptoms will not fully show because the people crying out can not do much else.

There is in Canada and the world an issue of such enormity that people need right now to act with wisdom and compassion. Yet an issue of such low awareness that the cries can't be deciphered. I am talking about the 50,000 Canadians who every year have their lives and the lives of their loved ones put through hell and changed permanently by brain injuries. Injuries so severe that their talking, walking, sexuality, thinking and personalities are permanently physically changed. Changed in 99% of cases, for the worse.

Changes so profound yet so fundamental to the way a person functions as to make that brain-injured person a completely different human being.

One who frequently has lost much of his short-term memory, one who has often lost control of his impulses, one who has almost no understanding of what has happened to him or her, because the brain that could do for him the understanding is broken.

One who has little ability to communicate what has happened, because the brain that governs the thinking and speech is damaged.

One who lives in paralyzing week-to-week fear as more of the hundreds of manifestations of his damaged brain make themselves known to the non-injured parts of his brain.

One who lives in terror of those manifestations becoming known to others and of more realizations being recognized by him. One who fights, if he can, the awesome depression rushing in with the feeling of one's essence being suddenly, permanently gone.

One who soon becomes unemployed and unemployable. One who becomes separated and divorced. One whose shattered impulse-control leaves him prey to addictions—caffeine, tobacco, sugar, salt, monosodium glutamate, drugs, alcohol. One whose same new lack of control leads him to physical fights he would never have done before, to indecision or impulse decisions, to trouble with the law, to jail, one who can have a labyrinth of physical and emotional impairments governing his or her every move, yet appear normal.

Brain-injured people. The 50,000 per year in Canada are a recent phenomenon. Twenty years ago, they died. In the last 20 years, many are surviving the car accidents or industrial drops on their heads, but in those situations where they are not left say, quadriplegic, the damage stays contained inside their normal-looking heads behind normal-looking faces.

And off they go, out of the hospital to face an unenlightened world, facing it with a fractured intellect, a rewired personality and an emotional state beyond their broken capacity to control. Oh to be sure, medical information and updates on brain injuries have spun out at a phenomenal rate over the last 10 years. Toronto's Academy of Medicine contains volumes of updates in articles, lectures and medical releases done, since one giant work was completed in 1981. But I respectfully submit, medicine with its quantum leap forward has not kept pace with the symptoms, the facts and the behavior of brain-injured people as they have revealed themselves.

Making matters worse is the information explosion itself and any caregiver's inability to keep up-to-date. Doctors, psychologists, neuropsychologists, psychiatrists and neurosurgeons have not stayed, perhaps cannot stay, abreast of the information about brain injuries. Compounding this problem further is the appalling behavior shown by many professionals whose egos, territorialism and lust for greed in tapping into ignorance, have created a whole new marketplace for pimping under the guise of professional caring. And so the helpless brain-injured people suffer more, through hellish injustices perpetrated by the powerful and professedly all-knowing.

Perhaps lust for power has been the worst by-product generated by this wealth of confusion and misunderstanding about closed head injuries, a power-lust of the same type many came to see too late when it occurred before. The Bible's Genesis talks of man's fall when he pretends to be like God, to hold God's wisdom and to display that wisdom to the uninformed in an environment, that he knows has been shaped to breed ignorance.

I ask you, I plead with you, if not for the love of God, if not for respect for nature and its biological slug onward to make things better, if not for compassion toward fellow human beings in desperate need, then please for the goodness contained in every human being, help Canada's, the world's, brain-injured people. I sincerely believe that each of you has that goodness.

Just as light advances and darkness recedes, love expands while hate in all forms contracts. Love is the mindset needed to allow awareness to blossom into an enlightened understanding of the now poorly understood brain-injured person.

ALAN J COOPER

With that love as our beginning, awareness must be created on a massive scale.

To date, organizations have sprung up but are still struggling newborns, screaming for help: the Brain Injury Association of Toronto; the Ontario Brain Injury Association; the Brain Injury Association of Canada. Representatives from all 3 are here today.

Other organizations are starting. The Ontario Government initiated this spring a province-wide inquiry into traumatic brain injuries and the complex plight of the brain injured. The Ontario Government's Ministry of Community and Social Services included this year in its mission statement and funding, pro-active help to people with brain injuries. McMaster University is evolving new programs.

But the area is, I believe, so large, so sweeping in complexity as to represent a bigger frontier for man and woman than the frontier of the earth's oceans or outer space. We are trying to understand and help the highest and most influential form of life known—the human brain. For all our studying and understanding of it so far, we know and understand little of its inner workings. It remains to a great degree, a mystery.

In our fight to enlighten, to help, 2 principles stay critical—truth and love. May they be with us in guiding us forward on this urgent mission.

Thank you."

Toronto newspapers got wind of the sermon and famed journalist Jill Compton paid me a visit. She asked my permission to write about me and promised she'd first show me the copy for approval. She then broke her promise. My bi-sexual boss Billy Blake got hold of her column and phoned the church to get the smut on me. Its minister Godfrey had a bond with Blake and spilled all, adding in that I was an alcoholic like Godfrey's brother. My junior job was ruined.

As things further unwound, appeal lawyer Chintak told Stone of his exposure. I received that blown-up legal bill for $500,000, together with Stone's offer that he was prepared to forgive the bill, exclusive of the tens of thousands I had already paid to his partner Dour. Stone added the conditional assurance that sleazebag Lord Advertising, which had breached its 9 months severance contract, would not counter sue.

Another litigation lawyer, husband to a former employee, volunteered to read the judgment and without knowing any of the facts, told me the judgment was a good one. He counseled me not to appeal or take any action against Stone, and dictated a guilt laden acceptance of Stone's offer. As I would hear again, the husband said to put the issue behind me. I took Stone's offer, and the husband and wife stopped answering all calls.

Days later, a "thank you" letter came from one of Canada's brain injury associations for my sermon, and I had barely read beyond the "thank you" before the letter fell. The association was sponsoring 2 guest speakers from a U.S. institution that helped brain-injured people who suffered from injury-caused addictive or behavioral problems. I finally picked up the letter and sat down. On the final page was a full-page advertisement for the law firm that had, with conniving from erudite doctors, used every conceivable trick, distortion and outright lie to convince a Supreme Court that permanently and multiply brain-injured Alan Cooper was a liar, cheat and abuser of the legal system.

# TRYING TO SURVIVE
# POST-JUDGMENT

After that 1989, I would go to sleep on heavy Ativan for the next 4 years. The Canadian job market knew of my court case and people presumed a Supreme Court judgment could be none other than the right one. I tried to hang onto my lower paying job to protect James and Robert, but church minister Godfrey had already blurted to my boss.

In May of 1991, Maria left our young sons alone in a park after dark in Ottawa while she gabbed with a friend. I hunted frantically for J and R, finally finding our sons among big kids and fire-crackers. As neuropsychiatrist Dr. Day had predicted when I had met him, I would lose control of my patched-up circuitry, and have another catastrophic experience. Employment left and but for a few short gasps, did not return.

James and Robert were now aged 7 and 5, and had been directly cared for by Maria for 4 years. Through my career counseling experience, I secured a much-needed job for my wife. I was to become again prime caregiver for J and R, and now added school-parent work. I became representative for Toronto's gifted children and stayed a Boy Scout leader, Sunday school teacher and Board member of the local residents association. I pioneered a drive for a safety median on Oriole Parkway to make the street children-safe and represented Toronto in Canada's capital over the protest of violent American spillover on TV.

By now, however, Maria had grown more like her mother and interfered at every turn. She would yell at our tender children a "Now means now" but regularly make them too late for me to walk them to school, so that she could drive them there. She crushed our son's heart when Robert pretended to send her a surprise letter and she speared, "Waita go, Robert, you just ruined a 36 cent stamp." Maria arranged for her friend Jan McGoo to abscond with my children at lunch from school, without telling prime caregiver me. She kept my young sons late at her place of work. There she made a video to show how well she was mothering James, but did not bother to tell me she was going to be late and had her phones shut off. Later, mother Maria sunned herself asleep on a beach, while James struggled for his life to retrieve a lost set of water wings. I recalled earlier Maria's abandoning our baby Robert in the house while she had driven toddler James to nursery school, all the while knowing from her social work that doing so was gross negligence.

One night, Maria acknowledged my full prime care to our sons by thanking me "...for taking them back and forth to school." She gave me a birthday card with my age wrong, despite my son's correction. When I kept her abreast across 6 months about my innocence in a fender bender and winning the small court case, she feigned not hearing a word of it and had me excluded from her car insurance. She lavished out $100's for furniture from an expensive shop from which she had promised never to buy, because it had helped put my father out of business. She received water filters from her brother's friends and made structural changes in our home, without once consulting her husband.

Maria bitched about the cost of our car and asked why we had not bought a Toyota which I said were best for the money. I told her again that we had agreed to buy the Volvo for safety. She then ignored her agreement and jumped on the word "safety," memorizing the word so as not to have to grasp the principle. Maria removed the "Made in Canada" from our Volvo, and made her name and self appear Scandinavian. Truth, Maria said was credibility, and as she would posit aside, sooner or later all issues boiled down to money. In private, Maria hurled racist slurs on our Jewish and Irish neighbors and boycotted any business with Lithuanians; in public she lied with veneered professionalism. Maria labeled her brother the "Polish Prince," but let her parents think I had affixed the title.

## After Doctor Fisher

Doctor Fisher died in 1992 but the night-time Ativan kept coming. Sunday school teaching was destroyed by minister Godfrey's rumors, and Cub Scout leadership too was stopped. I taught creative writing for a couple of months in 1993 within the Toronto school system but during the teaching's second month in June, Maria carried out her plans announced 5 months earlier, and took James and Robert again to her mother's. Maria saw a top lawyer paid for by her sister, and left me for good.

Late that June of 1993, I fell back into alcohol but by July, I determined that I was going to give the big Tudor family home to James and Robert. Maria's actions forced me to see a lawyer who advised that I could claim support against Maria but I chose not to, and Maria began pressing me to claim for disability compensation under the Canada Pension Plan.

On July 1, 1993 I admitted myself to a detoxification unit. My AA sponsor was the old lawyer who believed I could not have had a wrong judgment, and therefore had no brain damage. But he was also a boss of the rehabilitation unit, and staff were directed not to believe me, either. Counselor Bill Barter seized my Ativan of 4 years, despite my protests to consult a doctor, and within 30 hours, I had multiple seizures. I woke up in hospital, with tongue and lips ripped from being safety pinned, and the seizures killed my driver's license. I spent the rest of the summer of 1993 in rehab, where workers under my AA sponsor called me a "...liar, cheat and a thief." I went 23 days without sleep.

It became impossible that August to obtain short-term social assistance. A neurologist at the detox's hospital took exception to my commenting on the gold hanging down his open chest and declared that I had never been brain injured or in a car accident at all. Social services received the doctor's document and I was refused any kind of help. Finally, I reached social worker Gwen Lang, an ex-American who sensed the smell of corruption. She spearheaded my going through 4 weeks of neuro-psychological and vocational assessment, and I was declared unemployable due to brain damage. For my disability, I was granted early access to Canada Pension of about $700 per month.

Maria agreed that, in lieu of her providing support, the Pension disability supplement for children would be directed to me. I used it to fund time and expenses with J and R, and its first lump payment I used to buy a rowboat for James and canoe for Robert. Maria further agreed that if the supplement were ever routed to her, she would forward the same amount to me. Maria added the aside that, not only was I not an asset, I was a liability and she could not understand why I did not just move 200 miles north, to live with my mother.

In the autumn of 1993, I landed an apartment in a cellar near the matrimonial home. Soon Maria confided my most intimate secrets in her first language to landlady Jadwiga, all the while saying I should stay at arm's length from my landlady. Maria knew of Jadwiga's own marital break-up from an alcoholic husband. In months to come, when I received an AA medallion for another year's sobriety, Maria slipped to Jadwiga the confidential news. With shock, I received my landlady's lecture-laden congratulations.

Despite the 4-week tests confirming my permanent unemployability, I embarked in 1994 on an 8-year try to become once again employed. While continuing to send out hundreds more job applications, I went back to school, this time with 4 weeks of tests confirming my permanent brain damage. With help from the disability program at the University of Toronto, I got myself again into United Church Ministry school, and with student loans and an academic workload of 40%, slugged my way through the courses.

After another year, my own church's Discernment Committee failed me. They judged my personality too deranged to be a minister but refused to put it in writing. By now it was the spring of 1995 and I had invested thousands of student loan dollars and a full school year of 90-hour weeks. Maria was known to my Discernment Committee through her Clair Park Church executive and she wrote to the Committee an innuendo under a caring camouflage, that Alan's problems were "one day at a time." That poison would catch up with my trying again years later, the ministry. My 11-year-old son James would be my sole solace. "That's just them, Daddy" he would tell me. "In many ways, you are already more of a minister than they can know." Ironically, 7 years earlier, the Supreme Court had been convinced by opposing Gauze that I could be a minister if I tried.

Sometime during the period after the judgment had come down in 1989 and Maria's going back to her mother's in 1993, I had swum 4 miles across a northern Ontario lake in a charity marathon. I had also speed-walked the 25th annual New York Marathon in 1994, to help raise awareness of brain-injured people and the types of things we could still do. For a while later on, I served on the Board of the Toronto Brain Injury Association but resigned when my changed personality again conflicted with others. However, I did get a chance to meet another good person in the system, so with the previous Gwen Lang, the count of advocates was now up to 2. Ruth Crandle's spirit still lives on with me as one who took the time to try to understand a brain-injured person. In 1996, Ruth cut red tape to get me sponsorship for my presentation to the International Brain Injury Association Symposium in Dallas.

The decade after the 1989 judgment saw me lose my few remaining good friends. Tané Yoshimara stopped communicating after the summer of 1996, when he lectured me on my duty to forget my goddamn brain injury and support my children. Manfred in Germany had long gone. Patricia Langlois left after I supposedly insulted her. Some others, such as Angelo Colucci, who said he had lied for me to support court theatrics, I wish had never been friends. I had communicated my indignation about Angelo Colucci to Maria while still living with her, but she had only pretended to understand. Weeks later, she had accepted a Colucci dinner invitation, fully knowing I had refused.

After Maria's leaving, James and Robert were still there but Maria restricted me to seeing them only once on Saturday. Maria was breaking the law in denying greater access but knew the system, knew I had no money and knew I was soft. My sons and I tried to make the best of it and let ourselves feel the love we had for one another.

AA sponsor Camden continued projecting his own lying life on me and believed that my main problem was the same as his, alcohol. Once that problem was gone, he thought, and once I owned up to being a rascal like him, I would soon be working again. At one point in a 1995 AA meeting, he hollered "Got a job yet?"

Maria, too went on living her lie, westernizing her first name to have it read "Marie." Earlier, when it had suited her to have me perceived as brain damaged, she had phoned Dr. Fisher to claim I had sent Robert on a dangerous toboggan ride where he had bumped his head. She had also used similar tactics to ensure I was punched by a cab driver, and then had lied about the details. Now, Maria gave James long pants to wear at his track meet. James' peers and teacher queried why and I tried to support my son. He placed 3rd and his peers let him know he could have done better. Maria also stopped my initiatives of the Toronto Children's Chorus for J and R, and Robert's piano lessons. But she was less successful in stopping my getting our sons into the Toronto schools' gifted program, despite her lying and denying my 6 months related spadework.

I tried another shrink, Rosak, but he dwelt on his own rage over the injustices done to me and was astonished that I had thought to have children, when so brain injured. As for my personality, it conflicted with another volunteer Board, the downtown Toronto Chaplaincy, and I departed. I met the odd girl but failed sexually, even later with Viagra. Companionship I could not do and women freaked on hearing "brain injury." Nights had nightmares but my injured brain remembered few. One was of Robert stuck in my wife's back seat, while Maria drove out of a river. In my dream, she ignored my yells from afar, pulled out the car, cheered and was oblivious to drowning our son.

In the years that followed, Maria had a man living with her on weekends and she petitioned in 1998 for divorce. With what I could muster, I tried to retain a marital lawyer but was refused 3 times—each lawyer heard of the Supreme Court judgment and revered Stone, and so believed neither brain injury nor me.

I finally retained lawyer Sandra Dempster, an American who did not understand Canadian university subsidies. Without my approval or knowledge, marital lawyer Dempster agreed to Maria's request for me to set aside $25,000 as "college for the kids." I heard about Dempster's agreement, in concert with a litany of lies written by Maria about me. My separated wife included a concoction that her employer's insurance company wanted my huge prescription charges off her drug plan. I spent all night retrieving documentation to prove Maria's lies wrong, as well as point out to my lawyer that my son James had been compensated a full $12,000 in 1993 for a school playground accident. Robert, too, had been compensated. Those amounts, in addition to Maria's agreed-upon selling of the marital home after my sons' simultaneous high school graduation, were to have funded their university. Somehow, the playground accident sums had gone missing, leaving James and Robert with little knowledge of them and Maria with a weak memory of everything, particularly her agreement to sell the house upon our children's graduation.

My marital lawyer Dempster chose to read the Supreme Court judgment on me, and confirmed to me that I was a liar. She said I should try volunteer work. Like the Judge, Dempster knew nothing of my being Boy Scout leader, Sunday school teacher or anything else of my background. Her secretary was typing all my hand-printed input and was illegally charging me $160 per hour for so doing. My retainer was eaten up in days.

When it came time to settle, Maria agreed in writing that I could continue to receive the Canada Pension children's supplement in lieu of support, but then breached contract, the moment the divorce had gone through. It became clear why Maria had not wanted to register the home mortgage that she had promised me. I tried to assign the mortgage for what little money it would afford me but Maria refused to sign the acknowledgment of debt. She told the assignee's lawyer that she acknowledged the debt but would not do anything to help Alan.

I wrote a letter of protest to Maria and copied her lawyer. She countered by illegally charging me with harassment. She then lied to my sons and told them I was trying to steal their Canada Pension support money, "which they needed for their school future."

Maria illegally stopped access to my sons, concocting a lie that she feared for their safety. She secretly sold the matrimonial home, made a fortune and moved to an unknown location. I tried to see J and R at school but even there, Maria abused her senior social work position and lied to its Vice-Principal, stopping my seeing them on the pretense of safety. For over 2 years, I did not hear one word from J and R. Maria also lied to my own mother about the harassment and the lie spread among my family.

After 17 trips to court over 2 years, the harassment issue was dismissed as a civil matter and the Crown Prosecutor agreed to throw it out, provided I would not sue the Crown. I guessed Maria knew that I could legally sue her for mischief, but she also knew that I would not sue, because of James and Robert. She also knew that no lawyer believed I was brain injured and therefore not me, because the Supreme Court had ruled I was malingering.

I did finish a Master of Religious Education, though my chosen courses made the degree more one of sociology, with every option pertaining to how people were spiritually shaped. In one of the courses, instead of my being a mock minister in moot church, I chose to be a multi-faith chaplain in Toronto's Don Jail. As with my counseling, years earlier to fired people, the job in downtown Toronto's jail would be rewarding and I found no circumstance where I could not be of help to someone else. I did a second Masters, this one in Education, and became immersed in how children learn. I was intrigued with the role that spiritual development, that is the growth of conscience and a sense of right and wrong, plays in such learning and how religiosity shunts such growth. I had even written a thesis on it in my earlier Master of Religious Education and received an A-plus.

After the MRE and Master of Education degrees, I spent another 2 full years trying to find a job but had no luck. I went back for long term disability to my Ministry employer at the time of the car accident and found I qualified but was past the statute of limitations date. Then in 2001–2002, I ploughed into a Bachelor of Education to get certification to teach. The disability department urged me to take the course more slowly than my peers but I refused. I worked 100 hours per week, got an A average but failed the practicum, because of my closed brain injury.

In the 2002–2003 school year following, under disability appeal I again took the practice teaching as well as the internship and teacher's test, but was then held up 3 months by the University of Toronto and Ontario College of Teachers, before being certified to teach. The hold-up damaged my chances of getting a job before my teaching practice became stale-dated but the licensing body back-dated its certification to January 2003, to protect itself.

In June of 2003, I job interviewed with the Toronto School Board and the interview went so well that one of the 2 Principals interviewing, said "You got it!" to my choice of school area and grade. A week later, after references had been checked, I received a 2-sentence letter from the TSB, advising that I had been turned down for a job anywhere in its jurisdiction. The letter came June 19th and I was to receive convocation on June 20.

When I arrived for the Teachers' College convocation, wearing the academic robe and shawl draped over my arm, none other than my failing supervisor Katy Bard was the one on center stage, to don the shawl over my head. As I climbed the stairs to the stage and faced the Associate Dean, I bowed enough for Katy Bard to don the shawl over me. The Associate Dean congratulated me, saying, "*You're* sure to get a position".

She was mistaken.

# NOVEMBER 20TH 2003

The Hospital is of all places, Flanders. For 18 months, it has balked at giving me testing, because its old file is still contaminated by the original prejudices of G.P. Dr. Jensen and opposing Doctor Malthrop. Neuropsychologist Sari is feeding me back recent test results.

"Memory is a poor word, Mr. Cooper, since it conveys many things. People such as yourself can seem fine on our old tests but meanwhile your life is falling apart. People test 'Superior' but can't hold a job. There are significant problems relating to your frontal lobe, compared to other areas where intelligence is high. Word retrieval, for example, is weak."

"I have tremendous difficulty absorbing new names, and lose them even after learned."

"We test more your episodic memory and don't really test that more specific function."

"I even call my sons, James and Robert, by the wrong names."

"The left frontal lobe, if uninjured has a monitoring system for catching such mistakes. Your strategic use of memory is governed again by that frontal lobe which directs the executive parts of the brain. It probably now takes you an hour to do what you used to be able to do in 10 minutes. I would be surprised if you don't face indecisiveness when faced with critical decisions. Psychologists used to recommend more junior jobs but the problem is that people like you are still intelligent and don't find those lower jobs fulfilling. That causes *more* stress. Our tests even today are not really relevant to your circumstances and we want to refer you to a new institute in Toronto, one of only 5 in the world for coaching with your problems."

---

## December 2003 in Adam Stone's
## Canadian Government Office

"And why do you presume, Alan, that I still want to become Canada's Prime Minister?"

"We're not in court, lawyer Stone. You may drop the sophistry."

"Our Paul Martin is Canada's favorite for years to come."

"Paul Martin is hated by former PM Chrétien and people underestimate vindictiveness."

"Well, Canadians hate Toronto and that's where I'm from."

"Ottawa. You're from here, you went to law school here, you're fluently bilingual and you have merchandised yourself that way. But you're not on stage now, Adam Stone. There's no one else here. You will not be Canadian Prime Minister unless you co-operate."

"That sounds like a threat."

"Forget your specialty, Mr. Stone, and think about criminal law. You will lose more than your upcoming New York job. You will be disbarred. You will have a criminal record."

Adam Stone pauses to stare straight at me with the skills of a seasoned litigation lawyer. He thinks he still has me.

"Alan, I can understand your bitterness for things not going your way, but it is time to put the past behind you and move on."

I hear again the echo of what I have heard twice before.

"Spare the platitudes, Mr. Stone."

"It will cost you an enormous amount of money to defame a senior government person."

"Save your threats for the court. We fully anticipate counter-action."

"...We?"

"The royal we."

"...You have no case."

"Your firm forced me to take those psych tests with Central Trust, and you and I discussed them immediately before the trial. When I asked you what would happen if the other side raised them in court, you told me they would be dismissed as an aberration."

"And that is precisely what we tried to do."

"No, Adam Stone. When the other side sprung them in court, you jumped to your feet and stonewalled Judge Carter. You reduced her to a loss for words, tears and temporary adjournment. With your agile tongue and start-up shout 'Look here!', you led the Judge to believe that you had not concealed evidence from the Supreme Court, but that I, your defenseless brain-injured client, had kept it from you. Then in her judgment, Her Ladyship Nanette Carter concluded that a devious Alan Cooper had duped his lawyer Adam Stone by concealing those bogus psychological tests done by hack shrink Pin. You broke the law. You committed a criminal act by communicating that your client had done what you did yourself."

"I had to protect my client from those test results."

"You had to protect yourself. Those tests were for my immediate recall of numbers, not for my difficulty in absorbing and retaining new linguistic information. You didn't understand the difference but pretended before the trial you did."

"What you're suggesting, Mr. Cooper, is preposterous."

"True, too. Its preposterousness and your subsequent, preposterous manipulation of the appeal lawyer are also true."

"You're not suggesting..."

"You directed me in your office, to see 'Canada's best appeal lawyer' Chintak, and you then communicated with him in the interim. When I met him, he already knew of your untruthful and criminal damage of me to protect yourself. He repeatedly said that he knew you well and would have no part in working to your detriment. He also said there were no grounds for appeal. It was a setup."

"You were free to go to anyone you wished."

"You had pre-fed Chintak and manipulated my going to see him."

"You're paranoid."

"Nice try, Stone, but it won't work. You're caught now and even your killing me won't stop me. Only your agreement."

Stone is assuming a negotiating position familiar to himself.

"So, you have come with terms?"

"You already knew that."

"Oh? How?"

"Twenty years of litigation law and an I.Q. of 150."

"Where do you get your 150 from? I am not aware of that number myself."

"The number is just below your ego, and your ego is easy to see."

"...So, how much do you want?"

"10 years."

"T...you'll never put me in jail, Cooper. You'll be there first."

"Didn't you mention threats a few minutes ago, Mr. Stone? In any event, you continue to focus on yourself. I'm speaking of G.P. Dr. Steve Jensen, the pimp who pushed us all into court in the first place."

"Oh? How so?"

"After 6 months at trial, ostensibly on behalf of me, you remain as ignorant of goings-on as ever."

"I listened to whatever you had to say."

"You listened to my wife and she was already out to dump me. She had married me for better or better, in health and in health."

"She spoke well to me on your behalf."

"She spoke calculatingly to you. She lied about my drinking to M'Lady whom she knew was the widow of an alcoholic husband. My wife had already researched the marital indivisibility of any proceeds I was to get. She had the hots for you."

"Why me?"

"Because your social standing was a rung up from mine and several up from her own. She already had her 2 bright and beautiful sons—Scottish-Polish border collies as she called them—she had her center-hall house in Chaplin Estates, her Volvo and her grand piano. She had her momentum. She even admitted one day to her designs on you."

"You knew all this? Why did you not say so?"

"No one was listening, let alone believing me. Your partner, Dour thought me a total malingerer because of her."

"Dour?"

"He asked my wife at our first meeting with him to describe the accident. She calmly described a clear night of good weather, excellent visibility and no traffic. When stunned I was then asked to describe the pre-accident conditions, I loudly said 'No! The night was black, the visibility almost non-existent and the traffic heavy in a long, slow-moving chain, coming north and facing us.' I added to Dour that I had said to my wife 'You drove in this?' in response to her driving a year earlier under the same conditions. All the while I was describing the true conditions to your partner Dour, my wife Maria kept interrupting me, saying 'Oh yes, that's how it really happened, oh yes, yes'. Dour then lowered his glasses, took a long distrusting stare at me and from that second on, stopped believing any word I said.

While I was describing the true conditions to your partner Dour, he did not have the traffic report and did not bother getting it, even for Discoveries years later. Many more years later, you were being coaxed to trial with the other side's knowing of its lia-bility but not admitting to it, until in trial."

"And Dr. Jensen, what of him?"

"He personally, single-handedly spent hours on the phone with each specialist, telling every one that I was malingering before I met the specialists. Dr. Jensen was lying to prejudice them. I found out from one of them, Dr. Will my dentist, years later. Will then nixed his file."

"Why? Jensen was your doctor, your G.P.!"

"I had inherited him when my chosen G.P. Dr. Brethren had sold him the practice. Jensen's brother is a lawyer whose backyard was down the street from mine. Jensen's lawyer brother spied on me for 4 years and reported news back to Dr. Jensen."

"Why didn't you tell me?"

"I did, Mr. Stone, but my wife interrupted me and you chose to listen to her delivery. I also asked you why Regal Insurance, a facility insurance company, had spent more money on detective fees with its 2 agencies than its total $500,000 liability. But num-bers, as we know, baffle you."

"Two agencies?"

"The second working for the illegal cadre of insurance compa-nies above Regal Insurance's head. That cadre knew that if a brain injury victim remained intelligent but nevertheless severely brain damaged, a concept it hoped the Supreme Court would not grasp, then a legal precedent would be established such that hundreds of millions of dollars would be doled out in the 5–10 years ahead. It's the sort of scenario where the cadre would be willing to bribe the victim's G.P. for hundreds of thousands."

"And launder the money through his brother?"

"You're a little late, litigation lawyer Stone. You actually went to Jensen before trial and proudly returned, proclaiming that you had persuaded Jensen to come around. Jensen then appeared in court to be on my side, when his damage had already been done.

You played right into the other side's hands. It wasn't just numbers you were hopeless with."

"Why do you say numbers?"

"Because you refused to reflect on why Regal Insurance had spent more than the maximum it could lose. And because you couldn't count across a calendar year."

"Calendar?"

"Seven days, Mr. Stone. December 27th to January 2nd is 7 days inclusive, not 5. Seven days of my being incoherent in hospital. Opposing lawyer Gauze knew that but was not about to help you in court. Seven days constitute 'severe' brain injury, not the 'mild' you arrived at with 5 days. Severe, Mr. Stone, the same diagnosis 100% of the time from a hematoma in the brain, the same diagnosis when my pupils are now of a different size. Severe 100% of the time for each of those reasons, Mr. Stone. Even you can handle that number. You knew none of this and did not even mention my pupils' sizes in court."

"You'll never get away with this, Mr. Cooper. You'll still be seen as a greedy malingerer."

"We're ready for you, Mr. Stone. If I lose, you lose; if you kill me, you lose."

"Kill you? This is Canada!"

"That's right, Stone. And you want to be Prime Minister by 2012."

Stone's face is turning from me. His eyes are looking longingly at the rich wood in his Ottawa office. He will soon be leaving Ottawa for richer wood in New York.

"Money?"

"The long-term disability insurance to which I was entitled but for which your law firm never applied."

"Possibly."

"But first, Jensen. Then Malthrop."

"...Doctor Malthrop? He was just doing his job for the opposition."

"He misrepresented himself to doctors as working for me. As he did along with opposition detectives, to headhunters, professors and other people who knew and had known me."

"...How much from Malthrop?"

"10 years for Jensen and a like number for Malthrop. To say nothing of hack shrink Pin."

"10 years! For a crime that long ago? Impossible."

"Difficult, like your becoming Prime Minister."

"You don't seem brain injured to me, Mr. Cooper."

"Nice try, Stone, but even you know that not to be true."

"But will others?"

"You can try, Stone, and hope for more ignorance."

"Is that all, Cooper?"

"No. Regal Insurance is finished, the illegal cadre is exposed and opposing law firm Timpson Cable loses its hold on Canada's personal injury business."

"Too tall an order, Mr. Cooper. You ask too much."

I am not asking too much. In fact, I am not asking at all. This December 2003 meeting with lawyer Adam Stone is fantasy, and I think I put it in, to lend some sense of relief from the gruesome truth. Stone is still in the media, a Canadian household name, Dr. Jensen remains in practice, living in his massive Lawrence Park mansion, and opposing Dr. Malthrop has recently been seen at a brain injury seminar, in a scrum with medical lawyers.

Now back to reality.

# 3:00 p.m., April 7, 2004

"Dr. Sari makes clear, Mr. Cooper that she believes your brain damage not to be caused by your recent hit on your bike, but by your earlier brain injury of 1981. She labels that 1981 brain injury as severe and your bike one as mild."

The lawyer talking has just reviewed the report done by neuropsychologist Dr. Sari, the one she highlighted to me in Flanders Hospital on November 20, 2003.

"Severe? The Flanders Hospital neuropsychologist labels my December 27, 1981 brain injury as severe?"

After over 22 years of hearing my 1981 brain injury misdiagnosed in court and elsewhere as "mild," a neuropsychologist from the same hospital is now labeling it "severe."

"Yes, in fact Dr. Sari very specifically characterizes the problems you have, as related to a left frontal lobe injury of the kind you sustained in your 1981 car accident."

Lawyer Anthony Luke is confirming to me that my brain injury of December 27, 1981 was "severe" and the multiple impairments I am still experiencing over 22 years later are as a direct result of that severe 1981 brain injury. I am in his office. Lawyer Luke works for the law firm that is considered the best in Canada for handling brain injury claims. But that law firm is Timpson Cable, the one that duped a Supreme Court into thinking that my brain injury was mild, the same brain-injury-specialist law firm that fooled a Supreme Court Judge into concluding that my permanent, severe and diffuse brain damage did not exist at all but was being faked by a malingering, money-mongering me.

# 2006 AND ON

I would love to trust but fear I have not enough trust left. It is now 25 years since I was struck by a crazed driver on the wrong side of the road. I incurred a hematoma to my left frontal lobe, and a diffuse rupturing across my entire brain. A broken blood vessel winds down my left temple. My speech is mucked, my mouth viscous and my palate numb—as are my toes, fingers, tongue and outer lips. I void over 5 liters per day and am forever dehydrated. I am almost impotent. Short-term memory is precarious and retrieval worse. My words and letters get mixed. I have little sense of smell. When I get dressed, I balance along a wall and put on my shoes sitting down. I look at my sons' photos and twice get their names wrong. I've been fired 9 times since the brain injury, failed by 2 professional schools and kicked out of 4 organizations. Sports and the Mendelssohn Choir left long ago as did my home, wife, children, all relatives, all friends. My personality is mis-wired.

Textbook head injury symptoms. All that Supreme Court Carter's judgment stated were fake. I have been crushed by the state and all apparati related thereto.

I live in grinding poverty and relentless loneliness. I have lost millions in salary. Student loans linger. I live with an old stove and tiny fridge, with each food visible to minimize dependence on memory. At night I don't sleep but toss on a still sore clavicle. Fresh stress stews each day and I walk alone vast distances to hold anger in tow. The future looks charcoal…but I have lived on.

The lie carries its own momentum and I now feel what I can best do is write against that lie and lies like it. There are now millions of brain-injured people, who cannot write or express much at all. For many millions more, they face misunderstandings and the abuse that goes with such confusion. They are left both misunderstood by exasperated loved ones and prey to so-called experts in an area where so much is as yet unknown. The need to have brain-injured people communicate the intertwining complexities of brain damage, as only brain-injured people know and feel those complexities, is urgent. Never again should a brain-injured person have to undergo what I have undergone, in a true story you now know.

# ABOUT THE AUTHOR

Alan J Cooper knows first hand the multiple effects of a brain injury, brought to light in this true story.

A world famous psychiatrist pleaded with Alan to write about the brain injury's aftermath, saying that in the doctor's European and North American experience, only Alan could communicate clearly and comprehensively, the total picture from a patient's point of view. The world famous doctor was talking about not only the neurological fallout but also the behavior of Alan and surrounding doctors, family, lawyers, courts and senior people, before and after the author was struck by a wild driver.

Since his brain injury, Alan J Cooper has written for Toronto newspapers, has taught creative writing within the school system and has spoken publicly. He also speed-walked the 25th New York Marathon in 1994 on behalf of brain-injured people globally, and presented to the world brain injury conference in Dallas in 1996. He has been written up in Toronto's national newspaper, *The Globe & Mail.*

Alan has continued his philanthropy after his catastrophic accident, serving on a number of Boards dedicated to helping those less fortunate, and has been a career counselor to people who have lost their jobs. Alan devoted a full university year to helping prisoners in Toronto's notorious Don Jail.

Prior to his brain being crushed, Alan Cooper was a senior private and public sector executive, and frequent interviewee on radio and television. Outside of work, he sang as baritone in the world famed Toronto Mendelssohn Choir. He holds 5 degrees from the University of Toronto, including 2 Masters, the first examining how values affect human behavior, the second a Master of Education, focusing on the need for learner autonomy and a teacher's role as catalyst.

Alan has already completed an outline for a second book, a fiction novel unveiling the damage being done to North American society by perversions of religion.

## OTHER WHITE KNIGHT BOOKS

| | |
|---|---|
| **Adoption** | A Swim Against The Tide, *David R.I. McKinstry* |
| **Biography** | The Life and Times of Nancy Ford-Inman, *Nancy Erb Kee* |
| **Education** | From Student to Citizen, *Prof. Peter Hennessy* |
| **Health** | Prescription for Patience, *Dr. Kevin J Leonard*<br>Brain Injury, *Alan J. Cooper* |
| **Humor** | *By David R.I. McKinstry:*<br>• An Innkeeper's Discretion BOOK ONE<br>• An Innkeeper's Discretion BOOK TWO<br>Will That Be Cash or 'Cuffs?, *Yvonne Blackwood* |
| **Inspiration** | "Oh My God. It's ME!", *Dr. Sheryl Valentine*<br>*By Rev. Dr. John S. Niles:*<br>• The Art of Sacred Parenting<br>• How I Became Father to 1000 Children<br>*By Darlene Montgomery:*<br>• Conscious Women, Conscious Lives ONE<br>• Conscious Women, Conscious Lives TWO<br>• Conscious Women, Conscious Careers<br><br>Happiness: Use It or Lose It, *Rev. Dr. David "Doc" Loomis*<br>Sharing MS (Multiple Sclerosis), *Linda Ironside*<br>Sue Kenney's My Camino, *Sue Kenney* |
| **Personal Finances** | Spent Smarter, Save Bigger, *Margot Bai*<br>Don't Borrow $Money$, *Paul E Counter* |
| **Poetry** | Loveplay, *Joe Fromstein and Linda Stitt*<br>Two Voices, A Circle of Love, *Serena Williamson Andrew* |
| **Politics & History** | Islam, Women and the Challenges of Today, *Farzana Hassan*<br>Prophets of Violence, Prophets of Peace, *Dr. K. Sohail*<br>Turning Points, *Ray Argyle* |
| **Reference** | Self-Publishing, *Bill Hushion, Peter Wright*<br>The Complete Guide to Becoming A Firefighter, *Kory Pearn* |
| **Self-Help** | *By Dr. K. Sohail:*<br>• The Art of Living in Your Green Zone<br>• The Art of Loving in Your Green Zone,<br>• The Art of Working in Your Green Zone, *with Bette Davis*<br>• Love, Sex and Marriage, *with Bette Davis* |
| **True Crime – Police** | "10-45" Spells Death, *Kathy McCormack Carter*<br>Life on Homicide, *Former Police Chief Bill McCormack*<br>The Myth of The Chosen One, *Dr. K. Sohail* |

**Visit our website www.whiteknightbooks.ca or request catalogue.**

## RECOMMENDED READING FROM OTHER PUBLISHERS

| | |
|---|---|
| **History** | An Amicable Friendship (Canadiana), *Jan Th. J. Krijff*<br>Pro Deo, *Prof. Ronald Morton Smith* |
| **Religion** | From Islam to Secular Humanism, *Dr. K. Sohail* |
| **Biography** | Gabriel's Dragon, *Arch Priest Fr. Antony Gabriel* |